Enabling Technology for Neurodevelopmental Disorders

This cutting-edge volume explores how technological tools can be designed, engineered, and implemented to assess and support individuals with neurodevelopmental disorders from diagnosis through to rehabilitation. Tanu Wadhera and Deepti Kakkar and their expert contributors focus on technological tools as equalizers in Neurodevelopmental disorders at every stage, the importance of demand-specific design, and how we can best engineer and deploy both invasive and non-invasive individual-centered approaches that support and connect individuals. Considering the perspectives of patients, clinicians, and technologists, it explores key topics including design and evaluation of platforms for tech-tools, automated diagnosis, brain imaging techniques, tech-diagnostic frameworks with artificial intelligence (AI) and machine learning, sensing technology, smart brain prosthetics, gamification, alternative communication devices, and education tools and interactive toys. Outlining future challenges for research, *Enabling Technology for Neurodevelopmental Disorders* is useful for scholars and professionals in psychology, technology, engineering, and medicine concerned with design, development, and evaluation of a range of assistive technological tools.

Tanu Wadhera is Assistant Professor at Department of Electrical and Instrumentation Engineering, Thapar Institute of Engineering and Technology, Patiala, Punjab, India. She earned her Ph.D. degree in Electronics and Communication Engineering and has a total of six years of research experience, with four years at National Institute of Technology, Jalandhar, Punjab, India. Her research interests include AI, Assistive Technology, Behavioural Modelling, Biomedical Signal Processing, Cognitive Neuroscience, and Machine Learning.

Deepti Kakkar is Assistant Professor at Department of Electronics and Communication, National Institute of Technology, Jalandhar, Punjab, India. She has a total academic experience of 15 years and has guided more than 40 postgraduate engineering dissertations and over 30 papers international Journals and Conferences. Her recent research interests include Cognitive Neuroscience and Neurodevelopmental disorders.

Enabling Technology for Neurodevelopmental Disorders

From Diagnosis to Rehabilitation

Edited by
Tanu Wadhera and Deepti Kakkar

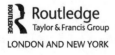

Routledge
Taylor & Francis Group

LONDON AND NEW YORK

First published 2022
by Routledge
4 Park Square, Milton Park, Abingdon, Oxon OX14 4RN

and by Routledge
605 Third Avenue, New York, NY 10158

Routledge is an imprint of the Taylor & Francis Group, an informa business

© 2022 selection and editorial matter, Tanu Wadhera and Deepti Kakkar; individual chapters, the contributors

The right of Tanu Wadhera and Deepti Kakkar to be identified as the authors of the editorial material, and of the authors for their individual chapters, has been asserted in accordance with sections 77 and 78 of the Copyright, Designs and Patents Act 1988.

British Library Cataloguing-in-Publication Data
A catalogue record for this book is available from the British Library

Library of Congress Cataloging-in-Publication Data
A catalog record has been requested for this book

ISBN: 978-0-367-76116-5 (hbk)
ISBN: 978-0-367-76118-9 (pbk)
ISBN: 978-1-003-16556-9 (ebk)

DOI: 10.4324/9781003165569

Typeset in Bembo
by Taylor & Francis Books

Contents

Figures

Tables

Contributors

Prof. Dr. Srinivasan Venkatesan is heading the Department of Clinical Psychology at All India Institute of Speech and Hearing in Mysore, India, for the past 20 years. His primary focus and interest lie in interventional assessments and therapeutic methods for the population of children and adolescents with disabilities and disorders. He has authored several books and publications, apart from guiding Ph.D. scholars on these topics.

Dr. Jesse M. Redlo is an Adjunct Professor in the Saunders College of Business at the Rochester Institute of Technology (RIT). In this role, he teaches courses in using technology to manage the flow of information within organizations. In addition, Dr. Redlo is an Adjunct Professor at St. John Fisher College where he teaches courses in American Studies, focusing on topics such as inequities, social justice movements, and community activism. Dr. Redlo contributes to the research community as an author of multiple book chapters, journal articles, and editorials. Outside of academia, Dr. Redlo is a community activist, helping to advocate for and facilitate community youth programming and more equitable access to education. Dr. Redlo can be reached at jredlo766@gmail.com.

Dr. Harpreet Kaur Dhir received her BA in multiple subjects from University of Redlands, CA and MA in Curriculum and Instruction from California Polytechnic University, Pomona. Her experience includes teaching for the past 28 years at the Ontario-Montclair Unified School District and Hacienda La Puente Unified School District, being an advisory board and a faculty member at the Art Center College of Design, and teaching at California Polytechnic University, Pomona. Currently, she contributes to the American College of Education as a member of the Advisory Board representing post-graduate students. She is currently a human rights advocacy coordinator for her district and can be reached at hkaurdhir@gmail.com.

Rizwana Azeez career spanning roughly two-and-a-half decades saw him in various capacities as a teacher, principal, professor, and finally as a researcher. The experience as a teacher and a school principal realized the need for understanding individual incapacities and the impact on child mental health. Adding on to this understanding he pursued a master in Psychology, an M.

Phil in learning disabilities and finally a PhD that enabled him to have thorough knowledge of cognition and language processes thus guiding children to strengthen their weaknesses. Later on, experiences as an Asst. Professor guided him towards research, and he took up his position as a senior Psychologist at the Epidemiology Research Unit, Holdsworth Memorial Hospital Mysore. Presently, Azeez is engaged in psychological assessments, training team members and health facilitators, preparing modules for intervention, conducting intervention for various groups, and contributing to scientific literature.

Dr. Iyer Kamlam has submitted his thesis for the award of Ph.D. degree in psychology from the University of Mysore, India. His research was in the domain of developmental neuropsychology. He is interested in and focused on assessment and cognitive training related to children with neurodevelopmental disorders and their families. Furthermore, he intends to utilize the latest statistical and digital techniques for pursuing research along with the same domains.

Dr. Tanu Gupta is presently serving as a Clinical Psychologist at Department of Psychiatry, AIIMS, Jodhpur. She earned M.Phil in Clinical psychology from IHBAS and obtained PhD (Clinical Psychology) from AIIMS, New Delhi. She has been awarded Doctoral fellowship from Indian Council of Social science Research, New Delhi and senior research fellowship from Indian Council Medical Research, New Delhi. She has worked as faculty with National Institute of Mentally Handicapped (NIMH), regional center, New Delhi. She has worked in collaboration with many international agencies such as National Institute of Health (NIH), USA and Brown University, USA. She has actively participated in various national and international conferences and workshops, writing book chapters and publishing articles in peer-reviewed journals. Her specific areas of interest are cognitive behavior therapy, child and adolescent psychotherapy, and stress management.

Dr. Pratibha Gehlawat is currently working as Associate Professor, Dept. of Psychiatry, AIIMS, Jodhpur. She did her MBBS at University College of Medical Sciences, University of Delhi and MD Psychiatry from Pt. B.D. Sharma, UHS, Rohtak, Haryana. She has over ten years of experience in the field of Psychiatry. She has a keen interest in Neurodevelopmental disorders. Other interest areas include Mood and Anxiety disorders, Child and Adolescent Psychiatry, mental wellbeing of college students, Consultation-Liaison Psychiatry and Medical Teaching. She is a Life Fellow of the Indian Psychiatric Society. She has done various projects in child and adolescent Psychiatry and has a number of publications in national and international journals to her credit.

Dr. Md. Asad Khan is an Associate Professor in Biochemistry, Faculty of Dentistry. Beside this position, Dr Khan served as Assistant Professor in Biochemistry, Faculty of Dentistry and Scientist in the Department of Biosciences, Jamia Millia Islamia, New Delhi, Assistant Professor, Department of Biochemistry at

Narayan Medical College at Sasaram and J. N. Medical College, Aligarh Muslim University. Dr. Khan has also received a Post-Doctoral Fellowship from the All India Institute of Medical Sciences, New Delhi. He has published more than 30 research articles in various international journals, book chapters and books and presented at international and national conferences/symposium. He has honored as DST-Young Scientist award and International Travel grants for research. Currently, his research interests have been focused on Nanotoxicology, Nanotechnology, Nanomedicine, and Polymers Chemistry.

Dr Sana Nafees has research experience in the field of carcinogenesis, cancer chemoprevention, molecular basis of chemical carcinogenesis, molecular biology, the role of free radicals in tumor promotion, progression, prevention of chemically induced toxicity in *in vivo* as well as *in vitro* systems. She has skills related to cell culture, cell handling, as well as animal handling. In addition, her expertise of handling techniques like Real-Time PCR (RT-PCR), Western blot and Immunofluorescence are an added advantage. Her post-doctoral experience at Jamia Millia Islamia based on *in vitro* and her Ph.D. expertise on *in vivo* models. She proved her credentials with her publication record.

Sapumal Ahangama is a lecturer at the University of Moratuwa, Sri Lanka. He holds a Ph.D. (National University of Singapore) and B.Sc. Eng. (Hons) (Moratuwa). His research interests include topics in financial technology (FinTech), entity resolution and data modelling of user behaviour.

Indika Perera is a senior lecturer at the University of Moratuwa, Sri Lanka. He holds a Ph.D. (St Andrews, UK) MBS (Colombo), MSc (Moratuwa), PGDBM (Colombo) and B.Sc. Eng. (Hons) (Moratuwa). His research interests include research topics of software architecture, software engineering; technology-enhanced learning, UX and immersive environments. He is a Fellow of HEA(UK), MIET, SMIEEE and a Charted Engineer registered at EC (UK) and IE(SL).

Ms. S. De Silva is a graduate student at the Department of Computer Science and Engineering, University of Moratuwa, Sri Lanka. She has research experience in Biomedical, Machine Learning and Data Mining. E-mail: ktsdesilva.15@cse.mrt.ac.lk

Ms. S. Dayarathna is a graduate student at the Department of Computer Science and Engineering, University of Moratuwa, Sri Lanka. She has research experience in Biomedical, Machine Learning and Data Mining. E-mail: sanuwaniudara.15@cse.mrt.ac.lk

Dr. D. Meedeniya is a Senior Lecturer in the Department of Computer Science and Engineering at the University of Moratuwa, Sri Lanka. She holds a Ph.D. in Computer Science from the University of St Andrews, United Kingdom. Her main research interests are Software Modelling and design, Bio-health informatics, Data Engineering, and Recommender Systems. She is a Fellow of

HEA(UK), MIET, MIEEE, and a Charted Engineer registered at EC (UK). E-mail: dulanim@cse.mrt.ac.lk

Radhika Malhotra received a B.Tech degree in Electronics and Communication from Maharishi Markandeshwar University, Mullana, Ambala, India and an M. Tech degree in VLSI Design from Kurukshetra University, Kurukshetra, India. Currently, she is a Research Scholar in National institute of Technology, Jalandhar, India. Her research interests are Biomedical Image Processing, Artificial Intelligence, Classification, Prognosis, and Survival Prediction of Neurodevelopmental Disorders.

Dr. Barjinder Singh Saini did his BTech and MTech in Electronics and Communication Engineering in 1993 and 1996, respectively. He did his Ph. D. in Signal Processing of Heart Rate Variability in 2009 at NIT Jalandhar. He has a total academic experience of 24 years, and at present he is Professor in Electronics and Communication department with Dr. B. R. Ambedkar National Institute of Technology, Jalandhar, India. He has more than 60 publications in various international journals and more than 40 publications at international conferences and book chapters. His recent research interests include Signal and Image Processing, Medical Image Analysis, Microprocessors, and Microcontrollers.

Dr. Savita Gupta did her BTech and MTech in Computer Science Engineering in 1992 and 1998, respectively. She did her Ph.D. in Computer Science Engineering from Punjab Technical University, Jalandhar, India in 2007. She has a total academic experience of 28 years, and at present she is Professor in Computer Science Engineering department with UIET, Panjab University, Chandigarh, India. She has more than 50 publications in various international journals and more than 40 publications at international conferences and book chapters. Her recent research interests include Signal and Image Processing, Network Security, Medical Image Analysis, Cognitive Enhancement, Machine Intelligence, Wavelets-based Signal and Image Processing, and Wireless Sensor Networks.

Dr G. Malar has dual graduation in rehabilitation sciences (B.R.Sc.) and special education (B.Ed.Spl.Ed.–HI) from Bharathidasan University, Tiruchirapalli, Tamil Nadu and Karnataka State Open University, Mysuru, Karnataka, respectively; and post-graduation in rehabilitation sciences (M.R.Sc. specializing in hearing impairment) from the latter. Since October 2020 she has been engaged as a post-doctoral fellow at the All India Institute of Speech and Hearing, Mysuru, Karnataka, carrying out research for development of adapted academic screening materials for children with communication disorders. She has also contributed to non-formal human resource development by serving as a resource person at more than 75 workshops/seminars/conferences.

Dr. S. P. Goswami holds a Ph.D. in Speech and Hearing and also a PGDHRM and MBA in Health Care Management. He is the first Speech and Hearing professional to receive the prestigious CV Raman fellowship from UGC, Government of India as Visiting Scholar at College of Applied Health Sciences, Department of Speech and Hearing Science, University of Illinois at Urbana-Champaign, USA. Presently he is working as Professor and Head Department of Speech-Language Pathology, formerly worked as Head Telecenter for Persons with Communication Disorders, Academic Coordinator, Clinical Services, AIISH, Mysore. He has more than 19 years of academic, clinical, research, and administrative experience. He works in the area of aphasia, ageing and neuro-cognitive communication disorders in adults and the elderly. He has completed more than 22 research projects and is presently working on five projects funded by national and international bodies.

Anshu Khurana is pursuing her doctoral degree in the Department of Computer Science and Engineering from Delhi Technological University. She is working as TRF in the Department of Computer Science and Engineering. She completed her M.Tech in Computer Science and Engineering from M. D. University in 2010. She served as contractual faculty in the Department of Information Technology in Delhi Technological University. Her area of interest lies in Nature-Based Optimization, Text Classification, Machine Learning, Evolutionary Computing, and Soft Computing.

Anudruti Singha is currently studying for an MSc in Communication and Multimedia Engineering as well as working as a research assistant in the domain of signal analysis and signal collection efficiency at FAU Erlangen. He is recent B.Tech Biomedical graduate (class of 2021) form the Vellore Institute of Technology. Recently he got into M.Sc. Communication and Multimedia Engineering at University of Erlangen-Nuremberg. His research ambitions are mainly in Signal Processing, Wireless Power Transmission, Optical Systems and Intelligent Systems Development to produce small-scale devices which possess attributes such as high signal processing and communication capability.

Om Prakash Verma, member of the IEEE (class of 2011), received his B. E. degree from the Malaviya National Institute of Technology, Jaipur, India, his M. Tech. degree from the Indian Institute of Technology Delhi, India, and his PhD degree from the University of Delhi, India. From 1992 to 1998 he was with the Department of Electronics and Communication Engineering, Malaviya National Institute of Technology, Jaipur, India. He joined the Department of Electronics and Communication Engineering, Delhi Technological University in 1998. Dr. Verma is a Professor of Delhi Technological University Delhi and currently working as Principal, G. B. Pant Govt. Engineering College Okhla, Delhi since April 2017. His present research interests include Data Engineering, Machine Learning, Evolutionary Computing, and Image Processing.

Dr. Anurag Sharma received his Ph.D. from NIT, Jalandhar. He currently works at GNA University, Phagwara handling Academic Matters and General Administration and solving technical problems. He works on behalf of autistic children, providing technological interventions. He has guided more than 20 M.Tech Students on diverse research topics. He has published more than 80 research papers in international journals (SCI, SCOPUS), at conferences and in national journals in the fields of Autism, Optical Communication, and Wireless Communication Research.

Dr. Shallu Sharma is a Project Scientist at the National Brain Research Centre (NBRC), Manesar, India. She completed her Ph.D. at Panjab University, Chandigarh, India. She received her Masters of Technology in Electronics Engineering from YMCA University of Science and Technology, Faridabad, India, in 2015 and Bachelor of Technology degree in Electronics and Communication Engineering from Kurukshetra University, Kurukshetra, India, in 2012. Her research areas include various subjects such as Advanced Digital Signal Processing, Digital Image Processing, and Artificial Intelligence. She is involved in typical research for exploring the remedies for Computer Vision Problem using 'Machine Learning' techniques and their implementations on bio-medical images for the detection of diseases.

Dr. Sumit Kumar is currently working as an Associate Professor in the School of Electronics and Electrical Engineering at Lovely Professional University, Jalandhar, Punjab, India. He has received his Doctorate from the Department of Electronics and Communication Engineering at Indian Institute of Technology (ISM), Dhanbad, India and Master of Technology from Guru Jambheshwar University of Science and Technology, Hisar, India. Dr. Kumar earned his Bachelor of Technology from Kurukshetra University, Kurukshetra, India. He has 12 years of research experience in various fields of Electronics Engineering. His research areas include Nanoelectronics, Photonics, Artificial Intelligence, and Computer Vision.

Preface

Enabling Technology for Neurodevelopmental Disorders: From Diagnosis to Rehabilitation demonstrates how technology drives the healthcare domain more than any other force, and in the near future, it will continue to grow in dramatic ways. Our book provides a crucial platform covering the emerging technology across different stages, i.e., from diagnosis to intervention and supportive stage to improve the condition and lifestyle of individuals on the spectrum of neurodevelopmental disorders (NDDs). Basically, NDDs manifest in early childhood and mature with the age of the individual. They encompass a cluster of conditions such as intellectual disability, communication, and learning deficit, autism spectrum disorder (ASD), attention-deficit/hyperactive disorder (ADHD), and visual and motor disorders. The disorder diagnostic/intervention methods have grown exponentially across a range of disciplines, including clinical, psychological, neurological, and technological. Among the stated methods, the technology-based innovations have shown tremendous potential in formulating the diagnostic, therapeutic schemes, prognostic procedures, and support programs which are proving beneficial both to NDD-affected individuals and clinicians.

Our book will reveal how innovative technology can accelerate the designs and formulation of diagnostic, therapeutic, adaptive, and supportive tools to reduce the progression of NDDs and drive revolutionary change in the capabilities of those affected by them. The considerations, concepts, and challenges of experts, researchers, and practitioners related to design, development, and testing of assistive technology devices is provided in detail with their respective solutions and conclusions. The book aims to: (i) explore innovations and inventions in technology that aim to intelligently catalyze rapid change in what is achievable in the field of NDDs; and (ii) to reflect how any technology-based method alone or in combination with other technology tools holds the potential to reduce the effects of NDDs. Our intention is to bring together the perspective of people affected by NDDs (and their parents) and promote and support the conversion of their thoughts into feasible products using intelligent technology, so that in the near future we will be able to cope with disability by delivering products that can turn disability into ability.

The book examines how the viewpoint can be blended with technology to convert thoughts into accessible products to meet the needs of people on the autism spectrum. The advances and research challenges in developing tech-based tools (within a laboratory or from laboratory to manufacturing units), learning programs (such as games), and multimodal systems (such as human-machine interactive systems) are brought forward from different domains. The objectives of these are:

- To demonstrate the feasibility of individual-centered technological approaches and cutting-edge methods, namely implantable brain devices, biosensors and neural engineering which can be developed in the near future.
- To explore the methodological challenges in designing, evaluating, developing, and employing *technology* for individuals with NDDs.
- To prove technology as an equalizer for individuals with NDDs.

In line with the book's objectives, the selected chapters are very meaningful in their attempt and ideology to understand the versatile nature and engineering viewpoint of technology in finding an interdisciplinary approach for young children on the autism spectrum. Each chapter in the book covers technology-enabled themes, discussing the current role and future of technology in different NDDs. The first chapter can be read as a primer to grasp baseline information about NDDs and role of technology relating to them. The chapter highlights the various forms of assistive technology and the impacts, challenges, issues, and opportunities for their ethical use on specific clinical conditions, especially regarding demand–supply and awareness-application gaps among the potential beneficiaries, caregivers, and healthcare providers in the country. The following chapters provide a well-defined route to exploring the book's theme in more detail and providing state-of-the-art-technological tools to enlist accurate, effective, and potential tools that can target the individual-specific behavioral traits, as well as intervening to address certain abnormalities. It will reveal how the clinical and research communities are formulating different practices, future standards, and metrics in tech-based devices, considering real-time challenges in designing, testing, evolving, and employing tech-tools for NDDs.

The second chapter discusses use of educational technology to improve learning for individuals with NDDs. Two case studies, wherein teachers worked continually with students and where technological interventions increased student success to mark the significance of technology, are discussed. In addition, a theoretical framework is provided for integrating technology constructively into teaching practice to help individuals, particularly those with different disabilities. Finally, the conclusion is drawn where the actionable recommendations for professional teaching practice are provided for future study frameworks. The third chapter discusses technological advances in the diagnosis and rehabilitation of learning disabilities. The review reflects that for the potential of technology to be realized, attitudes towards technology as a remedial measure need to change. In the fourth chapter, a description of technological instruments available to teaching autistic pupils is provided, which investigates the use of virtual reality (VR) in developing the education of children with ASD. The fifth chapter discussed the needs and challenges in e-interventions/telehealth for children with ASD and different NDDs from an Indian perspective. The sixth chapter discusses how sensors, convenient options, advanced assessments, and electronic devices are among the improvements that can change clinical consideration. An approach is proposed to manage patients with consistent, sporadic, or fluctuating issues. The chapter summarizes the contemplation of NDD offering an accomplishment in foreseeing risks and representation for disorders. The next chapter delves into the educational habilitation of children challenged with neurodevelopmental disorders. It details the versatility of assistive technology in enabling them to learn and grow along with their typically developing peers in inclusive learning environments, with a focus on the target of creating learning environments that support harmonious interactions and instruction. In the following chapter an overview of available technology-driven interventions such as brain interface, gamification, and VR are elaborated for ADHD. It concludes that there is a strong need to conduct well-designed and structured studies to strengthen the existing evidence. The following chapter is provided by the same team of authors who discuss the role of technology in enabling precision medicine for individuals affected with NDDs. The focus is on the application of technology, including artificial intelligence, High Performance Computing, machine learning, etc. to redirect large genomic and clinical datasets to facilitate improved diagnosis, intervention, and clinical outcomes.

In the tenth chapter, a review is given to provide insights on computational psychiatry to bridge the gap between data-driven and theory-driven approaches. The chapter reveals that the contrasting benefits and limitations of data-driven and theory-driven approaches have led to hybrid approaches that have higher future potential. In the eleventh chapter, the diagnosis of Alzheimer's Disease using Functional and Structural Neuroimaging Modalities is discussed. The three main architectures, namely, Capsule Network, Dense Net, and Inception V3 as the learning models, were considered and compared. The optimized Inception V3 model has shown high accuracy results of 96.1% and 95.5% for MRI and PET data, respectively. The twelfth chapter focuses on autism rehabilitation with webVR using text classification and proposes a software which comprised two games – "CASO" and "ATLAS" – to treat fear, social interaction and attention span of an autistic child with age four to 18 years.

The following chapters explore the usage of more advanced algorithms such as deep learning algorithms in the analysis of NDDs. The thirteenth chapter provides a systematic review of supervised brain tumor segmentation using deep learning-based approaches. The chapter addresses the most common problems in brain-tumor segmentation and offers potential solutions. In the fourteenth chapter, the author provides a deep brain stimulation-based model and set of spectral EEG features for faster detection and prognosis of Parkinson's Disease (PD). The chapter also provides deep insight into how the electric dipole generated from neurons can help in PD diagnosis. The fifteenth and final chapter proposes a hybrid deep model with convolutional neural networks placed in a concatenating framework, for identification of one of the major

NDDs, namely ASD. The author explores MRI images from a standardized dataset called ABIDE and identifies ASD with an accuracy rate of 84.5%. Thus, the automated detection and prognosis section demonstrates the potential of deep learning approaches in NDDs.

In summary, our book manages to provide ample theoretical knowledge about novel methodologies and ideologies that can complement the existing techniques by providing numerous solutions and approaches to translate such ideas into real possibilities. In addition, readers can find the key pointers to enhance their research and contributions in the NDD domain and related areas. A big thanks to all the authors for making the book worthwhile by sharing their ideas, making their contributions, and offering us support throughout. We are thankful to the Editorial Advisory Board and a team of reviewers for providing feedback that helped to give shape to the book. Special thanks go to Helen Pritt, Publisher at Routledge, Taylor & Francis, for her guidance and cooperation from editing the material to the publication stage of the book.

1 Assistive Technology and Neurodevelopmental Disorders

An Indian Perspective

Srinivasan Venkatesan

Introduction

The term "neurodevelopmental disorders" (NDD) is a newcomer in psychiatry and clinical psychology. NDD is increasingly replacing earlier terms used to designate a constellation of childhood and adult clinical conditions. There is no agreed definition for its diagnosis. Developmental disorders were first included in the DSM-III (American Psychiatric Association, 1980). The "neuro" prefix occurred in DSM-5 (American Psychiatric Association, 2013) with conditions like intellectual disability (ID), autism spectrum disorder (ASD), and attention deficit hyperactivity disorder (ADHD) under them. Some experts add schizophrenia and bipolar disorder to the list. The latest revision of the International Classification of Diseases (ICD-11) is expected to re-designate all these conditions supposed to be sharing a genetic basis.

The NDD is identified or classified based on genotype, molecular, or organic causative evidence rather than overt behavioral or phenotype symptoms. A host of molecular factors including genetic mutations, obstetric insults, congenital brain lesions, synapse connectivity, neural networking, heritable genomics, microglia, immune dysfunction, neurotoxicants, pesticides in the food chain, infectious disease, metabolic dysfunction, prenatal, perinatal and postnatal events, and abnormal nervous system development are linked to their onset, causation, and occurrence. The genotype-phenotype correlations are difficult to establish owing to the multiple factors that play a role in their eventual clinical outcomes. Technology is perpetually improving, attempting to understand the molecular etiology of NDD. To what extent it is possible to translate them into clinical practice continues to be just anybody's guess (Parenti et al., 2020).

Assistive and Adaptive Technology

What was hitherto screened, identified, diagnosed, or labeled on outwardly observable-measurable behavioral phenotype and molar parameters is now researched on a genotype and molecular level. More than paper-pencil developmental tests, neurological examination, observation of random behavior patterns, the use of technology-assisted tools like cranial ultrasounds, brain

DOI: 10.4324/9781003165569-1

magnetic resonance imaging, neurophysiological tests, and genetic tests have become routine. It is not for diagnosis alone. Even treatment and remediation schemes are explored at the level of gene therapy or correction, neural mechanisms, psycho–physiology, bio–signals, artificial intelligence, virtual reality, machine learning, wearable devices, mobile apps, tablets, robots, gaming, computerized tests, videos, gaming, television, DVDs, PDAs, and so on. All this is a move away from traditional anti-psychotic or psychotropic medication, cognitive behavior therapy, speech and learning therapy, stimulant and non-stimulant mono-therapy, integrative neurology, and others (Venkatesan, 2019).

Assistive technology (AT) is any item, piece of equipment, software, or product that is used to increase, maintain, or improve the functional capabilities of persons with disabilities (PWD). They can be acquired commercially off-the-shelf, modified, or customized to suit a given user. Examples vary from communication boards, prosthetics, special switches, keyboards, and pointing devices to screen readers, curriculum aids, walkers, wheelchairs, braces, power lifts, pencil holders, eye-gaze and head trackers, mounting systems, and positioning devices. Some more examples include Braille Books (or Dot Books), Braille Smartwatches, Smart Canes, Tactile Diagrams, mobile devices like tablets and smartphones, text-speech conversion, and word predictor tools. Smart gloves help the speech and hearing impaired to interpret other people's conversations by converting their words into text in the watch they wear. There are also apps to help with reading, writing, note-taking, building self-control, meditating, or undertaking math. A protective headgear ensures physical protection for people with epilepsy or head-banging (as in Lesch-Nyhan Syndrome). Parallel bars help to overcome balance problems and develop equilibrium and strength. A relief cushion in a wheelchair protects against developing pressure sores. Ramps and handlebars help to scale heights. A talking watch helps to tell time. Gaze-based AT is used not only for entertainment, gaming, and recreational activities but also for making drawings, literacy training, internet surfing, and developing social interactions. The operations of household gadgets are easily done using gaze-based technology. Bio-feedback instruments help to regulate their behaviors (Borgestig et al., 2016; Venkatesan and Hariharan, 2019).

Some AT instruments ameliorate the quality of life in PWD by helping in daily living activities. Exoskeletons are wearable mobile machines powered by electric motors, hydraulics, or pneumatics to enable limb movements or lift weights. AT can assist or augment cognitive processes like attention, memory, self-regulation, navigation, emotion-recognition, and sequential activities planning. Specific examples are abbreviation expanders, alternate keyboards, audiobooks and publications, electronic math worksheets, graphic organizers, speech-recognition programs, speech synthesizers, talking calculators, spell checkers, and pictionaries (Johnson et al. 2009). A distinction is made between hard and soft technologies. The former refers to tangible AT devices, while the latter covers human areas of decision making, strategies, training, concept formation, and service delivery. ATs are also classified based on their purpose to improve access (telephones and counters at wheelchair height, Braille markings in elevators), education, employment, or recreation. AT devices are different from AT services. The device refers to an item, piece of equipment, or product system. Services are to using them as part of therapy or interventions (Ravneberg and Söderström, 2017). AT is a generic term that includes assistive, adaptive, and rehabilitative devices for PWD and includes the process in selecting, locating, and using them. One way of classifying them is:

- Communication Aids like Speech and Augmentative Communication Aids, Writing and Typing Aids;
- Computer Access Aids like Alternate Input and Output Devices, Accessible Software, Universal Design;
- Hearing and Listening Aids;
- Transportation and Mobility Aids like ambulance aids, scooters, and power chairs, wheelchairs, vehicle conversions;
- Environment Aids like environmental controls and switches, home-work-place adaptations, ergonomic equipment;
- Daily Living Aids like clothing and dressing aids, eating and cooking aids, home maintenance aids, toileting, and bathing aids;
- Prosthetics and Orthotics;
- Seating And Positioning Aids;
- Educational and Learning Aids like cognitive aids, early intervention aids, etc;
- Vision and Reading Aids; and
- Recreational and Leisure Aids like sports aids, toys and games, travel aids.

Peterson, Prasad, and Prasad (2012) highlighted the absence of an international consensus on a classification system for AT and called for several professional groups to use a common language to define and describe the technology. If there is one way of Assistive Technology Device Classification based on the American with Disabilities Act, there is another based on the International Classification System of Functioning, Disability, and Health, or the International Classification of Diseases-11.

Uses

AT is beneficial for PWD as it promotes their independence and reduces the stress of the people around them. It enables them to have greater control over their lives, interact with others, and participate fully in life. In turn, all this increases their self-motivation, turns them accountable, provides new opportunities, or expands learning and life experience. There is a common misconception that AT is "cheating." The apprehension that its users become overly dependent upon them or that they can later never live without them is widespread. It is argued that they become unmotivated and then rely solely on technology to succeed, especially when surrounded by negative community attitudes, poor social acceptance and the prohibitive cost of the aids or appliances. It is argued that individuals who are permitted to use them are getting an unfair advantage. The issue is more about equity than equality. Some teachers resist the use of AT in the pretext that it involves more work for them. Another erroneous notion is that their use will "fix" all the problems of PWDs. The wheelchair, for example, does not make the paraplegic walk-it is just an enabling device. AT is not intended to replace regular practices. No AT solution can be a perfect fit for one and all. One might need a high-end or low-end device. Some argue that AT is expensive. Some of them are expensive-but many are free. Disability is an outcome of an interaction between the person and an environment with barriers that hinder their participation on an equal basis. AT can reduce or eliminate such barriers. Obtaining such devices is not always possible, owing to product and service-related barriers. Some obstacles to AT are lack of awareness about the availability of such products and services, absence of government legislation, deficient policies and national programs, or their prohibitive cost, the lack of availability of such products and services. The challenges to optimal AT depend on availability, accessibility, affordability, adaptability, acceptability, and quality (Atanga et al., 2020).

Assistive Technology Assessment

An assistive technology assessment (ATA) is often a prelude and starting point for their use by PWD. ATA is a continuous collaborative process, wherein a team of multidisciplinary professionals determines what technologies would improve an individual's performance, participation, and independence. The method considers the strengths and weaknesses, physical and cognitive abilities, activities to be performed, sensory status (vision and hearing), and the social-cultural environment where they are to be undertaken. The areas that are typically considered for NDD, for example, during these assessments, are spelling, handwriting, reading, math, written expression, recreation, seating or positioning, seeing, listening, self-care, and mobility. The list of potential team members could include the child, family, teacher, and therapist. The team meets regularly at fixed dates, locations, or timing. There are usually a facilitator, timekeeper, and recorder who minutes each meeting. Through brainstorming, discussions, and eventual consensus, AT alternatives are worked out at regular intervals. For example, a student with NDD having handwriting difficulties with a regular writing instrument might require pencil grippers, a portable word processor, wrist or arm supports, an enlarged keyboard, or voice recognition software. Another child with an expressive speech disorder might need manual signs, picture symbol boards, photograph cards, voice output devices with single messages, or multiple levels with dynamic displays. Students with visual impairments might need text enlargement in copy machines, word cards are written in more extensive form, use of markers for text, peer reading, audio recorded text materials, talking word processors, and screen reading software. At the end of an ATA, a report is generated with key elements such as the person's disability, the specific types of device being recommended, its cost, training and maintenance, service, or repair requirements.

Applications

As products, technology-enabled devices or equipment were listed in the preceding. Technology serves both as means as well as end process solutions for PWD. Technology Enabled Care Services covers telehealth, telecare, telemedicine, telerehabilitation, tele-consulting, teleservices, telecounseling, teletherapy mental health, and others. Each of these terms has a distinct meaning and the context for which they have to be used. For example, telecare for elderly PWD living in community care might have well-distributed alarms or pendants with detectors or sensors installed around them that get activated to ensure their safety or security. These devices can be linked to a telehealth mechanism, wherein emergencies like the onset of fits, an acute psychotic episode, or a drop in blood sugar levels can be reported to the nearest caregiver facility. Wherein mobile phone technology and Apps are used, there can be even greater flexibility to access these services. A cloud computing-assisted GPS and GPRS can help to make safe walking services for people with dementia, intellectual disabilities, and autism (Bowser, 2020; Wang, Gu, and Wu, 2020).

While there is consensus on possibilities, opportunities, and challenges in tele-based services for children across conditions and disciplines like occupational therapy, pediatrics, child neurology (Lo and Gospe Jr., 2019; Sarsak, 2020), there is still insufficient evidence of their impacts. There is a need for stringent measures on license regulations, credentialing service providers, and monitoring their costs against returns in India. AT-Enabled devices for use in the context of NDD require closer scrutiny. For example, there are reports on social skills immaturity owing to premature exposure and use of mobile robots or devices by children (aged under five years) with a diagnosis of NDD (Coutinho et al. 2020). A question often posed is whether there can or need to be AT devices-based applications focused exclusively on various clinical phenotypes of NDD? Is it needed to design devices separately for diagnostic conditions like ASD, ADD/ADHD, ID, and others? Or is there a standard underlying solution that can address all NDD? In general, the thumb rule is that mobility aids help those with locomotion problems, just as hearing aids help those with auditory disabilities. Cognitive aids help people with challenges in higher mental functions. A few investigators have searched for AT solutions specific to conditions under NDD such as Retts Syndrome, Downs Anomaly, Fragile X, Angelman, Cornelis de Lange, Kluver Bucy, PKU, OCD, schizophrenia, and others (Stasolla and Ciarmoli, 2020). There are also some conditions under NDD, for which no specific AT is available. Examples under this variety are Cri du chat, Patau, Edward, Cornelia de Lange, Kluver-Busy Syndromes, and others. It is not certain whether such syndrome specific attempts at AT applications would yield meaningful results. A tentative review of such research is given below:

(a) **ADD/ADHD**

Lindstedt and Umb-Carlsson (2013) attempted an evaluation of a model of intervention to promote community participation in everyday life settings consisting of cognitive AT for adults with ADHD. The results showed a higher frequency of involvement and satisfaction over one year of study. On-task focus improved with an AT device (Watchminder-2) to prompt the self-monitoring of individual students to increase academic engagement (Rich, 2009). Others have used similar prompting devices to aid such students complete their tasks by using digital smart glasses, gaming devices, table-top activities, video-modelling, iPad-based tools or other apps.

(b) **Reading/Writing Difficulties**

For children with reading difficulties or learning disabilities, gadgets involving AT such as pencil grips, specially lined paper, spell checkers, word prediction software, and audiobooks have been tried. It helps scaffold their reading-writing through the use of text-to-speech, and speech-to-text apps. Of course, the use of these technologies require extensive support, training and acceptance within the learning-teaching environment. One of the greatest challenges that poor readers experience is that they have deficits in many subject areas that are covered in the reading text passage. In such instances, an audio or video preview covering the words or vocabulary in the text can ease their oncoming reading task (Perelmutter, McGregor, and Gordon, 2017).

(c) **Autism Spectrum Disorders**

Personal FM Systems or remote microphone technology were tried on children with ASD (Schafer et al., 2016). Hetzroi et al. (2002) used AT for symbol identification by children with Rett syndrome showed a steady learning curve across six types of meaningful referents: real name, song, storybook, food, verb, and communication (Hetzroni, Rubin, and Konkol, 2002). Another attempt to use AT-based programs to support choice strategies by a sample of Rett's children showed increased performance and decreased stereotype behaviors during intervention phases (Stasolla, 2015). AT as a "supplementary program" with micro-switches and eye-tracking devices is recommended (Amoako and Hare, 2020), although caregivers reported challenges in the routine daily use of such devices (Alabbas and Miller, 2019). Most case studies on Fragile X Syndrome have used AT solutions like tickle box and mobile technology for improving decision making, supporting choice opportunities, promoting adaptive responses and to reduce hand mouthing in a useful, affordable, and effective manner (Perilli et al., 2019).

(d) **Intellectual and Developmental Disabilities**

Mechling (2007) summarizes available literature between 1990 and 2005 on AT as a self-management tool for prompting students with intellectual disabilities to initiate and complete daily tasks. It is found that picture prompts, tactile prompts, auditory prompts, and computer-aided systems were found to be useful tools to promote adaptive behaviors as well as reduce challenging behaviors in these children (Stasolla and Ciarmoli, 2020). Research reviews on the use of AT on students with Downs Syndrome have found beneficial improvements in their independence, performance, and social interactions (Al-Moghyrah, 2017).

(e) **Schizophrenia**

Some people with schizophrenia have a hard time with executive functions, including attention, memory, planning, sequencing, concept formation, strategizing, and problem-solving. Voice or sound recording devices have been used to track movements with less pressure and more control to enhance their self-management strategies. For example, a reminder watch sends a cue when it is time to take medication, begin exercises, eat food, or seek an appointment for the next consultation. A ball blanket is a heavy cover that fits snugly on the body to have a soothing effect on anxiety and fear. It can also facilitate sleep and relaxation (Devlin, Nolan, and Turner, 2019).

(f) **Bipolar Disorder**

Surveys have shown that a wide range of AT devices and solutions have been tried in bipolar disorders. Smartphones are used to monitor symptoms, forecasting forthcoming episodes (Busk et al., 2020), track mood-related triggers and cycle of symptoms. They help indicate when to seek consultation or maintain a digital cognitive diary of irrational and negative thoughts or breathe to relax. The use of bullet-pointed sheets help the users to keep daily records of mood swings, and goal tracker books help to set targets at the beginning of the week and reward themselves for good behavior. The Anger Thermometer App allows users to level up or down depending upon their mood (Mattson, 2017).

(g) **Multiple Sclerosis:**

Mobility is a characteristic challenge in most persons affected by multiple sclerosis. They need mobility devices like canes, crutches, quad or four-legged canes, walkers, wheelchairs, stairlifts, and scooters to secure better balance and support. Kitchen aids are used when there is limited hand, wrist, and forearm strength. Bathroom aids like a shower chair, grab bar, and nonskid bath mats make bathrooms accessible and safer for these persons. Electric toothbrushes with a big handle and toothpaste in a pump dispenser can become part of their accessories to get over their weak grip. Velcro-fitted footwear and zipper pull in place of buttons, large keyboard, touchpad, ergonomic mouse, joystick, or trackball devices can replace regular tying input devices for these persons. Weakness in the leg muscles makes it hard to go up and downstairs, rise from a chair, or walk. An ankle-foot brace can help keep the ankle stable and toes from dragging. AT solutions are required in at least half of the population of persons affected by multiple sclerosis having cognitive impairments related to memory, attention, executive functions, speed of information processing, and visual-spatial difficulties (Squires, Williams, and Morrison, 2019).

(h) **Dementia**

AT and robotics are useful for increasing autonomy and independence in persons with dementia. Electric calendars, schedulers, medication reminders, GPRS-enabled locators, picture phones, and remote-controlled devices are recommended. Memory Glasses is a wearable context-aware memory aid and reminder system in the form of a pair of spectacles that help in anomias and agnosias. There is an intelligent garment in the vest form that monitors posture, body temperature, EKG, respiration, EMG, and physical activity. Designer clocks help these patients to distinguish between day-night. Talking Mats is a popular app that allows people with dementia to communicate feelings by selecting symbols and pictures. GPS location and tracking devices help to alert when the patient tends to go astray or wander. Safety devices such as night lights with sensors automatically turn on as one passes through them (Thorpe et al., 2016).

Admittedly, there is no definitive list about which clinical conditions fall under the rubric of NDD. There can be many more clinical conditions like fetal alcohol spectrum disorder, motor coordination disorder, traumatic brain injury, communication, speech and language disorders, epilepsy, cerebral palsy, neuromuscular disorders, disorders of conduct, and emotion in the preceding. In short, it appears that the complete nosology of childhood and adolescent psychiatry gets included in this list!

Measures on AT

Within the AT devices, how effectively and efficiently AT users with disabilities can function in different contexts and environments determines the product or service usability. Device usage is not a one-time, all-or-nothing proposition. The decision process recurs over time. On one side, traditional psychometric and administrative measures have been developed and used to attempt AT outcomes assessment. On the other side, there are opinions that one must move outside or away from such approaches to pursue better ways. Several questions on how AT impacts PWD concerning their education, employment, and ability to live independently. What are essential needs met by the use of AT devices for the PWD? Usability Scale for Assistive Technology (USAT), The Quebec User Evaluation of Satisfaction with Assistive Technology (QUEST 2.0), The Psychosocial Impact of Assistive Devices Scale (PIADS), Assistive Technology Outcomes Measurement System (ATOMS), Family Impact of Assistive Technology Scale (FIATS), Social Cost Analysis Instrument (SCAI), Assistive Technology Device Predisposition Assessment (ATD-PA) are some popular instruments used in the field.

Ethical Issues

AT can provide assistance to ameliorate the QOL of the PWDs. There are critical ethical concerns related to the use or non-use of AT viz., beneficence, non-malfeasance, justice, autonomy, and fidelity. Beneficence is to do with ensuring that actions lead to good results that benefit others. Fidelity is to be honest, faithful, and trustworthy. Non-malfeasance refers to the principle of not causing harm to others directly or through avoidance of actions that risk harming others. Autonomy is to do with freedom of action and choice. Further, respecting the dignity of PWDs is essential for their well-being (Cook, 2009). A few examples of ethical issues in technology for PWDs are personal privacy, access right, and harmful actions resulting from IT use such as piracy, pilferage, or loss of information. Video-phoning might be perceived as an invasion of a person's privacy. When someone is sitting and talking to someone in front of the screen, anyone who walks past can be captured on screen against their will or without their knowledge. Not all households might have the option of a separate room or private area for technology-enabled interactions. The dignity of PWD is essential for their well-being (Venkatesan and Yashodharakumar, 2019).

A recommended route to the favor of AT for PWD is for states and countries to have a policy document combined with a political will. This has happened at many places in the west-not yet in India. Such an attempt is likely to provide an overarching vision, identify key themes to be addressed or prioritized, and ensure their implementation (Tangcharoensathien et al., 2018). The crux of the problem is that the need for AT is high, and demand is low owing to the widespread lack of awareness among the potential beneficiaries, their caregivers, and healthcare providers in the country. This situation is authentic for most low- and middle-income countries. Further, the product designs and financial constraints leave them poorly compatible with reaching the needy. There is a need to periodically publish updated directories on Assistive device producers, listing national and international mandates about their technical specifications, repair, and maintenance. For example, devices like motorized wheelchairs and tricycles are impossible in the hilly terrains of North-East India.

There is still no complete policy on AT for PWD in India. Such approaches have been in place since the 1990s in the United States, Australia, Brazil, and Norway, with periodic advancements and revisions (Dove, 2012). In fact, in some quarters, there are calls for developing an international framework for AT that could guide the development of policies, systems, and service delivery procedures worldwide. AT is being raised as a human right with a foundation in the UNCRPD. For optimal AT provision, many other elements are also essential. These elements include: good quality AT products have to be available at affordable prices, end-users should know that some products, devices, solutions, and services are available along with professional advice and supports. Follow-up mechanisms have to be ensured. Infrastructure for maintenance and repairs has to be in place. Funding mechanisms are to be ensured (de Witte et al., 2018).

In contemporary times, engineers, and technocrats have entered the arena of NDD. The traditional clinic-based diagnosticians and therapists are taking a back seat. Multinational biotech genomic companies are in the fray, offering drugs or next-generation treatments to repair critical genes linked to NDD. These offerings are not without their risks and uncertainties, pending approval for the candidate drugs from regulatory authorities. Technology proliferation in everyday life, owing to the pervasive presence of the internet, the rise of mobile and touchscreen devices, and various software apps have posed doubts whether they all serve as boon or bane for NDD. The children with NDD are wired to experience and use technology at home and in school frequently. They are observed to show the Mozart Effect. Technology is not a single unique entity. Thus, it is unlikely to have a single unique effect. As with food affecting physical development, the effects of technology will depend on the type of technology used, how much, and for how long. Any temporary effect of technology use, albeit significant, is unlikely to be specific to technology itself.

Assistive Technology: the Indian Scenario

Whereas the history of AT in the west dates back to the early 1900s, formal and legal mandates were accorded only with the enactment of the Tech Act (1988) was the first instance to define and provide federal funds for assistive devices in the United States. The ear trumpets were precursors in the 17th century to the later 20th-century hearing aids. Louis Braille came up with the ingenious binary writing system for the blind in 1824. During the 1920s, a "stair throne" (precursor to modern-day stairlifts) was devised to carry the overweight King Henry VIII up and down twenty steps in the Whitehall Palace. The wheelchair (1933), walking frame (1949), and the "sip-and-puff" device (1961) to aid bedridden patients to switch on-off lights or television were invented later. Speech-generating devices (the 1970s), the Prosthetic Limb (1980s), Accessibility Software (1990s), and Prehensile Robotics (2000) are modern-day inventions seeking to culminate in autonomous cars. The Assistive Technology Act (2004) has replaced the earlier version.

Robust research on AT or authentic sources for tracing or tracking its history lacks in the Indian context. Artificial Limbs Manufacturing Corporation (ALIMCO) is a government sector entity that is deemed the largest producer of assistive devices. Punarbhava, Swavalamban, and Accessible India Campaign (2015) provide a cyberspace gateway or portal to find information, discuss issues, network, or look for assistive devices. A Center for Assistive Technology and Innovation was established in the same year in the country. Lower limb orthosis is by far the most widely prevalent device in the Indian market, despite complaints by its users of pain while squatting, kneeling, sitting cross-legged, kneeling, walking in mud, or while riding a bicycle. Despite the availability of AT in the global market, their availability and access in the Indian markets are far from satisfactory. The reasons are not far to fathom. Some AT developed in the West might be expensive, not customized to suit local conditions, or be relevant and applicable to the country. In an institutional audit undertaken on the current status of various AT facilities available for PWD at libraries in Delhi, India, it was found that there were negligible facilities for deaf/hearing impaired and locomotor impaired users (Sanaman and Kumar, 2014).

In the contemporary scenario, several hundreds of start-ups have been initiated by capitalists in collaboration with technical experts, clinicians, disability NGOs, and policy experts to work on AT's research and development. Conferences and conclaves are just beginning to be regularly organized to showcase products and solutions to increase awareness to empower PWD. The Indian market for disability-assisting devices and technologies, which runs through a thousand crore, is just beginning to be tapped. The ongoing thrust given by the Government of India on Make in India and Skills India is being taken advantage of to promote AT solutions for the disabled.

Key recommendations made in the prevailing scenario typically include the setting of an exclusive fund for AT by the Government of India, universal health coverage for PWD, provisions for encouragement for research and development by incentives for affordable and straightforward solutions. Another recommendation is to prepare periodically updated directories on available AT devices or solutions for the disabled in the country. The spread of AT requires 4G Internet connections are enabled across the country. Available AT leadership personnel, certificate or graduate programs that offer specialized training on the theme, knowledge about which child with special needs requires what device or service, what will be their outcomes, and how to make them available to the needy are all areas that need an urgent re-examination. A majority of AT devices are abandoned immediately or within the first year. It is also shown that an interdisciplinary approach to evaluating AT needs decreases the risk of equipment abandonment, although it does not entirely solve the problem. Four factors were significantly related to abandonment – lack of consideration of user opinion in the selection, easy device procurement, poor device performance, and change in user needs or priorities (Phillips and Zhao, 1993). Some distinguish between personal and technology linked factors in discontinuation of the use of such devices. Personal factors might be that the need was never felt for the device or that their opinions were not considered during the initial selection process. Technology factors might make the device too expensive, lacks good looks and safety, is malfunctioning or challenging to use, takes too much time, or has not had sufficient training. Rarely social-cultural or environmental factors like accessibility problems and stigma can lead to the abandonment of AT devices.

The Ministry of Social Justice and Empowerment, Government of India, identifies aids and assistive devices for mobility, daily living, seating, positioning, home and workplace accommodations, or to increase accessibility of persons with disabilities in the country. However, there is still no exclusive cell, hub, or law that is dedicated in the nodal ministry to safeguard or promote the use of AT exclusively in the Indian settings.

Impact Evaluation

Several factors of AT determine their relative impact in terms of effectiveness and retention across different conditions. Some such factors typically identified are operational support, physical support, psychological support, social support, cultural match, reduced external help, affordability, travel help, compatibility, effectiveness, and retention. In addition, factors like reparability, dependability, durability, operability, learnability, portability, flexibility, personal comfort, and acceptability are also crucial for the acceptance of AT devices or solutions. All this is not to discount the value or importance of consumer involvement on satisfaction with and use of the AT. The consumer's involvement in the pre-purchase decision-making process, their perceptions of feeling informed, and their degree of being satisfied with or use of the device is crucial. Research has shown that consumers highly value AT devices' impact on their independence, subjective well-being, and participation in work and school. In the case of children with disabilities, caregivers rated AT devices highly wherein they reduced, helped reduce the child's dependence, increased their mobility, improved self-care and social function (McNicholl, Casey, Desmond, and Gallagher, 2019).

While AT's benefits, especially for PWD, have been severally mentioned, among its shortcomings are mentioned factors like the ease of their use. Wherein it seems overly complicated to some people, this might discourage them from making the best use of them. Some people are uncomfortable with the idea of sensors, cameras, or other gadgets monitoring them in their own homes. It might be seen as an invasion of their privacy. Despite a comprehensive AT assessment, sometimes, sheer common sense might turn out to be practical. After a free tricycle distribution community program for school children with locomotion disabilities, a parent asked why bicycles were not given. The whole family could have used bicycles to drop the child at school and attend their works.

Is this all sound and no action or the proverbial search for a needle lost in a haystack? As stated by the World Health Organization, the identification or manifestation of an infant at risk for NDD is a complex interplay between genes, social and physical environment, modulation of gene transcription and expression (epigenetic mechanisms), infant brain plasticity, and effects of an early enriched environment. Will technology-enabled treatments or interventions for NDD bring about consequent effects on the organism at behavioral, cellular, and molecular levels? Are these devices being used merely as babysitters? Are these contraptions put into these children's hands by parents to be left undisturbed during their pursuits? There are already indications that technology-induced compulsive behaviors in children and adults have long-term behavioral repercussions, such as increased aggression, mood disturbances, fatigue, risk-taking tendencies, attention problems, and trouble in socializing on a real-time basis.

AT promises an exciting future. Driverless cars, mobility scooters, the Internet of Things, GPS-enabled mobility, Virtual Reality, Personal Robots, Robotic Exoskeletons (which allow people with paraplegia to stand and walk), wearable suits powered by motors, gesture-controlled devices, and others Still, several questions remain on the need, validity, and reliability of the construct of NDD. There is abundant evidence that NDD co-occurs rather than existing as single or separate conditions. Added to all this, are they just other new names to already pre-existing conditions. Diagnostic labels help no more than to stigmatize than understand people. They could even stifle the thinking of both those who are attached to and the practitioners who name them so. There is still a need for randomized controlled trials and long-term follow-up studies to understand the efficacy of treatments claimed for NDD. There are ethical issues involving children with NDD bio-medical research. On the positive side, the use of technology in NDD has helped students with special educational needs to continue their education, enhance mobility, achieve greater accessibility, and empower or enable them. As an intervention tool, technology use with children carries the risks of safety, security, and addiction.

In contemporary times, engineers and technocrats have entered the arena to address the enigma of NDD. The traditional clinic-based diagnosticians and therapists are taking a back seat. Multinational biotech genomic companies are on the fray offering drugs or next-generation treatments to repair critical genes linked to NDD. These offerings are not without their risks and uncertainties pending approval for the candidate drugs from regulatory authorities. Technology proliferation in everyday life, owing to its pervasive presence, has posed doubts about whether they all serve as boon or bane for NDD. The children with NDD are wired to experience and use technology at home and in school frequently. They are observed to show the Mozart Effect. Technology is not a single unique entity. Thus, it is unlikely to have a single unique effect. As with food affecting physical development, the effects of technology will depend on the type of technology used, how much, and for how long. Any temporary effect of technology use, albeit significant, is unlikely to be specific to the technology itself.

In summary, this chapter has attempted to define NDD and bring it close to AT. Throughout the discourse, the emphasis is placed on discussing available technology to specific problem areas within the various clinical conditions. It is noted how there are a demand–supply and awareness–application gap among the potential beneficiaries, their caregivers, and healthcare providers in the country. The implication for updating legal accommodations for AT in the context of persons with disabilities is recommended. As an intervention tool, technology use with children carries the risks of safety, security, and addiction. This chapter has delved into all these details with empirical and evidence-based supports.

Acknowledgment

The author wishes to thank the Director of AIISH, Mysore, Karnataka, India, for the permission granted to write this chapter.

References

Abbas, Norah Abdullah and Darcy E. Miller. "Challenges and assistive technology during typical routines: Perspectives of caregivers of children with autism spectrum disorders and other disabilities." *International Journal of Disability, Development and Education*, 66, no. 3 (2019): 273–283.

Al-Moghyrah, Homoud. "Assistive technology use for students with Down syndrome at mainstream schools in Riyadh, Saudi Arabia: Teachers' perspectives." *Journal of Education and Practice*, 8, no. 33 (2017).

American Psychiatric Association. *Diagnostic and statistical manual of mental disorders (DSM-III Edition)*. American Psychiatric Pub, 1980.

American Psychiatric Association. *Diagnostic and statistical manual of mental disorders (DSM-5®)*. American Psychiatric Pub, 2013.

Amoako, Annika Nina and Dougal Julian Hare. "Non-medical interventions for individuals with Rett syndrome: A systematic review." *Journal of Applied Research in Intellectual Disabilities*, 33, no. 5 (2020): 808–827.

Atanga, Comfort, Beth A. Jones, Lacy E. Krueger and Shulan Lu. "Teachers of students with learning disabilities: Assistive technology knowledge, perceptions, interests, and barriers." *Journal of Special Education Technology*, 35, no. 4 (2020): 236–248.

Borgestig, Maria, Jan Sandqvist, Richard Parsons, Torbjörn Falkmer and Helena Hemmingsson. "Eye gaze performance for children with severe physical impairments using gaze-based assistive technology—A longitudinal study." *Assistive Technology*, 28, no. 2 (2016): 93–102.

Bowser, Gayl. "Remote Assistive Technology Services: Many Things Are Remotely Possible." In *Assistive Technology to Support Inclusive Education*. Emerald Publishing Limited, 2020.

Busk, Jonas, Maria Faurholt-Jepsen, Mads Frost, Jakob E. Bardram, Lars Vedel Kessing, and Ole Winther. "Forecasting Mood in Bipolar Disorder From Smartphone Self-assessments: Hierarchical Bayesian Approach." *JMIR mHealth and uHealth*, 8, no. 4 (2020): e15028.

Cook, Albert M. "Ethical Issues Related to the Use/Non-Use of Assistive Technologies." *Developmental Disabilities Bulletin*, 37 (2009): 127–152.

Coutinho, Franzina, Gauri Saxena, Akansha Shah, Shantanu Tilak, Neelu Desai, and Vrajesh Udani. "Mobile media exposure and use in children aged zero to five years with diagnosed neurodevelopmental disability." *Disability and Rehabilitation: Assistive Technology* (2020): 1–7.

de Witte, Luc, Emily Steel, Shivani Gupta, Vinicius Delgado Ramos, and Uta Roentgen. "Assistive technology provision: towards an international framework for assuring availability and accessibility of affordable, high-quality assistive technology." *Disability and Rehabilitation: Assistive Technology*, 13, no. 5 (2018): 467–472.

Devlin, Hannah, Clodagh Nolan, and Niall Turner. "Assistive technology and schizophrenia." *Irish Journal of Occupational Therapy* (2019).

Dove, Marianne K. "Advancements in assistive technology and AT laws for the disabled." *Delta Kappa Gamma Bulletin*, 78, no. 4 (2012): 23.

Hetzroni, Orit, Corinne Rubin, and Orna Konkol. "The use of assistive technology for symbol identification by children with Rett syndrome." *Journal of Intellectual and Developmental Disability*, 27, no. 1 (2002): 57–71.

Johnson, Kurt L., Alyssa M. Bamer, Kathryn M. Yorkston, and Dagmar Amtmann. "Use of cognitive aids and other assistive technology by individuals with multiple sclerosis." *Disability and Rehabilitation: Assistive Technology*, 4, no. 1 (2009): 1–8.

Lindstedt, Helena and Õie Umb-Carlsson. "Cognitive assistive technology and professional support in everyday life for adults with ADHD." *Disability and Rehabilitation: Assistive Technology*, 8, no. 5 (2013): 402–408.

Lo, Mark D. and Sidney M.Gospe Jr. "Telemedicine and child neurology." *Journal of Child Neurology*, 34, no. 1 (2019): 22–26.

Mattson, Donald C. "Usability evaluation of the digital anger thermometer app." *Health Informatics Journal*, 23, no. 3 (2017): 234–245.

McNicholl, Aoife, Hannah Casey, Deirdre Desmond, and Pamela Gallagher. "The impact of assistive technology use for students with disabilities in higher education: a systematic review." *Disability and Rehabilitation: Assistive Technology* (2019): 1–14.

Mechling, Linda C. "Assistive technology as a self-management tool for prompting students with intellectual disabilities to initiate and complete daily tasks: A literature review." *Education and Training in Developmental Disabilities* (2007): 252–269.

Ok, Min Wook. "Use of ipads as assistive technology for students with disabilities." *TechTrends*, 62, no. 1 (2018): 95–102.

Parenti, Ilaria, Luis G. Rabaneda, Hanna Schoen, and Gaia Novarino. "Neurodevelopmental Disorders: From Genetics to Functional Pathways." *Trends in Neurosciences* (2020).

Perelmutter, Bogi, Karla K. McGregor, and Katherine R. Gordon. "Assistive technology interventions for adolescents and adults with learning disabilities: An evidence-based systematic review and meta-analysis." *Computers & Education*, 114 (2017): 139–163.

Perilli, Viviana, Fabrizio Stasolla, Alessandro O. Caffò, Vincenza Albano, and Fiora D'Amico. "Microswitch-cluster technology for promoting occupation and reducing hand biting of six adolescents with fragile X syndrome: New evidence and social rating." *Journal of Developmental and Physical Disabilities*, 31, no. 1 (2019): 115–133.

Peterson, Carrie Beth, Neeli R. Prasad, and Ramjee Prasad. "Assessing assistive technology outcomes with dementia." *Gerontechnology*, 11, no. 2 (2012): 259–268.

Ravneberg, Bodil and Sylvia Söderström. *Disability, Society and Assistive Technology.* Taylor & Francis, 2017.

Rich, Lindsay Paige. *Prompting self-monitoring with assistive technology to increase academic engagement in students with attention-deficit/hyperactivity disorder symptoms.* Hofstra University, 2009.

Sanaman, Gareema and Shailendra Kumar. "Assistive technologies for people with disabilities in national capital region libraries of India." *Library Philosophy and Practice* (2014): 0_1.

Sarsak, H. I. "Telerehabilitation services: a successful paradigm for occupational therapy clinical services?" *International Physical Medicine and Rehabilitation Journal*, 5, no. 2 (2020): 93–98.

Schafer, Erin C., Suzanne Wright, Christine Anderson, Jessalyn Jones, Katie Pitts, Danielle Bryant, Melissa Watson et al. "Assistive technology evaluations: Remote-microphone technology for children with Autism Spectrum Disorder." *Journal of Communication Disorders*, 64 (2016): 1–17.

Squires, Luke A., Nefyn Williams, and Val L. Morrison. "Matching and accepting assistive technology in multiple sclerosis: a focus group study with people with multiple sclerosis, carers and occupational therapists." *Journal of Health Psychology*, 24, no. 4 (2019): 480–494.

Stasolla, Fabrizio and Donatella Ciarmoli. "Supporting Adaptive Responding and Reducing Challenging Behaviors of Children with Rare Genetic Syndromes and Severe to Profound Developmental Disabilities Through Assistive Technology-Based Programs." *International Journal of Psychology and Behavioural Research*, 8, no. 1e (2020): 1–3.

Stasolla, Fabrizio, Viviana Perilli, Antonia Di Leone, Rita Damiani, Vincenza Albano, Anna Stella, and Concetta Damato. "Technological aids to support choice strategies by three girls with Rett syndrome." *Research in Developmental Disabilities*, 36 (2015): 36–44.

Tangcharoensathien, Viroj, Woranan Witthayapipopsakul, Shaheda Viriyathorn, and Walaiporn Patcharanarumol. "Improving access to assistive technologies: challenges and solutions in low-and middle-income countries." *WHO South-East Asia Journal of Public Health*, 7, no. 2 (2018): 84–89.

Thorpe, Julia Rosemary, Kristoffer V. H. Rønn-Andersen, Paulina Bień, Ali Gürcan Özkil, Birgitte Hysse Forchhammer, and Anja M. Maier. "Pervasive assistive technology for people with dementia: a UCD case." *Healthcare Technology Letters*, 3, no. 4 (2016): 297–302.

Venkatesan, Srinivasan. "Analysis of Themes and Issues in Neurodevelopmental Disorders." In *Emerging Trends in the Diagnosis and Intervention of Neurodevelopmental Disorders*, pp. 1–31. IGI Global, 2019.

Venkatesan, Srinivasan and Hariharan Venkatraman. "Application of bio-feedback in neurodevelopmental disorders.Chapter 11." In *Emerging Trends in the Diagnosis and Intervention of Neurodevelopmental Disorders*, pp. 211–235. IGI Global, 2019.

Venkatesan, Srinivasan and G. Y. Yashodharakumar. "Certification and Medico-Legal Aspects of Neurodevelopmental Disorders in India." In *Emerging Trends in the Diagnosis and Intervention of Neurodevelopmental Disorders*, pp. 281–306. IGI Global, 2019.

Wang L., Gu, D., and Wu, B. (2020) "Technology-Enabled Long-Term Care Services and Supports (T-eLTCSS) in Home Settings." In: Gu, D. and Dupre, M. (eds) *Encyclopedia of Gerontology and Population Aging*. Cham: Springer.

World Health Organization. 1992. *The ICD-10 classification of mental and behavioural disorders: clinical descriptions and diagnostic guidelines*. Geneva: World Health Organization.

2 The Use of Educational Technology to Improve Learning for Persons with Neurodevelopmental Disorders

Jesse M. Redlo and Harpreet Kaur Dhir

Introduction

Students with neurodevelopmental disorders face many obstacles both academically and socially. Technological shifts require educators to integrate technology into their teaching practices (Donovan, Green, and Mason, 2014), which adds layers of complexity to students navigating learning environments, thereby necessitating differentiated instructional methods (Redlo, 2020). Despite this complexity, technology can help to level the field for students with neurodevelopmental disorders. Technologies such as learning management systems (LMS), virtual reality, and educational games are particularly impactful. This chapter will detail two case studies, wherein teachers worked continually with students and where technological interventions increased student success. In addition, this chapter will provide a theoretical framework for integrating technology constructively into teaching practice to help all students, particularly those students with disabilities. The chapter concludes with actionable recommendations for professional teaching practice.

Case Studies

K-12 Student

The first day of first grade was full of anxiety for six years old Mike (a pseudonym). As the teacher began instruction, Mike sat at his assigned seat and began tapping his shoes against his desk. The teacher had learned from the kindergarten staff of Mike struggling to sit and focus on any task. So she decided to ignore the tapping and continue conducting the first 20 minutes of the class getting to know the students. However, tapping increased in intensity with feet stomping on the ground. The teacher noticed Mike repeating the same actions or words, making random noises, spitting around his area, and frequently falling to the floor or dropping his materials. Over the next few days, the teacher noticed him having difficulty tracking the text, and he only followed directions when individual guidance was provided by the teacher. Listening to stories and playing computer games were two activities where Mike's increased engagement was noticeable.

DOI: 10.4324/9781003165569-2

According to the psycho-educational report, Mike had been diagnosed with attention deficit hyperactivity disorder (ADHD). During an interview with the psychologist assigned to the case, Mike's mother shared that she enjoyed his imagination and her goal was for Mike to be happy. She identified his strength in the area of mathematics and problem-solving. The areas of weakness, according to the mother, were Mike's inability to complete tasks or read directions. Mike's mother informed the psychologist that he was able to express his feelings and was aware of the social challenges.

A discrepancy was noticed between the ratings assigned by Mike's mother and teacher. On his clinical and adaptive profile, his mother had rated him as at-risk in the areas of externalizing and internalizing problems along with behavioral symptoms. Whereas the teacher-rated these areas in the extreme caution range. Despite the challenges, Mike was within the average range of verbal and non-verbal skills. Regardless of having ADHD diagnoses, Mike was strong in auditory and visual processing along with his strength in math and writing.

Mike qualified to receive services offered through occupational therapy, Resource Specialist Program, and individual counseling. His Individual Educational Plan (included goals in the areas of reading, math, social-emotional learning, and other social goals to increase classroom participation with improved behavior. An occupational therapist recommended strategies of clear instructions, blocking irrelevant visual information, work assigned in smaller portions, and incentives. The recommendations were to be implemented within the mainstream classroom setting.

Mike enjoyed listening to stories and working on computers. Classroom desktop computers were a learning tool and a form of incentive for Mike to reinforce task completion and positive behavior. Mike began to use Google Classroom daily to design single-slide presentations. He would start the day by finding an image of an animal, copy the image and paste into the slide. For about a week or so, copying and pasting images of animals was all that Mike was interested in completing. He talked about the animals with other students and learned to wait patiently for his turn on the computer. Other students began to accept Mike as a friend, and he enjoyed the positive attention of his peers. His peers began to ask him about his picture for the day and began to work with him in choosing an image. Before long many of them began their own slide presentations about animals. Gentry et al. (2014) informed about the integration of technology as effective when leading to collaboration and creativity. Over time, Mike's teacher asked him to type a sentence to go along with the picture of an animal. Mike began to take interest in writing. He wanted to write and share his writing with his parents. A portfolio of his work began to develop in his Google Classroom account.

Integrating technology was a successful strategy for an ADHD student such as Mike. According to Göksün and Kurt (2017) informational literacy development was a critical part of developing the 21st-century skills of accessing information with a holistic perspective and using information creatively. Mike became accustomed to begin his slide design by looking for a picture of an animal and describing it using sentences. It became a routine task, and he understood the directions. Focusing on one image helped to block irrelevant visual information and the assignment consisting of selecting an image and writing to describe the image could be completed incrementally. His teacher was able to instruct him one on one in other subjects using computer time as an incentive after completing other assignments such as math.

Building an online portfolio of writing enabled the implementation of strategies recommended by the occupational therapist, led to an increased positive peer interaction where Mike was invited to play with peers during recess and increased achievement in overall academics. Mike's score in reading High-Frequency Words at the beginning of the year was only two words only. Three months later, the score increased to 16 and three months later, it was 28. In Basic Phonics Skills Test, Mike could only sound out the initial sound in August, the beginning of the school year. By November, he was able to sound out all the letters with consonant-vowel-consonant pattern. By February Mike could sound out the word and blend the sounds to form words. When given a grade-level passage to read, Mike's reading accuracy score in October was 0% which increased to 63% in January. His mathematical skills also increased from gaining 30% to 40% on average on tests to gaining 62% on a district benchmark test during the middle of the school year.

Integrating technology in Mike's daily schedule where he was engaged in not just playing games on the computer, but developing an understanding of writing to describe using a visual image, organizing a slide, and developing technology skills such as searching for information online, copying and pasting, and moving on to formatting using fonts and colors extended the skills to focus and complete tasks in the other academic and social areas. An increase in academic achievement was a result of daily structure organized around technology where the teacher could pull him away from the computer for individualized instruction. Göksün and Kurt (2017) confirmed a teacher needs to plan instruction that meets the learner's needs. Mike was willing to give the teacher his time in exchange for knowing that teacher will be giving him time.

Undergraduate College Student

The professor walks into an over-sized communication class at 2:00 pm and all looks normal for the first day: the students are sitting as spread out as possible and most of them are not speaking to one another. As the professor surveyed the room while preparing to begin instruction, one student, who will be referred to as John (a pseudonym to maintain anonymity), stood out from the rest. John appeared visibly anxious, exhibiting behaviors such as excessive pen tapping, wondering eyes, shaky hands, and fidgety legs. While a bit odd, plenty of students are nervous on the first day of college, so the professor thought nothing of it and proceeded with the lesson. When the next class day came, the professor realized John was different.

John, in addition to exhibiting all of his first day behaviors, began talking out of turn; not in a rude manner, but with fervor to be the first one to answer a question. The professor was confused and happy at the same time, as John was clearly passionate about the subject, but seemed to be ignorant of social cues. Fascinated by the behavior observed in the classroom, the professor reached out to a friend who was a psychologist, described the behavior, and asked the psychologist's opinion on possible explanations for the behavior. The psychologist informed the professor that John likely had Autism Spectrum Disorder, but could not say to what extent without interviewing the student. The professor was not overly familiar with autism but was concerned that lack of social cue awareness could create a significant learning obstacle in a communication course that focuses largely on both verbal and nonverbal communication methods in professional settings.

A related compounding issue with John was his unwillingness to work with peers. When the professor would ask students to work on an activity in pairs, John would insist on working by himself, which indicated a high degree of communication apprehension, which refers to someone having fear of interacting with others (Sawyer, 2020). The professor found this quite odd, given John had no issue answering questions during the lecture, but objected to the group activities. At this point, the professor realized a need to be more creative with teaching methods to reach John, so John would have a chance at meeting the course learning outcomes.

The communication course in question is predicated on teaching students skills sought after by employers in the workforce, which primarily revolves around a set of skills coined the four Cs: collaboration, communication, creativity, and critical thinking (McGunagle and Zizka, 2020). While John was probably in good shape with critical thinking and potentially creativity, evidently collaboration and communication were going to be problematic. The professor asked John to meet with them after class one day to gently probe for information. During this meeting, John revealed having a high degree of insecurity and anxiety around working with others, as a result of having a social anxiety disorder, as well as autism. The fact that John discussed this with the professor was good progress.

With this new information about John, the professor decided to make use of differentiated instructional principles to help John slowly to overcome his fears to successfully collaborate and communicate with peers. Through a series of metacognitive exercises, John engaged in critical self-reflection and began to see himself as being capable of more than he previously thought (Warman, 2020). After a few weeks of critical self-reflection and trying a series of shorter collaborative exercises, John got to a point where he could participate in the regular course activities. By the end of the semester, John became a more confident communicator and even obtained a cooperative educational experience for the following semester.

Theoretical Framework

The current classrooms are, in many cases, designed for receiving information rather than participating in learning through experiential lessons. John Dewey called this type of learning environment as learning by listening, considering reading for information as a form of listening (Dewey and Jackson, 1990). Students with special needs, faced with various conditions, are not served effectively within a passive system. The uniformity of methods and curriculum and attitude of passivity was especially viewed as ineffective or old by Dewey and Jackdon (1990).

The theory of constructivism establishes a foundation through which to evaluate and understand the best practices for integrating technology to meet the needs of the students with special needs. A branch of cognitivism, constructivism employs approaches designed for the purpose of engaging learners in social interactions preceding cognitive development (Clark, 2018). The tenets of constructivism include viewing a learner as a manifestation of mind, setting a context for experiences to occur and instructing through narrative-based sequential experiences. The tenets frame a path for the learners to construct meaning by unifying language, thoughts, and social actions (Bruner, 1986).

A Learner as a Manifestation of Mind

According to the principles of constructivism, instruction must be planned to address the human mind rather than the person (Dewey and Jackson, 1990). Increased intelligence results when cognitive growth is facilitated through educational experiences designed to transform a learner's mind (1990) leading to local and global participation (Ilica, 2016). The democratization of learning through an educational environment structured to provide positive experiences and which resembles practical life can develop cognition facilitating social and intellectual progress (Dewey and Jackson, 1990; Ilica, 2016).

An Experiential Context

A constructivist classroom is a social context over other environments such as political or religious (Boyte, 2017) where ideas are examined in a laboratory-like setting (Dewey and Jackson, 1990). For new truths to emerge, innovative ideas must be examined and applied for practical interests (1990). A constructivist context is not a place for promoting ideologies. Bruner (1996) differentiates between *observable worlds* and *possible worlds*. Possible worlds can be judged against the observables and logical proof but developing intuition-like imagination can precede the formal ability to prove individual understanding (1996). Learners, as a manifestation of mind, are perceived as evolutionary in their understanding of concepts and not simply passive subjects who receive and regurgitate pre-established doctrines (1990). In an educational setting, curriculum and methods used for all can be viewed as pre-established doctrine or inferred as an observable world where students with special needs struggle to develop an understanding of concepts through individual capacities. A manifestation of what they know might occur over time and not follow the logical paths appropriate for the mainstream population of learners.

Narrative-Based Sequential Experiences

Contextual experiences are activities where learners possess a sense of control, to varying degrees, over their abilities related to an assumed role. A narrative-based experience creates a social reality leading to contextual experiences through activities such as drama, role-play, debate, and simulations (Bruner, 1986; Halcrow, 2018). Social interaction is embedded in the context of time and space and consciousness of thoughts and feelings with an ability to engage learners emotionally (Bruner, 1986) acknowledging social interests to predominate cognitive development (Dewey and Jackson, 1990). Context is important for developing thinking skills. Bruner (1986) considered humans as products of biology and environment and therefore viewed learning to be an outcome of social exchanges preceding the development of cognitive processes. Cognition was influenced by social context and interaction (1986).

Knowledge is a form of personal interpretation developed through contexts available to the learner (Smith, 2016) consolidating a learner's psychology and the events of a narrative-based experience (Bruner, 1986). Experiencing role play situated in real-life builds a learner's character connecting a constructivist environment to developing an understanding of the content (Dewey and Jackson, 1990).

Differentiated Instruction

Differentiated instruction means tailoring instruction to meet individual students' needs with the primary goals being to improve learning outcomes, increase engagement, increase self-awareness, inspire a love of learning, and help students to learn more efficiently and with deeper understanding (Tomlinson, 2017). Differential instruction recognizes students are unique and might have vastly different learning styles. The VARK model encompasses the most common types of learning styles, which are: visual, auditory, reading/writing, and kinesthetic (Fleming, 2001). The VARK model is by no means an exhaustive list of learning styles and this discussion is particularly relevant when discussing learners with neurodevelopmental disorders, as depending upon the disorder the learner has, they are likely to gravitate towards a specific learning style. Without knowing the details of the disorders students might have, it is a best practice for teachers to practice differentiated instruction on a regular basis in their courses.

Differentiated instruction can be used by teachers in a multitude of ways - some of which use traditional approaches for in-classroom instruction and others using technology tools for virtual instruction. For example, in the classroom, when teaching vocabulary a teacher could give students a guided worksheet wherein they are prompted with page numbers to look up each term in the book, read the definition, and they write down a definition in their own words (Redlo, 2018). Another approach could be providing the student with a crossword puzzle wherein the definitions of the terms serve as clues and the students must fill in the vocabulary term to solve the puzzle - this doubles as an example of using games in the classroom (2018).

For virtual instruction, it is wise to use an interactive asynchronous online engagement tool, such as VoiceThread (Redlo and Gilbert, 2019). VoiceThread is similar to using a regular, online discussion board, except it allows the student to create text, audio, and/or video posts and comments, which crosses multiple learning styles in one activity (Redlo and Gilbert, 2019). VoiceThread is particularly easy to use when teachers are already using a LMS in their course, as VoiceThread can be integrated into the LMS, which means students do not have to access multiple websites.

Social Interaction in a Virtual Environment

As discussed in the theory sections of this chapter, social interaction is an integral element to successful student learning. Facilitating social interaction in the traditional, in-person classroom environment is often part of classroom management, which refers to strategies for organizing resources and activities for students – a skill that many primary school teachers are trained in (Donovan, Green, & Mason, 2014). Despite the connotation of classroom management pertaining only to the in-person classroom, it is also relevant to the online classroom through the use of LMSs. These help to make material more easily accessible to students in both independent and collaborative formats, which are linked with increased student performance (Donovan et al., 2014).

An LMS is a unique virtual environment, which is often new to all students, which means it can serve as an equalizer between students with neurodevelopmental disorders and those without, as nobody is starting with an advantage. It is also worth noting that teachers might need to provide tutorials and similar resources on how to use an LMS for students, particularly international students, where the students must learn English proficiency at the same time they are learning how to use new technology (Alsobahi, 2017). The virtual environment offers teachers a unique opportunity to design resources for students with disabilities as the primary consideration, instead of the typical after thought in the in-person classroom. When teaching online, a documented best practice is to make use of the Universal Design for Learning principles, which are predicated on making all learning activities accessible for learners of varying abilities through flexible instruction (Meier and Rossi, 2020).

Within an accessible, virtual learning environment, teachers can make use of readings, videos, interactive assessments, case studies, and games to engage students through multiple learning methods (Kiss and Redlo, 2020). The teacher can choose whether the aforementioned activities should be done in isolation or in teams to promote greater peer interaction. Moreover, instructors could support activity completion through use of videoconferencing software programs, such as Zoom, Skype, or Microsoft Teams, to name a few, wherein they can see and speak with students in real-time. The opportunities in a virtual environment are nearly endless.

Virtual Reality

The tenets of constructivism were present in Mike's example of how he progressed in skill development. The engagement in learning occurred when his mind was immersed into the digital tasks. Technology provided a vehicle to experience the real world through images and videos of animals. Mike made animal sounds becoming a part of the narrative himself and shared his views with his peers moving from an individualized digital context to social interactions. During recess, Mike ensured the safety of creatures such as worms on the playground putting them back in the grassy areas. The emotional response emerged from his experience of learning about animals using technology as a tool to interact with the topic of interest.

Increased emotional response to the subject was a sign of a student's positive experience via online sources. Technology served to reduce the anxiety associated with expressing one's ideas in a group setting. Initially, Mike's engagement with the topic of animals using online images was individualistic without the pressure of social expectations. According to Hadley et al. (2019), digital experience can provide a context where students assume a role to behave realistically without facing a sense of embarrassment amongst their peers. Students with neurological disorders such as ADHD or autism can interact within the context of virtual reality where students interact with avatars through immersive simulations (2019). In a contained virtual reality environment, simulation technologies create real world experiences (Smith, Prybylo, and Conner-Kerr, 2012) and role playing can lead to transitioning into social interactions outside the digital platforms.

Mike transitioned to social interactions over time as he shared his excitement about the images he found and his love of protecting the animals. The other students displayed interest in his conversations and began to invite him to join their play during breaks. His technology-based experience led him to social interactions while his mind stayed engaged with the same topic of animals. In a way he became a manifestation of his own mind applying his learning out into the playground while interacting with his peers socially. The principle of applied behavioral analysis establishes the foundation for considering immersive experience as the most effective treatment for students with autism spectrum disorder (Higbee et al., 2016). Learning through experience-based engagement, students learn to curb anxieties related to social interactions and increase self-efficacy by learning to regulate emotions (Hedley et al., 2019). Mike's example illustrates this progression from being distressed in a social setting, initially and developing his confidence to interact with others outside the individual digital experience. He became less anxious and developed skills of communication. Hedley et al. (2019) found virtual reality to improve conversational skills while increasing assertiveness through immersive experience.

Increased engagement through virtual simulations foster learning as player's role play and complete tasks with sustained attention, owing to visuals and sounds connected with digital games (Sukstrienwong, 2018). With the removal of potential social evaluation using technology (Hedley et al., 2019), some other features need to be considered for computer-based games to be effective for students such as embedded content, as little text as possible or highlighted text, vivid colors, clickable icons, and stimulates thinking (Sukstrienwong, 2018). The visuals and sounds are important to enhance interaction with images (Hedley et al., 2019). Neuroscientific research has found cognitive processes to be connected to music and language emphasizing the need for simulated experiences to use features such as rhythm, drama and role play (Halcrow, 2018). However, social learning precedes cognitive development (Clark, 2018), emphasizing the need for virtual simulated experiences to learn to interact with others.

Neutral Learning Networks

The integration of simulation technology and general use of computers in instruction is essential for students with special needs. The affective network involved in the learning process is employed when learning connects to an emotional experience (Scott and Temple, 2017). Emotional experience can range from distress to joy stressing the need for providing a positive learning environment appropriate to the needs of the students. For students with special needs, anxieties involved in learning in a social setting can be reduced through the use of virtual reality simulations. Experience-based learning can be engaging while situated in a digital context and where a student, overtime, can transition to a social context with increased confidence.

Along with emotions, brain functions include gathering and categorization of facts. The recognition network facilitates fact-based learning whereas the strategic network helps to organize and express ideas (Scott and Temple, 2017). Multiple digital tools and platforms can assist in gathering and organizing information freeing the path of students with special needs who might find organization skills to be a barrier in learning. According to neuroscience research, experience and experimentation leads to skill and confidence development (Halcrow, 2018). Experiential learning employs the affective network to engage with the subject emotionally making a case for integration of role play and simulation technologies.

Role of a Teacher and School

In order to use the necessary technologies for students to engage, a trained teacher is essential to cultivate the learning process consisting of the implementation of the three neutral networks. An expert teacher to instruct students with a range of disabilities needs to be a problem-solver and an innovator with deep content knowledge (Ruppar, Roberts, and Olson, 2017). According to the authors, building relations with students is a prerequisite to provide individualized instruction. Technology integration can only be successful if an instructor is trained in building a supportive environment for the learning process to occur.

Special education instructors need to be knowledgeable about teaching students with a variety of disabilities. Understanding not only the disability, but learning about a student's traditions and cultures can facilitate designing instruction relevant to the learner (Scott and Temple, 2017). Teachers with more training in curriculum and instruction are more effective in providing student support ((Barrio, Miller, Ojeme, and Tamakloe, 2019). They facilitate meaningful communication with students, manage accommodations, and develop positive relations with families (2019).

Technology can assist in designing instruction and environment so that the needs of the students can be met. Schools need to have an appropriate technology infrastructure to create inclusive programs (Barrio, Miller, Ojeme, and Tamakloe, 2019) where special needs students are provided instruction within the mainstream setting. A teacher has an essential role in integrating technology in instruction and holds high expectations for continued progress of students (Ruppar, Roberts, and Olson, 2017). Trained teachers, supported by their respected institutions, can integrate instructional methods to use technology to provide appropriate educational experience in addition to using non-digital instructional approaches.

The Use of Gaming to Engage Students

The use of gaming to engage students with education content, known as gamification, has existed for many years, but is receiving more attention in modern-literature (Wiggins, 2016). One could assert the notion of gamification stems from social development theory, wherein students can learn from a more knowledgeable other (MKO), traditionally thought to be a teacher (Vygotsky, 1980). Through a slight re-conceptualization of social development theory, one could posit the MKO could be an interactive game (Abtahi, Graven, and Lerman, 2017). The use of gaming to engage students has numerous benefits to multiple student populations, but these benefits are highlighted among groups of students with disabilities.

Games can help to take dense information and divide it into smaller sections, which might feel more manageable to learners, thereby increasing learner motivation (Young, 2016). When information is consumed in smaller pieces, it makes the overall topic potentially less scary and therefore more approachable to learners of varying ability levels. Evidence supports the use of games for learners with different ability levels as research indicators learners at all levels have increased achievement through the use of educational games and have reported enjoying the games in courses (Turan, Avinc, Kara, and Goktas, 2016). To help with the enjoyment factor of the games and to keep learners of varying ability levels form losing motivation, it is wise to not make the games competitive through the use of badges and leader boards, as the students will become too fixated on how they compare to their peers (Kiss and Redlo, 2020). When strategically implemented, following the best practice recommendations above, games are powerful methods of student engagement in courses across academic disciplines.

Conclusion/Recommendations

As discussed throughout this chapter, technology tools when created with accessibility in mind within education are here to stay, especially in consideration of their positive effects of helping students with neurodevelopmental disorders (Meier and Rossi, 2020). Some of these technology tools include LMSs, virtual reality, and gaming, to name a few. While educators might agree about these technology tools being valuable, the time has come for educators to go a step further to embrace technology and fully integrate these powerful technology tools into their teaching practices. Integrating technology into instructional practices might be easier said than done, as educators report a need for specialized training in this area (Redlo, 2020). In response to this need, with ended goal ultimately being to help educators meaningfully integrate technology tools into their instructional practices, educational leaders should prioritize providing ongoing training and support for teachers, select fewer, but more impactful technologies, and design training session which are hands-on to allow for me application to the teachers' instructional practices (2020). When these suggestions are followed and technology tools are integrated into instructional practices, all students are more likely to succeed, regardless of their disability status.

Further research implications include policy making and teacher training in implementing instructional methods compatible with inclusive education integrating technology. Innovative methods of teaching can guide students to progress overtime through experiencing concepts in constructivist classroom environments (Dhir, 2019).

In order to implement instructional practices necessary to meet the diverse needs of students, educational institutions need to include stakeholders in setting compatible policies which can help students to progress academically and socially. Along with the necessary policies and having access to technological tools, teacher training will also be essential in bringing appropriate instructional practices in classrooms. Technology, however advanced, remains a tool and not a complete method of teaching and learning. Methods which integrate instruction across disciplines are essential for implementing innovation in instruction with the goal of including all students in learning.

References

Abtahi, Y., Graven, M., and Lerman, S. (2017). "Conceptualizing the more knowledgeable other within a multidirectional ZPD." *Educational Studies in Mathematics*, 96(3), 275–287. doi:10.1007/s10649-017-9768-1.

Alsobahi, G. (2017). "What are Saudi students' perceptions toward using Blackboard as a learning-management system in United States universities?" Retrieved from ProQuest Dissertations and Theses database. (UMI No. 10263074).

Barrio, Miller, Ojeme, and Tamakloe. (2019). "Teachers' and Parents' Knowledge about Disabilities and Inclusion in Nigeria." *Journal of International Special Needs Education*, 22(1), 14–24. https://doi.org/10.9782/17-00010.

Boyte, H. C. (2017). "John Dewey and citizen politics: How democracy can survive artificial intelligence and the credo of efficiency." *Education & Culture*, 33(2), 13–47. Retrieved from https://docs.lib.purdue.edu/eandc/vol33/iss2/art3.

Bruner, J. (1986). *Actual minds, possible worlds.* Cambridge, MA: Harvard University Press.

Clark, K. R. (2018). "Learning theories: Constructivism." *Radiologic Technology*, 90(2), 180–182. Retrieved from www.radiologictechnology.org/content/90/2/180.full.pdf+html.

Dewey, J. and Jackson, P. W. (1990). *The school and society and the child and the curriculum: A Centennial Publication.* Chicago, IL: The University of Chicago Press.

Dhir, H. K. (2019). Planning curriculum for teaching thinking skills needed for 21st century education. In S. Robinson and V. Knight (Eds), *Handbook of research on critical thinking and teacher education pedagogy*, pp. 107–133. Hershey, PA: IGI Global. doi:10.4018/978-1-5225-7829-1.ch007.

Donovan, L., Green, T. D., and Mason, C. (2014). "Examining the 21st century classroom: Developing an innovation configuration map." *Journal of Educational Computing Research*, 50(2), 161–178. https://doi.org/10.2190/EC.50.2.a.

Fleming, N. D. (2001). *Teaching and learning styles: VARK strategies.* Christchurch: N. D. Fleming.

Gentry, J. E., Baker, C., Thomas, B. D., Whitfield, C., and Garcia, L. (2014). "Transforming Technology Integration: An Instrument to Measure Educator's Self-Efficacy for Modeling 21st-Century Skills." *National Teacher Education Journal*, 7(3), 31–38.

Göksün, D. D. and Kurt, A. A. (2017). "The relationship between pre-service teachers' use of 21st century learner skills and 21st century teacher skills." *Education & Science/ Egitim Ve Bilim*, 42(190), 107–130. doi:10.15390/EB.2017.7089.

Hadley, W., Houck, C., Brown, L. K., Spitalnick, J. S., Ferrer, M., and Barker, D. (2019). "Moving Beyond Role-Play: Evaluating the Use of Virtual Reality to Teach Emotion Regulation for the Prevention of Adolescent Risk Behavior Within a Randomized Pilot Trial." *Journal of Pediatric Psychology*, 44(4), 425–435. doi:10.1093/jpepsy/jsy092.

Halcrow, K. (2018). "Imitation and innovation: Harnessing the principles of music pedagogy for the writing classroom." *Literacy Learning: The Middle Years*, 26(3), 48–57. Retrieved from www.questia.com/read/1G1-554040665/imitation-and-innovation-harnessing-the-principles.

Higbee, T. S., Aporta, A. P., Resende, A., Nogueira, M., Goyos, C., and Pollard, J. S. (2016). "Interactive computer training to teach discrete-trial instruction to undergraduates and special educators in Brazil: A replication and extension." *Journal of Applied Behavior Analysis*, 49(4), 780–793. https://doi.org/10.1002/jaba.329 and http://digitalcommons.kennesaw.edu/glq/vol53/iss3/7?utm_source=digitalcommons.kennesaw.edu%2Fglq%2Fvol53%2Fiss3%2F7&utm_medium=PDF&utm_campaign=PDFCoverPages.

Ilica, A. A. (2016). "On John Dewey's philosophy of education and its impact on contemporary education." *Journal Plus Education/Educatia Plus*, 14(1), 7–13. Retrieved from www.uav.ro/jour/index.php/jpe/article/viewFile/627/688.

Kiss, E.A. and Redlo, J.M. (2020). "Meeting the need: Creation of an online infection prevention course by the Golisano Institute for Developmental Disability Nursing for direct support professionals during COVID-19." *Journal of Intellectual Disabilities*. doi:10.1177/1744629520962617.

McGunagle, D. and Zizka, L. (2020). "Employability skills for 21st-century STEM students: The employers' perspective." *Higher Education, Skills and Work-Based Learning*, 10(13), 591–606. https://doi.org/10.1108/HESWBL-10-2019-0148.

Meier, B.S. and Rossi, K.A. (2020). "Removing instructional barriers with UDL." *Kappa Delta Pi Record*, 56, 82–88. doi:10.1080/00228958.2020.1729639.

Redlo, J.M. (2018). "Using differentiated instructional strategies to promote student success" [Conference session]. 2018 Faculty Senate Professional Development Week, June 2018, Monroe Community College, Rochester, NY.

Redlo, J.M. (2020). "Faculty perceptions of effective online teacher training: A phenomenological approach" (Publication No. 28024115) [Doctoral Dissertation, American College of Education]. ProQuest Dissertations Publishing.

Redlo, J.M. and Gilbert, A.M. (2019). "Tools for interactive online teaching" [Conference session]. 2019 Professional Development Week, June 2019, Monroe Community College, Rochester, NY.

Ruppar, A. L., Roberts, C. A., and Olson, A. J. (2017). "Perceptions about expert teaching for students with severe disabilities among teachers identified as experts." *Research & Practice for Persons with Severe Disabilities*, 42(2), 121–135. doi:10.1177/1540796917697311.

Sawyer, C.R. (2020). "Communication apprehension." In: *Oxford Research Encyclopedia of Communication*. Oxford: Oxford University Press.

Scott, L. and Temple, P. (2017). "A Conceptual Framework for Building Udl in a Special Education Distance Education Course." *Journal of Educators Online*, 14(1), 48–59.

Smith, N., Prybylo, S., and Conner-Kerr, T. (2012). "Using Simulation and Patient Role Play to Teach Electrocardiographic Rhythms to Physical Therapy Students." *Cardiopulmonary Physical Therapy Journal* (American Physical Therapy Association, Cardiopulmonary Section), 23(1), 36–42.

Smith, S. (2016). "(Re)counting meaningful learning experiences: Using student-created reflective videos to make invisible learning visible during PjBL experiences." *Interdisciplinary Journal of Problem-based Learning*, 10(1), 1–16. doi:10.7771/1541-5015.1541.

Sukstrienwong, A. (2018). "Animo Math: the Role-Playing Game in Mathematical Learning for Children." *TEM Journal*, 7(1), 147–154. doi:10.18421/TEM71-17.

Tomlinson, C.A. (2017). "How to differentiate instruction in academically diverse classrooms." Association for Supervision and Curriculum Development.

Turan, Z., Avinc, Z., Kara, K., and Goktas, Y. (2016). "Gamification and education: Achievements, cognitive loads, and views of students." *International Journal of Emerging Technologies in Learning*, 11(7), 64–69. doi:10.3991/ijet.v11i07.5455.

Vygotsky, L. S. (1980). *Mind in society: The development of higher psychological processes.* Cambridge, MA: Harvard University Press.

Warman, S.M. (2020). "Experiences of recent graduates: Reframing reflection as purposeful, social activity." *Veterinary Record*, 186(11), 347–347. doi:10.1136/vr.105573.

Wiggins, B.E. (2016). "An overview and study on the use of games, simulations, and gamification, in higher education." *International Journal of Game-Based Learning*, 6(1), 1–12. doi:10.4018/IJGBL.2016010102.

Young, J.E. (2016). "Can library research be fun? Using games for information literacy instruction in higher education." *Georgia Library Quarterly*, 53(3), 1–7. Retrieved from http://digitalcommons.kennesaw.edu/glq/vol53/iss3/7?utm_source=digitalcomm ons.kennesaw.edu%2Fglq%2Fvol53%2Fiss3%2F7&utm_medium=PDF&utm_campa ign=PDFCoverPages.

3   Technological Advances for the Diagnosis and Rehabilitation of Dyslexia

Rizwana Azeez

Introduction

A learning disability (LD) is a neurodevelopmental disorder (NDD), of which dyslexia is the most common, that adversely affect speed and accuracy of word recognition, consequently hampering fluency and comprehension. An estimated 5%–10% of the population suffers from this disorder globally (Benfatto et al., 2016), and an estimated 5%–17% are identified to have developmental dyslexia, as there is no specific rule for identification/or diagnosis and is viewed in relation to the approximate limit of normal reading ability (D'Mello et al., 2018; Jenneke et al., 2015).

Reading/learning disability falls under a continuum, and dyslexia might be seen as a barrier on this, with no obsolete limit (Adubasim et al., 2017). Research in recent decades has evidenced dyslexia as either a result or a consequence of an inability of pre-reading skills and inefficient/impaired functioning of brain regions required to learn the skill of reading warranting early identification and intervention to be the best style of curation (D'Mello et al., 2018).

Current psychometric methods do not sufficiently measure specific areas of underlying cognitive skills necessary for reading while placing excessive pressure on subjects to perform and respond explicitly within a given time period and evaluate correct responses as a measure of ability for diagnosis. Informal methods of diagnosis such as performance tasks, questionnaires and the like might result in the child being reluctant, avoidant or even might not know he/she has such a difficulty, thereby damaging his self-esteem and confidence (Benfatto et al., 2016).

Technology and Learning Disabilities

Diagnosis and rehabilitation approaches have been focusing on technological advances and educational interventions that are associated with brain changes. Research using technologies such as neuroimaging and eye tracking explain typical functioning of a human brain, highlighting deviations as atypical, reasoning out its differential functioning thus enabling both understanding and guiding treatment of neurodevelopmental disorder (America's children and the environment, 2018).

DOI: 10.4324/9781003165569-3

Neuroimaging studies tracking reading difficulties from childhood to adulthood in individuals with dyslexia have reported structural and functional dissimilarities of the brain (D'Mello et al., 2018). Such studies use blood-oxygen-level-dependent signals as a measure to understand the amount of blood in the brain which forms the index to functional capacities of the brain cells i.e. increases in blood levels denote an increase in neural activity and localizes specific brain regions to understand the neural circuits underlying a reading task (Arthurs, 2002).

Studies have revealed that left hemispheric networks such as frontal, temporo-parietal and occipito-temporal regions of the brain to be associated with skilled reading and language related tasks (Price et al., 2012). Although it is understandable that all networks of the brain work in concert for discrete reading, for operations such as phonological decoding, processing, visual word recognition, and perceptual processes, there are specific areas involved to ascertain meaning that develop and specialize throughout development, resulting in skilled reading ability (Dehaene et al., 2010).

Magnetic resonance imaging (MRI) has been considered a gold standard to imaging structural abnormalities of the brain as it provides exquisite, quantifiable high resolution information. MRI precisely measures gray and white matter volume that enables differentiation of typical readers and dyslexics. Studies using MRI report correlation of greater gray matter volume with skilled reading (Hoeft et al., 2007) and suggest that connections between cortical regions are orchestrated with separate parts of the brain into a successful interactive reading network that increases with increasing age (Yeatman et al., 2012) and predictive of typical reading outcomes (Meyer et al., 2014).

A similar technique is functional magnetic resonance imaging (fMRI), which detects subtle changes associated with language. Studies have reported increases and decreases in functional activation of areas of the brain involved in processes necessary for reading and/or reading-related tasks associated with reading behavior (D'Mello, 2018). Interestingly, a study on auditory processing intervention, focusing on phonological awareness, showed that phonological processing and other functions of the brain were significantly activated following intervention (Temple et al., **2003**).

Electrophysiological techniques such as event related potential (ERP) and evoked potentials (EP) are non-invasive and provide detailed neural activity associated to cognitive information processing. It provides qualitative and quantitative data regarding the differences between typical processing and differential processing (Karapetsas et al., 2011). Researchers study the P300 waveform to understand higher order cognitive processes and suggest that P300 evaluates as a temporal measure to attention, speed allocation, and working memory.

Apart from research, ERPs are also used in understanding the impact of interventional programs and reported that audio-visual intervention showed larger waveform amplitude (Kujala et al., 2001). It assessed executive functions impaired in individuals with reading disability and showed lower P300 waveform amplitude in poor readers (Karapetsas et al. ,2011) and increased P300 latency on lexical decision task (Miller-Shaul et al., 2004) and auditory stimuli (Zygouris et al., 2017) as characteristic features in individuals with reading difficulties.

Neuroimaging studies on children and adult dyslexics have consistently reported a reduction in gray matter, the strength of white matter, and functional activation of the left hemisphere, suggesting reading difficulty as a basis of differences in structural and functional neural networks responsible for reading in dyslexics but typical of normal readers (Paulesu et al., 2014). Therefore, structural differences throughout cortical networks of separate brain regions that can be summed up as reading networks such as reduced gray matter typically display functional differences, and poor white matter connections display phonological and orthographic impairment in dyslexics, which is not true in normal readers (Hoeft et al., 2007). This explains the overreliance on the right lateralized brain regions as a cause or consequence of hyper-activity between hemispheres (Gabrieli et al.,2009).

In addition, neuroimaging studies also report differences in functional and anatomical connectivity of the cerebellum resulting in differences in phonological processing, verbal working memory and semantics (Stoodley et al., 2012). In addition, pre-reading skills necessary to learn the skill to read exist even before an individual learns to read which are differed in children with dyslexia (Langer et al., 2017). Despite such evidences reported through MRI, fMRI, SPECT, PET, EP, or EEG techniques being helpful in research and to evaluate results of intervention, could not be of diagnostic value owing to the inconsistent findings with regard to learning disability.

Interestingly, similarity between neuroscience and poetry is that both view 'eyes' as a window to the soul. Mounting evidence from autism research reveals that individuals with Austism Spectrum Disorder (ASD) fail to orient themselves or spontaneously see what everyone else is seeing – a prerequisite for social and language learning. Eye tracking as a screening method enables predictions at individual level with accuracy within a minute of tracking time, thereby reducing stress (Rayner et al., 2003; Clifton et al., 2007), as compared to traditional methods. Results from eye tracking prove to be accurate, efficient, and non-invasive, promising diagnostic utility and might be considered as an effective tool to understand processing demands of the functioning brain engaged in reading in children with LDs (Benfatto et al., 2016).

Many other studies report eye tracking to enable one to understand/study the underlying processing strategies while perceiving information through eye movement patterns and obtaining accurate, precise, moment-to-moment online spatial information in real time. Eye tracking measures such as first fixation duration measure early processing, while dwell time duration is an index to late processing. The author in a review observed reading ability matched that of beginning readers with longer fixation durations, increased regression, and shorter saccades in dyslexics typical of beginning readers (Rizwana, 2019).

Machine learning and predictive modelling enable detection at individual and group level of discrepancies with higher sensitivity and specificity, thereby making eye tracking a viable tool to screening LDs (Modak et al., 2019). Although eye movement might not directly pinpoint areas of deficit brain functioning, they are promising biomarkers/behavioral biometric signatures that aid diagnosis (Itti et al., 2015).

Furthermore, eye movement patterns of dyslexics exhibit frequent smaller saccades, longer fixation duration, and higher regression for linguistic tasks, which was inversely proportionate to word length and word frequency (Hutzlerr et al., 2004) and normal eye movement patterns for non-linguistic tasks bringing about explicit differences between dyslexics and normal readers, thereby suggesting that atypical eye movement patterns were an index to impaired visual-perceptual mechanisms and visual-attention processing thereby reflecting processing difficulties of linguistic information (Rizwana, 2019). Studies have shown that dyslexics process a smaller number of letters, hence process words, owing partly to visual attention span deficits resulting in processing fewer letters at each fixation. Eye tracking methodology is cost effective, relatively inexpensive, and non-invasive and adds quantification and precision to measure of social behavior in an objective way during evaluation of NDDs (Wang et al., 2015).

Technology for Rehabilitation

For an individual to produce harmony between self and environment adjustment with the environment is a paramount continuous process resulting in adept behaviors. On similar line, LD seems to result as an adaptational difficulty which is otherwise necessary in daily living and societal life (World Health Organization, 2009); is the single largest category receiving special education (Bender et al., 2013 and an ever increasing prevalence (5%-17%) between three and 17 years identified as learning disabled. The core etiology is assumed to be neurobiological associated with major weaknesses in executive function. A meta-analytic and factor-analytic review suggested weaknesses in core areas of executive functions (inhibition, working memory and cognitive flexibility) (Dickstein et al., 2006).

Furthermore, reading requires precise coordination of occulomotor processes and cognitive mechanisms as prerequisites to skilled reading. Any deficits in either of the processes accounts for dyslexia (Olulade et al., 2013; Stein et al., 2014). In other words, attentional processes have to be allocated effortfully as against basic processes necessary for reading, owing to occulomotor impairments, thereby impacting speed, accuracy, and comprehension in dyslexics (Thiagarajan et al., 2012). Thus a high incidence of learning disability accentuates the importance of remediation and rehabilitation.

Robots on one end have known to enhance rehabilitative processes as it can be used to asses performance before, during and after an intervention and high plasticity of the central nervous system in early stages of development on the other provide targeted consistent outcomes (Schneps et al., 2013).

Eye movement recording during reading and oculomotor rehabilitation are viable options (Paolozza et al., 2014; Ball et al., 2013). The authors reported that by training in fixation, saccades, and tracking for two months, children with LDs showed improvement in eye movement, enabled quicker, fluent, and less effortful reading outcomes, resulting in reduced word identification impairment and improved oculomotor control. Eye movement analysis showed oculomotor deficits in children with LDs, suggesting daily eye movement-based exercises could improve basic visual micro-mechanisms necessary for language fluency (Jafarlou et al., 2017).

Importantly, inclusive education offers equality to all by providing equitable opportunities for children with differential abilities enabling learning on similar lines with non-disabled peers initiating the idea of a plethora of teaching-learning strategies in an equitable manner and a shift in attitudinal barriers, making education for children with disability a shared responsibility (Ahmad et al., 2015). Research suggests phonological deficits as a characteristic feature and training this ability would be beneficial (Falth et al., 2013; Torgesen et al., 2001). A promising option for training in phonological deficit areassistive technologies (AT), which supports reading and writing made available on smart phones and tablets.

ATs are tools, strategies, and services designed and recommended to compensate, work around, or match individual needs, enabling individuals to function with ease in their customary environment which otherwise was difficult. Rehabilitation plans and programs coordinate with selection, design, customization, application, maintenance, and repairs of AT (Wong et al., 2012).

AT, a derivative of information and communication technology (ICT), has been instrumental in educational delivery and management facilitates acquisition and absorption of knowledge on the one hand and provides extraordinary opportunities on the other in developing countries like India to a great extent. Furthermore, electronics, word processors, electronic type writers, handheld calculators, and computers offer tailor-made programs and help to circumvent a wide range of specific disabilities to make information accessible across irrespective of the kind or extent of disability.

Application of assistive devices (AD) such as text-to-speech and speech-to-text is easily accessible and compensates decoding and writing impairments. Assimilating and communicating text is another AD that enables individuals to convey their thoughts and ideas and to take part in all kind of classroom activities. Moreover, children are familiar with and feel comfortable using them (Itti et al., 2015).

Although a majority of studies show beneficial effects of using AT, children with reading disability become better readers and writers, although research focusing on LDs and AT per se seems to be limited (Perelmutter et al., 2017). However, interventions based on word processors, multimedia, and hypertext can be customized and effectively tailored to individual needs. Multifunctional apps enhance decoding ability and motivation, improve reading ability, and bridge the gap between the disabled and non-disabled children, allowing children with difficulties to manage easily, thereby increasing listening and comprehension ability, thus not only compensating but promoting reading skills (Lindeblad et al., 2017). However, although AT shows evidence of positive effects on reducing disability − it is not self-evident, in other words, although children become good at assimilation and communicating text, they still lack the capacities of reading and writing in the traditional way, and some children are still handicapped in the absence of such technology.

In addition, developing a universally designed learning (UDL) environment fundamentally alters teaching and learning processes, a framework based on neuroscience with a focus on educational outcomes. It is flexible, supportive, goal-oriented with accessible/alternate methods and materials (Hall et al., 2012; Meyer et al., 2014). It provides multiple means for expression, action, ways of strategizing, motivating, engaging, sustaining interest and persistence, and improving learning (Roseth et al., 2017).

Thinking readers are devices that work on improving reading and providing variable reading strategies (Dalton et al., 2002). Web-based reading tools add curriculum-based assessment and provide an interactive digital reading environment. Strategic readers support and interact digitally, enabling teacher-student topical discussion, curriculum-based monitoring and track student progress. E-learning is another instructional approach that does away with conventional methods, is learner-cantered, self-regulated, collaborative, and supported by the trainer, offering great potential for lifelong learning. Using a POD as a reading device significantly decreases inefficient saccades and improves reading rate, producing fewer errors. Previous eye tracking studies have shown that shorter line width (as evident in POD) decreases reading time and regressive saccades while increasing retention. Thus e-readers such as PODs are affordable with easily adaptable electronic text to individual needs thus reinventing reading and ceasing reading skill as be a barrier for children with LDs (Schneps et al., 2013). These devices are accessible and flexibly designed to meet students' need. UDL environments foster a general approach to using technology in learning, improving comprehension and creating tailor-made intervention based on individual need.

Recently, studies have reported hemisphere-specific stimulation resulting in significant improvement of literacy skills (Swanson et al.,2009). Also, a computerized grapheme-phoneme-correspondence game provided a new learning environment to learn letter-sound correspondence in isolation, then syllables before learning words, reporting better reading skills in comparison to conventional phonic remediation technique. The participants continued to be good readers on par with their typically growing peers (Saine et al., 2011), and the same results were replicated (Kyle et al., 2013).

Digital technology provides a pedagogical approach to meet ever-growing demands. ICT tools provide varied opportunities suiting each individual's learning demands to pursue education, access employment, enable independent integrated functioning and confidently spend time in social settings and leisure. The innovative systems encompassing ICT, UDL, and AT address the emerging educational demands and increase, maintain, and/or improve the functional capacities of impairment (Hall et al., 2015).

Furthermore, the proximity of hand-held devices produces attentional bias (Reed et al., 2006), shields visual perception, and enhances sensitivity to text because holding a device in a hand can alter allocation of attention, regulate oculomotor dynamics, shield attention from visual interference (Davoli et al., 2011; 2012) and improve distributed attention. Subsequently, e-readers, strategic readers, or thinking readers and the like have opened new avenues/possibilities, making it easier for children with dyslexia in compliance with suggestions by researchers that alternate treatment of text such as alterations in font (O'Brien et al., 2005; deLeeuw et al., 2010), rearrangement in physical format (Schneps et al., 2010), or masking to isolate an item (Geiger et al., 1987) have produced small but beneficial effects. It maximizes attentional focus to detail, minimizes distraction (Davoli et al., 2011; 2012) and significantly improves word decoding and increases comprehension. Although these devices slow attentional shift and reading speed, they have been beneficial for individuals with poor visual attentional span that diminishes sensitivity to the number of letters perceived at one glance, which is a strong characteristic of dyslexia (Schneps et al., 2013).

Nonetheless, three aspects should be kept in mind before planning remediation and educational interventions. *Comorbidity* such as math and speech disorders, ADHD or ASD with pre-existing learning disabilities add to the complexity of assessment, intervention, and treatment efforts. *Demands of language* such as orthographic decoding or grapheme-phoneme-correspondence of a language places heavy demands on the child; bilingualism impacts the skill necessary to decode a specific writing system(Das et al., 2011), and finally *socioeconomic status* (SES) stands as a strong predictor for reading disability (Romeo et al., 2017).

Therefore, early identification facilitates successful rehabilitation of the structural and functional differences of a dyslexic brain through brain plasticity. Studies report empirical evidence that quantifiable brain changes occur through appropriate remediation (Aylward et al., 2003; Hoeft et al., 2011). While the underactive left hemispheric temporo-parietal and inferior frontal cortices have shown increased activation in children with dyslexia (Gaab et al., 2007), improvement in phonological processing in adults with dyslexia was evident through remediation (Eden et al., 2004; Krafnick et al., 2011).

Importantly, oral language ability was reflected in increased activity in the right-hemisphere, reflecting alternate strategies utilized in children or adults with dyslexia (Temple et al., 2003), suggesting greater right-hemispheric prefrontal activation and white matter connectivity with brain regions, enabling greater reading gains (Hoeft et al., 2011). This indicates that alternate pathways to reading improvement might be a promising, possibility through remediation. Studies reported increased gray matter volume and strong white matter connections in brain regions as a result of remediation (Keller et al., 2009; Romeo et al., 2017).

Tools for mathematical calculations such as electronic mathematics worksheet assist children to arrange, ally, and route basic mathematics calculations such as addition, subtraction, multiplication, and division. The speech synthesizer enables aligning problems in the correct order, symbols, operational keys, and/or numbers through loud reading (Neeraja et al., 2016).

Listening devices such as recorders allow oral presentation repeatedly for processing information, enabling comprehension and memory. It can be used whenever such information is needed. AT for memory and organization such as personal data managers are software packages that can be loaded on electronic devices help to children with organizational and memory problems. Free-form databases allows storage and retrieval of notes or pieces of information whenever needed and can be stored as reminders; prewriting organizers and graphic organizers are useful tools in generating topics and/or content in academic projects and assignments, where ideas might be presented as graphic bubbles which can be moved to construct a standard outline, thus enabling increased participation (Neeraja et al., 2016).

Furthermore, electronic books (e-books) a multisensory technological resource, provide exposure to vocabulary, phonological awareness, and concepts about print as an opportunity to access new learning methods and positive learning outcomes in children with low reading capacities, helping them to overcome their insecurities regarding their learning capacities and enhancing self-esteem and self-confidence. E-books help individuals with reading difficulties to stay focused for longer, providing multiple representation of information in the form of text, voice, pictures, and animation and effectively supporting a child's language and literacy development (Shamir et al., 2012).

Multimedia is another technology that supports learning and can replace written text with audio or add audio and pictures to written text. The cognitive theory of multimedia learning (Mayer et al., 2005) posits that learning impacts differently with different types of multimedia. Audiovisual channels maximize learning enabling retention and the fruitful transfer of knowledge. A meta-analysis also showed that individuals learnt better with audiovisual presentation of information in comparison to traditional text and picture presentation on paper (Ginns et al., 2005; Knoop-van et al., 2018).

Neuropsychological studies suggest that intervention through remediation programs could improve the differential abilities of children with dyslexia, suggesting that remediation programs should mainly focus on strengthening visual-perceptual skills, audiovisual, phonological, and working memory processes. Phonological training (Tijms et al., 2003), classical phonic instructions (Galuschka et al., 2014), and working memory (Loosli et al., 2012) interventions are reported to have strengthened the aforementioned processes.

Nonetheless, proof-reading, grammar checkers, and the like identify and correct grammar, capitalization, and word usage; speech synthesizers enable reading and hearing of a spoken word from the text simultaneously (Neeraja et al., 2016). Speech recognition systems enable children with LDsto speak through a microphone which might be displayed on the monitor; MicrosoftWord is the easiest and most common tool for reading passages, facilitating a change of font size, copying and pasting text, and changing formatting as per individual needs,while speech synthesis is a reading engine where the child reads back what they hear.

Furthermore, variable speech control is a form of tape recorder that presents text at the pace of the child's needs thereby improve comprehension. Optical character recognition can be connected to a speech synthesizer, enabling typing or reading aloud text as per the specific needs of the child; it can also be used to scan printed materials and present it on the monitor, making it easier for children with reading disabilities to read, edit, and comprehend (Raskind et al., 2000).

The global embrace of computers has enabled children with LDsto get the appropriate tools for an independent, successful time at school or employment with enhanced quality of life and various interventional opportunities at different levels, assisting both the teacher and the taught. The use of technology for intervention, especially hand-held calculators, computers, data processing systems, electronics, individualized computer programs, and microcomputers tailored to individual needs, learning styles, and academic levels, seem to have the potential to answer the visual, auditory, and perceptual deficits found in learning disabilities and to support the heterogeneous population according to their specific disabilities and/or recommended tools.

Early childhood educators and parents pay special attention to integrating traditional training methods with multisensory technological resources for remediation in language and emergent literacy programs in order to compensate the disrupted cognitive processes in children with learning disabilities. These provisions of technology and computers could be incorporated with traditional training in order to make remediation more purposeful, meaningful, and interactive, thus enabling rehabilitation practices in the child's natural environment, motivating the learner and keeping him/her engaged in learning in a relatively shorter period of time and the parent or teacher motivated in teaching children with LDs.

Choosing the Right Technology

A large population of 'at risk' children do not get early diagnosis as having LDs and often lack assistance. AT bridges this gap by helping children to learn in the way they understand at their own pace in their own environment. Attitudinal barriers that view AT as rehabilitative or remediational devices are the most difficult to change (Prabhu et al., 2017), owing to misconceptions, fear of the unknown, labelling, and stigma, often resulting in isolation of the individual with disability.

Although there is no hard and fast rule in choosing technology, one has to be cautious choosing the right one. Selection of AT should depend on the individual child, the skill problem, the extent of impairment, the degree the technology could compensate the impairment, the setting, and the task the child wishes to achieve. In addition, a tool that compensates for a child's disability might or might not be helpful to another child with the same disability (Raskind et al., 2000). Although it is true that assistive devices are easily accessible, cost effective, and available and/or dispensable, one has to be cautious and keep in mind the nature of demand that AT places on the individual, the kind and extent of disability, and available resources.

However, a multidisciplinary approach might ensure the functional faultless use of technology, but one has to be aware of not becoming carried away or excessively impressed by the shapes and designs of the technology.

Challenges Using AT for Children with LDs

There is no doubt that technology circumvents the impaired ability, helping individuals towards independence, assisting individuals in learning a specific task or material, and providing immediate feedback and individualized learning, while measuring progress. However, a major challenge of technology is its use in the classroom, selecting an appropriate device, availability and evaluating its efficiency against the needs of a child. A few disadvantages of technology could force the individual to abandon the same because the device was either not as useful as intended to function, made them stand out of the group, was difficult to repair or follow commands, needed too much assistance, or did not address the actual need arising from the individual's disability or indecision of the students, parents, or teachers to choose the precise device.

In developing countries like India, availability of AT is scarce, often not provided by the school or government, there are different polices, available only in urban areas, and high costs sometimes place the child with disabilities, the parent, and the teacher either with no access or with the wrong choice of tool suiting the pocket or availability and seldom the need of the child. Also, the training of teachers, parents/caretakers, and children, access to management, and the incorrect application of devices hamper the selection of the right technological device for a child. Moreover, a lack of trained professionals, support, flexibility of training options, disabled-friendly hard- and software resources, support structures, policies, attitudinal barriers, finances are major challenges.

It is therefore important to first determine a child's specific problem, identify his/her strengths that could be developed, and involve the child during the selection process to understand how the assistive device works and to determine if it would be usable in a specific setting, including storage and the right equipment needed. It is important for a child to choose a device that works for them, is easy to handle, learn with, and operate, making for an enjoyable and productive learning process.

Noteworthy is the economic impact associated with specific LDs. In addition, many parents of children with LDs live in denial and waste precious time in spending large amountsof money on hypothetical cures and tuition classes as a remedial measure, reflecting parental anguish, especially in the lower SES strata. Hence it is important to understand the economic burden of this hidden disability in order to enable decision making and guide tangible interventions (Karande et al., 2019).

A multisensory approach along with teacher-aid towards teaching-learning practices in the classroom could foster the integration of children with LDs, making learning an achievable task and reducing stress both for the teacher and taught. Governments, stakeholders, and policymakers might have to work together in reframing the Persons with Disabilities Act (2005) addressing, recommending, and providing assistive devices to children with disabilities, irrespective of economic and social status. Devices and software need to be designed to suit a wide range of specific needs, languages, cultures, and curricula, sponsored by software companies and corporate and social responsibility funds that might reduce costs and increase availability.

Focused and repeated faculty development programs need to be organized that could address the major attitudinal challenges and enable a broader perspective of viewing technology to improve/compensate a particular weakness than just as a remediation tool. The provision of equipment, aids, devices, and medical and neuropsychological evaluation should be provided free or at minimal cost at school level through public-private partnerships, which would reduce direct, indirect, and tangible costs ,thereby cutting the economic burden for families with children with LDs.

Summary

Practical wisdom and research conclude that learning disabilities are a disorder of cognitive and perceptual styles with intact intelligence but less cognitive flexibility. Information to treat such children must be presented in a way that matches the individual's learning style, making learning and comprehension easier. An LD is an imperfect ability to listen, think, calculate, and speak. Although these LDs are incurable, such individuals might learn to manage or even overcome their difficulties successfully with the support of appropriate assistive technology, with support from parents and the school environment, teachers, and peers, to improve their potential (Raskind et al., 2000).

In addition, studies suggest that training children with dyslexia using non-linguistic, audiovisual stimuli improves language function and thereby reading (Keyale et al., 2011). Assistive technology, the internet, and virtual reality are powerful tools fostering inclusive education and the additional capacity to construct an individual's learning environment, experiences, and shared activities with individual outcomes. These enable a child to complete an everyday task, maintain or improve functioning, enhance academic achievement, improve memory and organization, and finally foster social acceptance (Neeraja et al., 2016). However, one has to remember that while these technologies enhance basic skills and enable children with disabilities to achieve specific tasks with greater ease, they might make specific demands on the learner as they might have to learn specific commands to make a piece of software operational or undergo specific and frequent training. Moreover, although certain devices are educationally oriented, they focus little on diminishing the disability, eventually resulting in the individual feeling handicapped in the absence of the technology.

Advanced technologies enable independent learning, reduce dependence, open new avenues to equal educational opportunities, allow individuals to work alongside peers and participate in recreational and community activities, develop strengths, and minimize/eliminate weaknesses. The use of ATs becomes imperative as it promotes a sense of belonging, increases self-esteem and confidence, enhances interactive participation, and improves motivation.

In addition, multimedia provide information in various forms such as written, spoken, or visualization, enabling sensory information to be processed both through audio and visual channels. Furthermore, eye tracking technology has shed light on the possible differences in learning strategies, cognitive load from multimedia learning, and underlying learning processes (Knoop-van et al., 2018).

Technological advances can enable precise, moment-to-moment, online, real-time diagnosis, entailing rehabilitation and remediation of children with learning disabilities, easing the process of learning, compensating weaknesses, or enabling evaluation; this reassures parents and teachers and heightens educational gains and employment opportunities. However, the findings in some areas also signify inadequate knowledge and skills, a lack of confidence in using technology, and attitudinal barriers as major challenges. Last but not least, one has to accept that for all technological advances to be beneficial and effective, the reassuring, encouraging, and consoling human touch is vital to instil confidence and hope, motivating both the learner and the stakeholder.

References

Adubasim, I. C. J. and Nganji, J. T. (2017) *Dyslexia-A Learning Difference*. Autism Open Access 7: 203.

Ahmad, F. K. (2015) "Challenging Exclusion: Issues and Concerns in Inclusive Education in India." *Researchpaedia*, 2(1): 15–32.

America's Children and the Environment. 2018. *Health Neurodevelopmental Disorders*, third edition.

Arthurs, O. J. and Boniface, S. (2002). "How well do we understand the neural origins of the fMRI BOLD signal?" *Trends in Neurosciences*, 25(1):27–31.

Aylward, E. H.et al. (2003). "Instructional treatment associated with changes in brain activation in children with dyslexia." *Neurology*, 61(2): 212–219.

Ball, K, Pearson, D. G., and Smith, D. T. (2013). "Oculomotor involvement in spatial working memory is task-specific." *Cognition*, 129, 439–446.

Bender, W. N. (2004). *Learning disabilities: Characteristics, identification and teaching strategies* (5th ed.). Boston, MA: Pearson.

Benfatto, M. N. et al. (2016). "Screening for dyslexia using eye tracking during reading." *Plosone*, 11(12): e01655088.

Clifton, C, Staub, A, and Rayner, K. (2007) Eye movements in reading words and sentences. In: van Gompel, R.(ed.)*Eye Movements: A Window on Mind and Brain*. Amsterdam: Elsevier, pp. 341–372.

D'Mello, A. M. and Gabrieli, J. D. E. (2018). "Cognitive neuroscience of dyslexia." *Language, speech and hearing services in school*, 49, 798–809.

Dalton, B., Pisha, B., Eagleton, M., Coyne, P., and Deysher, S. (2002). *Engaging the text: Reciprocal teaching and questioning strategies in a scaffolded digital learning environment* (Final report). Washington, DC: U.S. Department of Education, Office of Special Education Programs.

Das, T., Padakannaya, P., Pugh, K. R., and Singh, N. C. (2011). "Neuroimaging reveals dual routes to reading in simultaneous proficient readers of two orthographies." *NeuroImage*, 54(2), 1476–1487.

Davoli, C.C., Brockmole, J. R. (2011) "A bias to detail: how hand position modulates visual learning and visual memory." *Memory and Cognition*, 40(3), 352–359. doi:10.3758/s13421-011-0147-3.

Davoli, C. C. and Brockmole, J. R. (2012) "The hands shield attention from visual interference." *Attention, Perception and Psychophysics*, 74: 1386–1390. doi:10.3758/s13414-012-0351-7.

de Leeuw, R. (2010) *Special Font For Dyslexia?*(Master's thesis). Twente: University of Twente.

Dehaene, S. et al. (2010). "How learning to read changes the cortical networks for vision and language." *Science*, 330(6009): 1359–1364.

Dickstein, S. G., Bannon, K., Castellanos, F. X., and Milham, M. P. (2006). "The neural correlates of attention deficit hyperactivity disorder: an ALE meta-analysis." *Journal of Child Psychology and Psychiatry*, 47(10): 1051–1062.

Eden, G. F.et al. (2004). "Neural changes following remediation in adult developmental dyslexia." *Neuron*, 44(3): 411–422.

Falth, L. et al.(2013). "Computer-assisted interventions targeting reading skills of children with reading disabilities–a longitudinal study." *Dyslexia*, 19: 37–53.

Gaab, N., Gabrieli, J. D. E., Deutsch, G. K., Tallal, P., and Temple, E. (2007). "Neural correlates of rapid auditory processing are disrupted in children with developmental dyslexia and ameliorated with training: An fMRI study." *Restorative Neurology and Neuroscience*, 25(3–4):295–310.

Gabrieli, J. D. E. (2009). "Dyslexia: A new synergy between education and cognitive neuroscience." *Science*, 325(5938): 280–283.

Galuschka, K., Ise, E., Krick, K., and Schulte-Korne, G. (2014). "Effectiveness of treatment approaches for children and adolescents with reading disabilities: A meta-analysis of randomized controlled trials." *PLoS ONE*, 9(2):e89900.

Geiger, G. and Lettvin, J. Y. (1987) *"Peripheral vision in persons with dyslexia."* New England Journal of Medicine, 316: 1238–1243. doi:10.1056/NEJM198705143162003.

Ginns, P. (2005). "Meta-analysis of the modality effect." *Learning and Instruction*, 15: 313–331.

Hall, T., Meyer, A., and Rose, D. (Eds). (2012). *Universal design for learning in the classroom*. New York City, NY: The Guilford Press.

Hall, T. E., Cohen, N., Vue, G., and Ganley, P. (2015). Addressing learning disabilities with UDL and technology: Strategic readers. *Learning disability quarterly*, 38(2): 72–83.

Hoeft, F. et al. (2007). "Prediction of children's reading skills using behavioral, functional, and structural neuroimaging measures." *Behavioral Neuroscience*, 121(3): 602–613.

Hoeft, F. et al. (2011). "Neural systems predicting long-term outcome in dyslexia." *Proceedings of the National Academy of Sciences of the United States of America*, 108(1): 361–366.

Hutzler, F. and Wimmer, H. (2004). "Eye movements of dyslexic children when reading in a regular orthography." *Brain and Language*, 89: 235–242.

Itti, L. (2015). "New eye tracking techniques may revolutionize mental health screening." *Neuron*, 88(3): 442–444.

Jafarlou, F., Jarollahi, F., Ahadi, M., Sadeghi-Firozabadi, V., and Haghani, H. (2017). "Oculomotor rehabilitation in children with dyslexia." *Medical Journal of the Islamic Republic of Iran*, 31: 125.

Jenneke, C. A. W. et al. (2015). "Efficacy of working memory training in children and adolescents with learning disability: A review study and meta analysis." *Neuropsychological Rehabilitation: An International Journal.* doi:10.1080/09602011.2015.1026356.

Karande, S., D'Souza, S., Gogtay, N.Shiledar, M., and Sholapurwala, R. (2019). "Economic burden of specific learning disability: A prevalence-based cost of illness study of its direct, indirect and intangible costs." *Journal of Postgraduate Medicine*, 65(3): 152–159.

Karapetsas, A. V.and Zygouris, N. C. (2011). "Event related potentials (ERPs) in prognosis, diagnosis and 8 N. C. ZYGOURIS ET AL. rehabilitation of children with dyslexia." *Encephalos*, 48(3): 118–127.

Keller, T. A. and Just, M. A. (2009). "Altering cortical connectivity: Remediation-induced changes in the white matter of poor readers." *Neuron*, 64(5): 624–631.

Keyale, T.et al. (2011). "Plastic neural changes and reading improvement caused by audio-visual training in reading impaired children." *Pnas*, 98(18): 10509–10514.

Knoop-van, Campen, C. A. N., Segers, E. and Verhoeven, L. (2018). "The modality and redundancy effects in multimedia learning in children with dyslexia." *Dyslexia*, 24: 140–155.

Krafnick, A. J., Flowers, D. L., Napoliello, E. M., and Eden, G. F. (2011). "Gray matter volume changes following reading intervention in dyslexic children." *NeuroImage*, 57(3): 733–741.

Kujala, T. et al. (2001). "Plastic neural changes and reading improvement caused by audiovisual training in reading-impaired children." *Neurobiology Psychology*, 98(18): 10509–10514.

Kyle, F., Kujala, J., Richardson, U., Lyytinen, H., and Goswami, U. (2013). "Assessing the effectiveness of two theoretically motivated computer-assisted reading interventions in the United Kingdom: GG Rime and GG Phoneme." *Reading Research Quarterly*, 48(1): 61–76.

Langer, N. et al. (2017). "White matter alterations in infants at risk for developmental dyslexia." *Cerebral Cortex*, 27(2): 1027–1036.

Lindeblad, E. et al. (2017). "Assistive technology as reading interventions for children with reading impairments with a one-year follow-up." *Disability Rehabilitation Assistance Technology*, 12: 713–724.

Loosli, S. V., Buschkuehl, M., Perrig, W. J., and Jaeggi, S. M. (2012). "Working memory training improves reading processes in typically developing children." *Child Neuropsychology*, 18(1): 62–78.

Mayer, R. E. (ed.). (2005). *The Cambridge Handbook of Multimedia Learning*. Cambridge: Cambridge University Press.

Meyer, A., Rose, D. H., and Gordon, D. (2014). *Universal design for learning: Theory & practice*. Wakefield, MA: CAST Professional Publishing.

Miller-Shaul, S. and Breznitz, Z. (2004). "Electrocortical measures during a lexical decision task: A comparison between elementary school-aged children normal and dyslexic readers and adult, normal and dyslexic readers." *Journal of Genetic Psychology*, 165: 399–424.

Modak, M., Ghotane, K., Siddhanth, V., Kelkar, N., Iyer, A. and Prachi, G. (2019). "Detection of dyslexia using eye tracking measures." *International Journal of Innovative Technology and Exploring Engineering*, 8(654).

Myers, P. I. and Hammill, D. D. (1990). *Learning Disabilities* (4th ed.). Austin, TX: PROED.

Neeraja, P. and Anuradha, K. (2016). Importance of assistive technology in teaching children with learning disability in India. *International Journal of Applied Research*, 2(11), 283–243.

O'Brien, B., Mansfield, J., and Legge, G. (2005) "The effect of print size on reading speed in dyslexia." *Journal of Research in Reading*, 28: 332–349.

Olulade, O. A., Napoliello, E. M., and Eden, G. F. (2013). "Abnormal visual motion processing is not a cause of dyslexia." *Neuron*, 79, 180–190.

Paolozza, A. et al.(2014). "Deficits in response inhibition correlate with oculomotor control in children with fetal alcohol spectrum disorder and prenatal alcohol exposure." *Behavioural Brain Research*, 259: 97–105.

Paulesu, E., Danelli, L., and Berlingeri, M. (2014). "Reading the dyslexic brain: Multiple dysfunctional routes revealed by a new meta-analysis of PET and fMRI activation studies."*Frontiers in Human Neuroscience*, 8: 830.

Perelmutter, B., McGregor, K. K. and Gordon, K. R. 2017. "Assistive Technology Interventions for Adolescents and Adults with Learning Disabilities: An Evidence-Based Systematic Review and Meta-Analysis." *Computer Education*, 114: 139–163.

Prabhu, A., Olivier, M. and Uplanem, M. (2017). "Use of assistive technology in classroom assessment to achieve inclusive education and the challenges faced there in." *Scholarly Research Journal for Interdisciplinary Studies*, 4(32): 321–331.

Price, C. J. (2012). "A review and synthesis of the first 20 years of PET and fMRI studies of heard speech, spoken language and reading." *NeuroImage*, 62(2): 816–847.

Raskind, M.(2000). *Assistive Technology for Children with Learning Disabilities*. San Mateo, CA: Schwab Foundation for Learning.

Rayner, K., Liversedge, S. P., White, S. J., and Vergilino-Perez, D. (2003) "Reading disappearing text: Cognitive control of eye movements." *Psychological Science*, 14: 385–388.

Reed, C. L., Grubb, J. D., and Steele, C. (2006) "Hands up: attentional prioritization of space near the hand."*Journal of Experimental Psychology and Human Perception and Performance*, 32: 166–177.

Rizwana, A. (2019). "Eye tracking as a tool for diagnosing specific learning disabilities." In S. K. Gupta, S. Venkatesan, S. P. Goswami, and R. Kumar (Eds.), *Advances in medical technologies and clinical practice. Emerging trends in the diagnosis and intervention of neurodevelopmental disorders* (pp. 153–170)

Romeo, R. R. et al. (2017). "Socioeconomic status and reading disability: Neuroanatomy and plasticity in response to intervention." *Cerebral Cortex*, 28(7): 2297–2312.

Roseth, C. J., Johnson, D. W., and Johnson, R. T. (2008). "Promoting early adolescents' achievement and peer relationships: The effects of cooperative, competitive, and individualistic goal structures." *Psychological Bulletin*, 134: 223–246.

Saine, N. L., Lerkkanen, M. K., Ahonen, T., Tolvanen, A., and Lyytinen, H. (2011). "Computer-assisted remedial reading intervention for school beginners at risk for reading disability." *Child Development*, 82(3): 1013–1028.

Schneps, M. H., O'Keeffe, J. K., Heffner-Wong, A., and Sonnert, G. (2010) "Using technology to support STEM reading."*Journal of Special Education Technology*, 25: 21–32.

Schneps, M. H. et al. (2013). "Shorter lines facilitate reading in those who struggle." *Plosone*, 8(8): e71161.

Shamir, A., Korat, O., and Fellah, R. (2012). "Promoting vocabulary, phonological awareness and concept about print among children at risk for learning disability: Can e-book help?" *Read Write*, 25: 45–69.

Stein, J. (2014). "Dyslexia: the Role of Vision and Visual Attention." *Current Developmental Disorders Report*, 1: 267–280.

Stoodley, C. J. (2012). "The cerebellum and cognition: Evidence from functional imaging studies."*Cerebellum*, 11(2): 352–365.

Swanson, H. L., Xinhua, Z., and Jerman, O. (2009). "Working memory, short-term memory, and reading disabilities: A selective meta-analysis of the literature." *Journal of Learning Disabilities*, 42: 260–287.

Temple, E.et al. (2003). "Neural deficits in children with dyslexia ameliorated by behavioral remediation: Evidence from functional MRI." *Proceedings of the National Academy of Sciences of the United States of America*, 100(5): 2860–2865.

Thiagarajan, P. (2012) *Oculomotor rehabilitation for reading dysfunction in mild traumatic brain injury*. State University of New York, pp. 207–274.

Tijms, J., Hoeks, J. J., Paulussen-Hoogeboom, M. C., and Smolenaars, A. J. (2003). "Long-term effects of a psycholinguistic treatment for dyslexia." *Journal of Research in Reading*, 26(2): 121–140.

Torgesen, J. K., Alexander, A. W. and Wagner, R. K. et al. (2001). "Intensive remedial instruction for children with severe reading disabilities: immediate and long-term outcomes from two instructional approaches." *Journal of Learning Disabilities*, 34: 33–58.

Wang, S. et al.(2015). *Neuron*, 88: 604–616.

Wong, B. and Butler, D. L. (2012). *Learning About Learning Disabilities (4th ed.)*. Waltham, MA: Academic Press.

World Health Organization. (2009)"Assistive devices/technologies". Retrieved from www.who.int/disabilities/technology/en.

Yeatman, J. D., Dougherty, R. F., Ben-Shachar, M., and Wandell, B. A. (2012). "Development of white matter and reading skills." *Proceedings of the National Academy of Sciences of the United States of America*, 109(44): E3045–E3053.

Zygouris, N. C., Avramidis, E., Karapetsas, A. V., and Stamouis, G. I. (2017). "Differences in dyslexic students before and after a remediation program: a clinical neuropsychological and even related potential study." *Applied Neuropsychology: Child*. doi:10.1080/21622965.2017.1297710.

4 The Impact of Technology on Children with Autism Spectrum Disorder

Anurag Sharma and Hitesh Marwaha

1 Introduction

Autism spectrum disorder (ASD) is a pervasive illness in neurodevelopment indicated by abnormalities in social contact, communicating, and decreased needs and/ or repeated actions. The same as modern technologies change the lives of human beings in ways that we have not dreamed of, autism is likewise no exception. Actually, Colby (1973) used computers to educate pupils with ASD. To coach kids with ASD, technological interventions are extremely useful, as these interventions are readily customized, take time to style, and lessen therapist expenses.

The important goal of this chapter is to offer a review of distinct technical technologies like virtual reality (VR), therapeutic robots, speech program equipment, mobile interactive apparatus, and table/floor projectors to improve the lives of children with ASD. Different studies are presented by which these tools are utilized to help autistic children and their parents to enhance their own lives. The first section gives a brief description of specialized tools, which can be supported by more detailed descriptions from the following sections. The section after that investigates the use of VR in encouraging the education of children with ASD, while the final section is organized around enhancing the utilization of robotics in several areas of disabilities. The decisions and also the scope for future work will be ultimately addressed.

2 Diverse Technical Kits to Improve Educational Skills in Children with Autism

This section discusses technological instruments available for teaching autistic pupils, as assessed by Bekele et al. (2013). A thorough survey of specialized tools is provided in this chapter with the objective of solving numerous impairments of glaucoma.

VR can simulate an immersive, customized, and secure digital environment. It delivers the potential for users to detect social scenarios and comprehend different behaviour answers for a variety of simulated social interactions. Regardless of the massive potential of VR, no such facilities are usually implemented in learning centers.

DOI: 10.4324/9781003165569-4

Robotic technology has potential with children with ASD, as robots are less difficult to converse with than individuals, can replay games with boundless patience, and might also record more study knowledge, altering the manner in which ASD children learn new skills. The robots might be utilized to sense many conditions under which it would be suitable to swap any societal prompts. This might be configured appropriately and let children in a personalized environment to converse steadily (Tanu et al., 2018).

Among the primary improvements in speech, availability of VR can enhance the addition of instruction, expand the social circle, and finally increase liberty (Finn et al., 2005). Compared with language tutors, language remediation applications are readily available and user friendly. These language tools are not restricted by time or location and are also suitable for houses and learning facilities.

A comparatively recent paradigm of human computer interaction, the more Multitouch tabletop presents a collaborative interface to encourage interaction involving co-located users. The tabletop projector eases normal experiences and boosts demanding motor skills (Chen, 2012). It is also feasible to utilize floor projections to produce the immersive concepts, and many such games could be planned for people.

The next sections include an extensive description of the above tools alongside their study attestations.

3 Virtual Reality to Sustain the Education of Children with Autism

A series of computing technologies that enable VR are three-dimensional representations of realistic-looking worlds, to be produced and explored. It is a VR that allows simultaneous users to be more active at precisely the same time; it is also an environment for several users. The actual vision for VR layout was supposed to take the user away to an exciting fictional planet, but the real situation is somewhat different, and VR technologies are mostly used for realistic functions.

This section is divided into three sub-sections, and the use of VR in autism is addressed in the first sub-section. From the next sub-section, some scientific information to prove the usefulness of VR is examined and finally concluded.

3.1 Role of VR in ASD

VR ASD programs and awareness of the VR opportunities for children on the continuum began to emerge at the end of the 1990s (Strickland et al., 1996).

In VR, users can explore Victorian immersive surroundings themselves and communicate in real time with imaginary characters or objects at the same level as activities in the real world. Therefore, VRs make a genuine simulation of scenarios, allowing participants to appreciate the significance of the real world, which raises the chance of learning (Strickland et al., 1996). It is possible to track the ambient surroundings in VR (visual and audio) by programming and also to represent any condition without any limitations or expense. Children with ASD can make mistakes in VR and then learn new skills that build confidence among them which are essential in the actual world. If correctly constructed, VR will develop the social and motor skills of children with ASD who suffer in these areas (Mitchell et al., 2007).

3.2 Efficacy of VR for Children with Autism

Some of the analysis evidence to prove the efficacy of VR for kids with ASD is summarized in this section. Using VR for autism treatment was discussed by Cai et al. (2013), where a simulated dolphinarium was utilized for autism intervention. This interactive dolphinarium has allowed kids with ASD to act as dolphin trainers and learn to communicate with virtual dolphins by using hands signals. It was discovered that kids in this setting learned the fundamental movements effectively. The planned virtual dolphinarium is shown in Figure 4.1.

To be able to research stronger therapeutic paradigms, Bekele et al. (2013), revealed a brand new VR-based facial emotional expression systems which monitors eye gaze and bodily signals in autistic and normal children.

In comparison to their control group peers, it has been reasoned that there have been variations in how children with ASD apply the procedure to identify psychological faces (Tanu et al., 2019).

ASD and ten non-ASD children used VR in a study conducted by Yogeswara et al. (2013) A cartoon animation was created showing a narrative of grandma standing supporting two boxes and dropping a toy into every box, as shown in Figure 4.2. The purpose of the experiment was to investigate the effect of VR on kids with autism throughout the intervention plan. This experiment was designed to confirm cognitive activity, and it was discovered employing event-related potential (ERP) signs that better outcomes were listed by kids who were trained with VR than people trained with traditional procedures.

A novel VR-based eye monitoring model named Virtual Interactive System using Gaze-sensitive Adaptive Response Technology was designed by Lahiri et al. (2011). Throughout VR-based interaction, it is equipped to present one-on-one comments, depending on the complicated gaze patterns of a child. VIGART will offer that the "avatars" with constant details on the length of time that the child

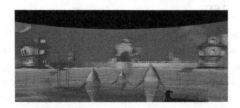

Figure 4.1

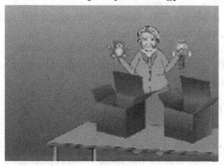

Figure 4.2

looks at them through interaction, and because of this, the "avatars" will adapt their mode of address to permit kids and VIGART to supply a greater level of interactivity. Using VR to create mutual care skills was proposed by Simões and Carvalho (2012), in which an avatar guides focus on a digital object on the Earth, which the youngster is expected to comprehend by paying attention to it.

The brain activity of the topic is monitored by ERP signs in real time, and a classifier attempts to recognize the target object. Courgeon et al. (2014) analyzed the simulation of shared attention with virtually presented people in a different report. An experiment where children with ASD communicate with virtual people and need to follow their disposition was designed. It has been demonstrated that children with ASD might use virtual avatars to find out objects or people and in less time than any other traditional procedure.

3.3 Concluding Comments

It is clear from the research described above that VR has an edge over traditional mechanisms of studying. But on a bigger scale, there is no persuasive proof that VR can convert learning in the digital world into the real world. Only time will tell if VR technology for children with ASD can enter mainstream usage of learning, social creativity, and communication and interaction.

4 Robots to Instruct Social Skills, Joint Attention and Motor Skills

For autistic children, robotic technology appears to be appealing to operate with. This section will explain the possible utilization of robots for kids with disabilities who are experiencing challenges mostly in social communication and motor skills in therapeutic practice. Social therapeutic robots are used as tools to educate children with ASD many unique skills. These tools might be impacted to be able to give children with ASD using regular, special, and individualized intervention solutions (Esubalew et al., 2013). For special educators working with ASD kids, robots are applicable, as they find programs in a variety of areas of disability, like learning interpersonal skills, learning motor skills, mutual focus, and communicating, etc.

From the next sub-section, some study data show how the usefulness of autonomous technology is addressed and, ultimately, in the next sub-section, concluding remarks are made.

4.1 Famous Bots

There are a variety of robots that scientists have built to manage autistic kids. In the next paragraphs, a number of the most usual robots used for autistic kids are discussed.

For kids with or without disabilities, the CosmoBot robot is utilized to facilitate rehabilitation and educational clinics. It is fabricated by AnthroTronix and can be created in a fashion which permits information to be accumulated about the child's results. Utilizing this, clinicians will examine the treatment's effectiveness and adjust the techniques accordingly (Brisben et al., 2013).

Paro, constructed by AIST, is an innovative interactive robot in the form of a baby seal. It reacts to petting, and assorted moods might be displayed. Rather than a dog or a cat, baby seal has been chosen as a model, as individuals are less comfortable with these creatures, and their moods are somewhat inconsistent. This robot was proven to be suitable for teaching children with ASD various moods, which might boost their social participation. The PARO robot used to teach social skills as found in Figure 4.3 (Riek, 2015).

At the University of Hertfordshire researchers developed and designed the Kinesics and Synchronization in Personal Assistant Robotics (KASPAR) robot. It has been designed to be utilized as a societal moderator, allowing kids with disabilities to communicate and socialize with other people and also to encourage them.

KASPAR has the capability to participate in quite a few societal situations, for example turn-taking, joint-gaze games, etc., where it is hard for kids with

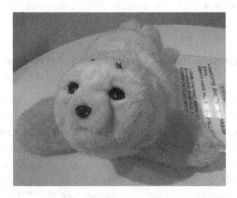

Figure 4.3

autism. The face of KASPAR can exhibit a number of expressions and contains movable nerves, nerves, and mind which might be handled by the teacher and can react to your child's touch (Cabibihan et al., 2013).

Pleo is a robot shaped like a dinosaur, as seen in Figure 4.4. It is about 21 inches long, 6 inches wide and 8 inches tall, and was designed to communicate feelings and attention through body gestures and speech patterns that people would quickly recognise (Kim et al., 2012). To express interest, disinterest, disappointment, happiness, agreement, and disagreement in children with ASD, Pleo's movements can be customized and synchronized with verbal commands.

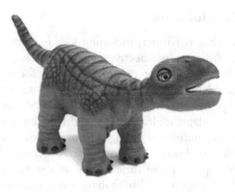

Figure 4.4

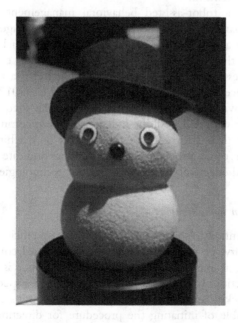

Figure 4.5

In a playful and relaxed mood, Keepon (Figure 4.6) is designed to assist and inspire kids to learn oral contact. The robot is structured to share feelings and attention with children in the easiest and most detailed manner (pronounced as key-pong) (Kozima et al., 2005).

The robot also functions as an embodied apparatus and reconciles the social link that children build in daily discussions. The main intention of this segment was to supply autistic kids with a few robots which were designed because of their own involvement. To construct their particular curative robots to prepare powerful actions, the teacher takes hints from them.

4.2 Social Skills Education

One such societal robot is Kismet, including kids in numerous activities like facial expressions, different perspectives, etc. (Breazeal, 2003). An elastic robotic method, it is capable of restarting mutual focus at predetermined intervals and reacting based on system dimensions, as was shown by Esubalew et al. (2013). In the process, six ASD and six non-ASD kids interacted with the robot. The robot adapts itself within an individualized method to provide support and drives, depending on the signs from the head motion of the baby, having the capability to boost skills in the first societal alteration in ASD. Children with ASD spend more time staring at the humanoid robot compared with non-ASD children. This analysis was encouraging and suggested that robotic tools are moving toward the ideal orientation to target and optimize mutual attention.

The impact of a robot-assisted behavioral management program, which operates in two manners – kids' decision-making and engagement – was discovered by Yun et al. (2014) to improve the societal potential of kids. In child-robot interaction, the robot can significantly reciprocateto compliments,interplay game and assesses the level of reactivity of children via recognition modules for cerebral face and signature attributes. Kim et al. (2012) analyzed, using three encounters with a person, video games and the Pleo robot, the social activity of children with ASD. All the kids are shown to communicate with the Pleo robot rather than with a game for humans or machines. Rather than human trainers or other procedures, these findings indicate that social skills could be improved effectively by utilizing robotic technologies.

4.3 Joint Attention Enhancement

One must pay attention to the actions in order to learn efficiently. Thus, shared curiosity is necessary, i.e. the act of measuring attentional concentration is the initial thing to be learnt (Diehl et al., 2012). The robot is utilized through child-robot interactions to guide the child's attention to a specific thing, so the youngster can quickly comply with the path of the robot's eyes. The baby is consequently capable of initiating the procedure for directing the eye of the robot and might also expand this activity in order to interact with the therapist

(Kozima et al., 2007). Imitation involves creating a backup of expressions by witnessing the moves of others. This plays an essential role in the shipping information from robot into the baby. Does a baby experience new body motions or fakes it, or feels societal atmosphere can be examined by a robot. A series of imitations help to set a cross-modal mapping mechanism for children (Kozima et al., 2005) and enhance hand-eye coordination and empowers children to spot the individuals around them as they can easily mimic their social co-workers. For interactive imitative play, autistic kids constructed a doll formed robot called Robota (Billard et al., 2007).

4.3.1 Motor Skills Training

Motor skills involve preparation and an inner model of the projected outside activity. Autistic children are usually deficient in gross and fine motor skills. The AuRoRa (AUtonomous RObotic platform as an Remedial tool for kids with Autism) project investigates how an independent mobile robot might be utilized as a therapeutic instrument in order to encourage kids with disabilities to take the initiative and use the autonomous 'toy' to become engaged in an assortment of different activities (Dautenhahn, 1999). Robin et al. (2009) analyzed children playing with a therapeutic robot and detected moves in hands and cooperative behaviour.

4.4 Conclusion

Robotic technology plays a significant part in the lives of kids with ASD, and it has a multitude of benefits for treating children with disabilities. Through different games and engaging activities, the robots might communicate and socialize with the kids as a way to instruct them desirable skills and elicit specific behaviours and to provide reinforcement and positive feedback regarding the completion of a job. Continuing research has to construct a base of concepts, tools, and methods which might boost the comprehension of child-robot interaction and invite experiments to be reproduced across research classes. This will need the joint efforts of experts from most of the areas in order to incorporate diverse sources of knowledge and skills.

5 Conclusion and Future Research

In this study, a variety of technical tools are explored to enhance the diverse skills of autistic children, but it has been noted that there is also a lack of efficient and adequate usage of these instruments in families or schools. The strong appeal of these tools is clear, and this will continue to inspire researchers. In the coming years, we expect the ability of teachers to introduce and explore these devices in their own schools to be fortified. These specialized apparatuses are very fascinating, if we can deal with the requirements of kids with ASD with a specific tool, but these tools require skilled employees to get maximum benefit from them.

References

Allen, D. et al. (2004). The Boardmaker Project, Retrieved from www.bctf.ca/Tea chingToDiversity/BC-projects/boardmaker.pdf.

Bekele, E. et al. (2013). "Understanding How Adolescents with Autism Respond to Facial Expressions in Virtual Reality Environments." *IEEE Transactions on Visualization and Computer Graphics*, 19(4): 711–720. doi:1077-2626/13.

Billard, A., Robins, B., Nadel, J., and Heyes, C. (2007). "Building Robota, a mini-humanoid robot for the rehabilitation of children with autism." *Assistive Technology*, 19(1): 37–49. doi:10.1080/10400435.2007.10131864.

Boccanfuso, L. and Kane, J. M. (2011). "CHARLIE: An adaptive robot design with hand and face tracking for use in autism therapy." *International Journal of Social Robotics*, 3(4): 337–347. doi:10.1007/s12369-011-0110-2.

Boser, K. I., Goodwin, M. S., and Wayland, S. C. (2013) *Technological tools for students with autism*. Paul H. Brookes Publishing Co.

Breazeal, C. (2003). "Emotion and sociable humanoid robots." *International Journal of Human Computer Interaction*, 59: 119–155. doi:10.1016/S1071-5819(03)00018-1.

Bricken, M. (1991). "Virtual reality learning environments: Potentials and challenges." *Computer Graphics*, 25(3): 178–184. doi:10.1145/126640.126657.

Brisben, A. J., Safos, C. S., Lockerd, A. D., and Lathan, C. E. (2013). "The CosmoBot System: Evaluating its Usability in Therapy Sessions with Children Diagnosed with Cerebral Palsy." Retrieved from http://web.mit.edu/zoz/Public/AnthrotronixRO MAN2013.pdf.

Cabibihan, J.J., Javed, H., Ang, M., and Aljunied, S. M. (2013). "Why Robots? A Survey on the Roles and Benefits of Social Robots in the Therapy of Children with Autism." *International Journal of Social Robotics*, 5(4): 593–618. doi:10.1007/s12369-013-0202-2.

Cai, Y., Chia, N. K. H., Thalmann, D., Kee, N. K. N., Zheng, J., and Thalmann, N. M. (2013). "Design and development of a Virtual Dolphinarium for children with autism." *IEEE Transactions on Neural Systems and Rehabilitation Engineering*, 21(2): 208–217. doi:10.1109/TNSRE.2013.2240700.

Chen, W. (2012). "Multitouch Tabletop Technology for People with Autism Spectrum Disorder: A review of the Literature," *Procedia Computer Science*, 14(1877): 198–207. doi:10.1016/j.procs.2012.10.023.

Colby, K. M. (1973). "The rationale for computer-based treatment of language difficulties in nonspeaking autistic children." *Journal of Autism and Childhood Schizophrenia*, 3: 254–260. doi:10.1007/BF01538283.

Courgeon, M., Rautureau, G., Martin, J., and Grynszpan, O. (2014). "Joint Attention Simulation using Eye-Tracking and Virtual Human." *IEEE Transactions on Affective Computing*, 14(5): 238–250. doi:10.1109/TAFFC.2014.2335740.

Dautenhahn, K. (1999). *ROBOTS AS SOCIAL ACTORS: AURORA and The Case of AUTISM*, In: Proceedings Third Cognitive Technology Conference CT'99, August, San Francisco.

Diehl, J.J., Schmitt, L.M., Villano, M., and Crowell, C.R.(2012). "The clinical use of robots for individuals with autism spectrum disorders: A critical review." *Research in Autism Spectrum Disorders*, 6(1): 249–262. doi:10.1016/j.rasd.2011.05.006.

Esubalew, T.et al. (2013a). "Robot-Mediated Intervention Architecture (ARIA) for Children With Autism." *IEEE transactions on neural systems and rehabilitation engineering*, 21(2): 289–299. doi:10.1109/TNSRE.2012.2230188.

Finn, D., Futernick, A., and MacEachern, S. (2005).Efficacy of language intervention software in preschool classrooms. Paper presented at the annual meeting of the American Speech Language Hearing Association, San Diego, CA.

Flores, M. et al. (2012). "A comparison of communication using the apple iPad and a picture-based system." *Augmentative and Alternative Communication,* 28(2): 74–84. doi:10.3109/07434618.2011.644579.

Giusti, L., Zancanaro, M., Gal, E., and Weiss, P.L.(2011) *"Dimensions of collaboration on a tabletop interface for children with Autism Spectrum Disorder."* Conference on Human Factors in Computing Systems; May 7–12; Vancouver, BC, pp. 3259–3304.

Grønbæk, K., Iversen, O. S., Kortbek, K. J., Nielsen, K. R., and Aagaard, L. (2007). "iGameFloor — A Platform for Co-Located Collaborative Games." In: *Proceedings of the international conference on Advances in computer entertainment technology,* pp. 64–71. doi:10.1145/1255047.1255061.

Hopkins, I. M. et al. (2011). "Avatar assistant: Improving social skills in students with an asd through a computer-based intervention." *Journal of Autism and Developmental Disorders,* 41(11): 1543–1555. doi:10.1007/s10803–011–1179-zICD-10. Retrieved from www.icd10data.com/ICD10CM/Codes/F01-F99/F80-F89/F80-/F80.1.

Jowett, E. L., Moore, D. W., and Anderson, A. (2012). "Using an iPad-based video modeling package to teach numeracy skills to a child with an autism spectrum disorder." *Developmental Neurorehabilitation,* 15: 304–312. doi:10.3109/17518423.2012.682168.

Kakkar, D. (2019). Diagnostic assessment techniques and non-invasive biomarkers for autism spectrum disorder. *International Journal of E-Health and Medical Communications (IJEHMC), 10*(3), 79-95.

Kim, E. S. et al. (2012). "Social Robots as Embedded Reinforcers of Social Behavior in Children with Autism." *Journal of Autism and Developmental Disorders,* 43(5): 1038–1049. doi:10.1007/s10803–012–1645-2.

Kozima, H., Nakagawa, C., and Yasuda, Y. (2005). Interactive robots for communication-care: a case-study in autism therapy. ROMAN 2005. IEEE International Workshop on Robot and Human Interactive Communication, 2005. pp. 341–346. doi:10.1109/ROMAN.2005.1513802.

Kozima, H., Nakagawa, C., and Yasuda, Y. (2007). "Children-robot interaction: a pilot study in autism therapy." *Progress in Brain Research,* 164–385.

Lahiri, U., Warren, Z., and Sarkar, N. (2011). "Design of a gaze-sensitive virtual social interactive system for children with autism." *IEEE Transactions on Neural Systems and Rehabilitation Engineering,* 19(4): 443–452. doi:10.1109/TNSRE.2011.2153874.

Meltzoff, A. N., Brooks, R., Shon, A. P., and Rao, R. P. (2010). "Social robots are psychological agents for infants: A test of gaze following." *Neural Networks,* 23(8): 966–972. doi:10.1016/j.neunet.2010.09.005.

Michaud, F. and Theberge-Turnel, C. (2002). "Mobile robotic toys and autism." In: *Socially Intelligent Agents, Multiagent Systems, Artificial Societies and Simulated Organization,* Vol. 3 (pp. 125–132). doi:10.1007/0-306-47373-9_15.

Mitchell, P., Parsons, S., and Leonard, A. (2007). "Using virtual environments for teaching social understanding to 6 adolescents with autistic spectrum disorders." *Journal of Autism and Developmental Disorders,* 37(3): 589–600. doi:10.1007/s10803–006–0189–8.

Miyamoto, E., Lee, M., Fujii, H., and Okada, M. (2005). How can robots facilitate social interaction of children with autism? Possible implication s for educational environments. Proceedings of the fifth international workshop on epigenetic robotics July 22–24, Nara, (pp. 145–146).

Modugumudi, Y. R., Santhosh, J., and Anand, S. (2013). "Efficacy of Collaborative Virtual Environment Intervention Programs in Emotion Expression of Children with Autism." *Journal of Medical Imaging and Health Informatics*, 3(2): 1–5. doi:10.1166/jmihi.2013.1167.

Murray, D. (1997). "Autism and information technology: therapy with computers." In: *Autism and learning: a guide to good practice* (pp. 100–117).

Pioggia, G., Igliozzi, R., Sica, M. L., and Ferro, M. (2008). "Exploring emotional and imitational android based interactions in autistic spectrum disorders." *Journal of Cyber Therapy and Rehabilitation*, 1(1): 49–61.

Postil, J. and Lloyd, L. (2012). "iPad Applications for Kids with Autism Spectrum Disorders." Retrieved from www.tacanow.org/wp-content/uploads/2012/11/iPad_and_ABA_Beginning_Handout.pdf.

Pressman, H. and Pietrzyk, A. (2011). "Free and inexpensive apps for people who need augmentative communication supports." Retrieved from www.centralcoastchildrensfoundation.org/draft/wp-content/uploads/2012/03/FreeandInexpensiveAACAppsFinal.pdf.

Prizant, B. M. and Wetherby, A. M. (2005). "Critical considerations in enhancing communication abilities for persons with autism spectrum disorders." In F. R. Volkmar, R. Paul, A. Klin, and D. J. Cohen, *Handbook of Autism and Pervasive Development Disorders* (3rd ed., Vol. 2, pp. 925–945). Hoboken, NJ: Wiley.

Ralston, K. K. (2013). Learning Grammar in a Suitable Way. Unpublished doctoral dissertation. University of Iceland.

Riek, L. D. (2015). "Robotics Technology in Mental Health Care." *Artificial Intelligence in Behavioral Health and Mental Health Care*, 185–203. doi:10.1016/B978-0-12-420248-1.00008-8.

Robins, B., Dautenhahn, K., and Dickerson, P. (2009). "*From isolation to communication: A case study evaluation of robot assisted play for children with autism with a minimally expressive humanoid robot.*" Proceedings of the 2nd international conference on advances in human-computer interactions, Cancum, Mexico. doi:10.1109/ACH.2009.32.

Rogers, Y. and Lindley, S. E. (2004). "Collaborating around vertical and horizontal large interactive displays: Which way is best?" *Interacting with Computers*. 16(6): 1133–1152. doi:10.1016/j.intcom.2004.07.008.

Shane, H. C. and Albert, P. D. (2008). "Electronic screen media for persons with autism spectrum disorders; Results of a survey." *Journal of Autism and Developmental Disorders*, 38: 1499–1508. doi:10.1007/s10803-007-0527-5.

Shane, H., Laubscher, E. H., Schlosser, R. W., Flynn, S., Sorce, J. F., and Abramson, J. (2012). "Applying technology to visually support language and communication individuals with autism spectrum disorders." *Journal of Autism and Developmental Disorders*, 42(6): 1228–1235. doi:10.1007/s10803-011-1304-z.

Simões, M. and Carvalho, P. (2012). "*Virtual reality and brain-computer interface for joint-attention training in autism.*" In: Procedures of 9th International Conference on Disability, Virtual Reality & Associated Technologies, pp. 10–12.

Strickland, D., Marcus, L. M., Mesibov, G. B., and Hogan, K. (1996). "Two case studies using virtual reality as a learning tool for autistic children." *Journal of Autism and Developmental Disorders*, 26: 651–659.

Tager-Flusberg, H., Paul, R., and Lord, C. (2005) "Language and communication in autism." In F. Volkmar, A. Klin, and R. Paul (Eds), *Handbook of Autism and Pervasive Developmental Disorders* (3rd ed., pp. 335–364). Hoboken, NJ: Wiley.

Tanu, T. and Kakkar, D. (2018). "Strengthening risk prediction using statistical learning in children with autism spectrum disorder." *Advances in Autism*, 4(3): 141–152. doi:10.1108/AIA-06-2018-0022.

(This reference sas per google scholar is revised and added as starting from "Kakkar" alphabetically)Tartaro, A. and Cassell, J. (2008). "Authorable Virtual Peers for Autism Spectrum Disorders." *Extended Abstracts on Human Factors in Computing Systems*. 1677–1680. doi:10.1145/1240866.1240881.

Tse, E., Greenberg, S., Shen, C., and Forlines, C. (2007). "Multimodal multiplayer tabletop gaming." *Computers in Entertainment*, 5(2). doi:10.1145/1279540.1279552.

Turner, S. and Pearson, D. W. (1999). Fast ForWord Language Intervention Program: Four Case Studies. *Texas Journal of Audiology and Speech Pathology*. Retrieved from www.scilearn.com/sites/default/files/imported/30314Abstract10.pdf.

Webber. (2013). "Introduction to hearbuilder." Retrieved from www.hearbuilder.com/pdf/HBWebsiteContent_WhitePaper_092713.pdf.

Whalen, C., Liden, L., Ingersoll, B., Dallaire, E., and Liden, S. (2006). "Behavioral Improvements Associated with Computer-Assisted Instruction for Children with Developmental Disabilities." *The Journal of Speech and Language Pathology – Applied Behavior Analysis*, 1(1): 11–26. doi:10.1037/h0100182.

Yogeswara, R. M., Kumar, S., Santosh, J., and Anand, S. (2013). "Virtual Technologies in Intervention Programs for Autistic Children." *International Journal on Emerging Technologies*, 4(1): 39–43.

Yun, S.-S., Park, S.-K., and Choi, J. (2014). "A robotic treatment approach to promote social interaction skills for children with autism spectrum disorders." 23rd IEEE International Symposium on Robot and Human Interactive Communication, pp. 130–134. doi:10.1109/ROMAN.2014.6926242.

Zarin, R. and Fallman, D. (2011). "Through the Troll Forest. Exploring Tabletop Interaction Design for Children with Special Cognitive Needs." Conference on Human Factors in Computing Systems; May 7–12, 2011; Vancouver, BC: pp. 3319–3322.

5 Telehealth for Children with Autistic Spectrum Disorder

Indian Need Versus Challenges

Iyer Kamlam Gopalkrishnan and Srinivasan Venkatesan

Caselet #1

Anirudh (a pseudonym), aged three years, a pupil at a pre-primary school in Bangalore, visited his pediatrician for a regular check-up. The pediatrician observed poor eye-to-eye contact and mild restlessness in the child. The child's parents were asked to contact the hospital's clinical child psychologist for further evaluation. Before the parents could get the child psychologist, COVID-19 hit the city, and the family left for their home in north-eastern India. Accessing a clinical child psychologist closer home was not feasible for them. They preferred to seek assistance from the child's hospital in Bangalore.

Caselet #2

Ridhima (a pseudonym), aged five-and-a-half years, attends a senior kindergarten, was diagnosed with mild autism spectrum disorder (ASD) at age 3.5 years. She was on early intervention therapy comprising speech and occupational therapy since her diagnosis. Presently, she lacks attention to activities at hand, slower information processing, and social skills at school. She was referred to a clinical child psychologist for further assistance. On assessment by the clinical child psychologist, she was average in her intellectual functioning, had very mild symptoms of ASD, and poor working memory skills. Cognitive training and developmental skills training were started. The child was seen once a week at the clinic for an intervention. After five sessions, the child moved to her grandparents' home and could not come to the clinic for further therapy.

Caselet #3

Pratap (a pseudonym), aged five years, attends a senior kindergarten and did the same, repetitive play activities, few friends, and repeated talk that teachers in school found challenging to deal with. On assessment by a clinical child psychologist, he was reported to have ASD. The family details the separation of his parents two years ago. The child is mainly at the day-care center six days a week, owing to the child's mother working full-time at a multinational company. The child requires behavioral and cognitive therapy. His mother finds it challenging to bring him into the clinic regularly, owing to her hectic office obligations.

DOI: 10.4324/9781003165569-5

In each of the examples mentioned above, there are issues of geographic isolation, lack of transportation, and shortage of trained professionals. Hence, evidence-based telehealth services for the rehabilitation of developmental skills of young children with neurodevelopmental disorders (NDD) are required.

ASD: the Nature and Burden of the Issue in India

The number of children experiencing "moderate to severe disability" owing to the "difficulties in functioning" approach in the core domains of vision, hearing, mobility, self-care, and communication is provided in the *World Disability Report* (World Health Organization, 2011). An estimated 200 million children or more in developing countries under the age of five years lack age-appropriate development of cognitive and socio-emotional development (Grantham-McGregor et al., 2007). India emerges, unfortunately, as the country with the highest estimate of children in the ages of three to four years with a lag in the development of some 17.7 million children, according to the latest study (McCoy et al., 2016). Many of the reasons for the poor development of children were reported to be due to infectious diseases, malnutrition, iron-deficient anemia, poverty, and the low availability of high-quality healthcare and educational resources (Walker et al., 2011).

In this background, one of the most widely prevalent NDDs in India (Arora et al., 2018) is autism spectrum disorder (ASD). The Diagnostic and Statistical Manual of Mental Disorders (DSM; 5th ed., American Psychiatric Association, 2013) defines ASD as deficits predominantly in social communication and interaction, originating in the developmental period. ASD affects the child and their families and is known to be an essential developmental disability. One meta-analysis on four community-based Indian studies showed a pooled prevalence of 0.11 in the age group of one to 18 years in rural settings, 0.09 in children up to 15 years in urban settings (Chauhan et al., 2019). Many studies have reported the burden (Arora et al., 2018), the challenges, and unmet needs of the families of children with ASD (Divan et al., 2012), depression, and burden on primary caregivers such as mothers of children with ASD (Singh et al., 2017). These numerous findings depict the public importance of this disorder for a developing nation like India.

What is Telehealth?

Various terminologies/domains exist with the use of information technology in the field of health. A broader domain is the recent emergence of telemedicine. The World Health Organization (2010) defines telemedicine as providing health using health information technology. Telehealth is another domain intricately connected to telemedicine but encompassing health and patient care with its broader application of technologies (World Health Organization, 2016). Telemedicine uses many systems or routes of delivery. For instance:

i With the help of high-speed internet, connecting remote places to tertiary care hospitals or clinics

ii Live consultations using audio and video systems connecting patients at home to the health provider

iii Assisting patients in remotely monitoring their health condition by connecting them to their monitoring centers

iv All e-health web-based services to the patients and their families over the internet

Thus, telehealth/telemedicine are e-health techniques to deliver treatment to people of remote areas and people for whom expert clinical care is complex (World Health Organization, 2016). A subtle difference exists between telemedicine and telehealth domains. Telemedicine is the clinical service provided by a registered medical practitioner. At the same time, telehealth is an all-encompassing term of use of technology for health and health-related services, including telemedicine.

The Ministry of Health and Family Welfare (2020a) considers many modalities of telehealth/telemedicine. Primarily the three modes of video, audio, and text-based are noted. Important guidelines for telemedicine in India are the context, identification of a registered practitioner and the patient, mode of communication, consent, type of consultation, patient evaluation, and management. Telemedicine should be appropriate and sufficient as per the context. One offshoot of telemedicine is telepsychiatry. Owing to an increase in using technology-based interventions in mental health (Sinha Deb et al., 2018), telepsychiatry is one of the essential delivery tools at the hands of a mental healthcare provider (Bada Math et al., 2020; Dinakaran et al., 2020). Guidelines for the optimal delivery of mental healthcare using information technology have been provided (Ministry of Health and Family Welfare, 2020b).

Telepsychiatry branches to telerehabilitation techniques as methods of intervention for the diathesis of NDD. Telerehabilitation methods are one of the ways of increasing the affordable use of technologies in the field of NDDs or other childhood disabilities/disorders (World Health Organization, 2016).

A mild variation of treatment delivery to telerehabilitation for NDDs is called "e-interventions." E-interventions are defined as adopting electronic information technology for medical assessments or treatments (Dean et al., 2009). It is the mode of adhering, designing, and delivery of treatment using computers, gadgets, and the internet. This form of treatment is being used more and more by mental healthcare professionals (Andersson, 2016). Barak et al. (2009) provide a complete understanding of various internet-delivery in psychotherapeutic and psychological treatments. They clearly and consistently enumerate the terminologies "web-based interventions" to incorporate:

i Web-based education services

ii Self-guided web-based therapeutic interventions

iii Human supported web-based therapeutic interventions

These subtypes of web-based interventions emphasize components of program content, use of multimedia, online activities, and support and feedback service. Using these components, each of the subtypes is defined elaborately (Barak et al., 2009). Hence technology could mean a wide range of electronically driven modalities, gadgets, and healthcare machines; we refer to computers and mobile apps to deliver treatment to children with NDD. Instructions offered through audio/video, internet-based, online, web-based, or mobile interventions will be referred to as telehealth herein in this chapter.

Telehealth in ASD: International studies

Many systematic reviews have been conducted in ASD (Jang et al., 2012; Wainer and Ingersoll, 2014; Knutsen et al., 2016; Sutherland et al., 2018), focusing on different age groups, varied definitions of telehealth, and assesses applicability to other professionals. The present review is focused on the age group of children between the ages of two and 12-and-a-half years children, their parents, and e-interventions for skills training and problem behaviors in ASD.

Method: The preferred reporting items for selective review and meta-analyses (PRISMA) (Moher et al., 2009) are used here to sample the selection of studies used in ASD with telehealth. The perusal of studies was according to the inclusion and exclusion criteria provided in Table 5.1.

Table 5.1 Inclusion and Exclusion Criteria for the Sampling of Studies

No.	Inclusion Criteria	Exclusion Criteria
1.	Any research article/book published in International Journals in the age group of 2–12 years	Opinion papers on telehealth
2.	Original studies published in English-language journals only	Telehealth on assistance for physicians caring for children with ASD
3.	Telehealth, defined as the use of video, web-based, internet-based, audio or texting, mobile apps, serious games were considered	Telehealth such as remote healthcare machines, robots, electronic records
4.	Telehealth for rehabilitation or psychotherapy	Telehealth encompassing pharmacological treatment/behavioral techniques
5.	Study objectives assessing telehealth of children with ASD and involving their parents	Studies with adolescents or adults on telehealth in ASD, involving teachers or other caregivers
No.	Inclusion Criteria	Exclusion Criteria
6.	Any year studies Full-text articles only	Telehealth on clusters/communities/groups
7.		Only e-assessment/e-analysis
8.	Articles on ASD only considered	Articles on other childhood mental disorders

Note: These criteria were for the sampling of studies in telehealth in ASD research.

Search strategy: Databases and search engines such as Google Scholar, PubMed were searched by using the terms "E-interventions for Autism Spectrum Disorder" "Telehealth in Autism Spectrum Disorders" "Web-based Interventions for Autism Spectrum Disorder" and using Medical Subject Headings terms "Internet-based Intervention for Autistic Disorder." First, the abstracts of all the studies/articles were assessed. These were limited to childhood (2–12.5 years) for ASD and their

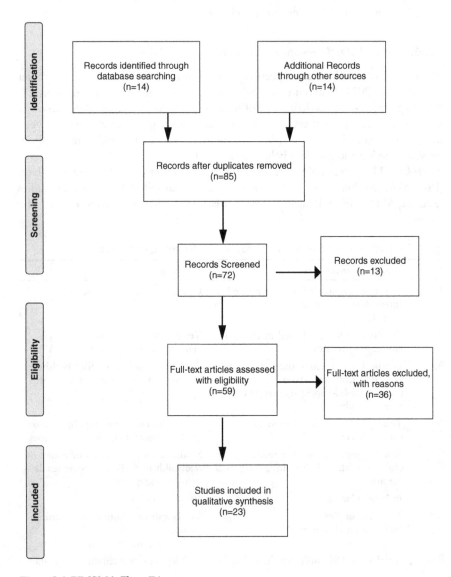

Figure 5.1 PRISMA Flow Diagram

mode of intervention. Furthermore, a snowballing hand search was conducted on the reference lists for relevant articles fitting the eligibility criteria. The list of studies cannot be claimed to be fully exhaustive or all-inclusive.

Data Management: Each full article was assessed to understand the study's objectives. Information pertaining to the age of the children, sample size, study design, the modality of telehealth, their duration, and treatment models were entered.

A narrative analysis of the studies in Table 5.2 reveals the clinical and demographic details of the sample. The objective mostly has been to assess the efficacy and gains obtained in training programs for children with ASD through telehealth conducted in various sites like U.S., U.K., Israel, Sweden from 2010 to 2020. The age group of the children is from two to 12.5 years. The sample size of the studies has been from two to 80 children and from two to 112 of their parents. Single case pre-posttest design, randomized control trials, and two comparative group designs have proven efficacious studies.

Language, communication skills, discrete trials for early intervention programs, parent training techniques and education, sensory skills, reciprocal initiation training in children has been undertaken. Significant reduction in problem behavior, user satisfaction, increase in parental knowledge, and education has been reported. Either evidence-based models of intervention have been adopted or developed explicitly for online mode of delivery. Nevertheless, techniques from early start Denver model (Rogers and Dawson, 2010), functional communication training Carr and Durand, 1985), pivotal response training (Koegal and Koegal, 2006), and ImPACT (Ingersoll and Dvortcsak, 2009) has been conducted using video tutorials, video two-way conferencing, Google Hangout and Skype platforms. Specific background measures for such telehealth services have been computer literacy in parents and accessibility to teleconsultation units. Most of the researchers have provided computers/laptops/iPads with secure access to the program or game. This has been backed by the availability of research support to troubleshoot issues of these programs.

Further, studies have motivated parents by giving them extra booster sessions of coaching and education on interventions in face-2-face (F2F) sessions as an adjunct to e-intervention. A minimum of three to six sessions has produced results of significance with varied objectives. In some studies, participants have received regular clinical therapy for six to 12 months and then transferred to the telehealth mode of intervention for the maintenance of gains. These factors might have helped to reduce attrition rates and improve gains for online remote interventions.

This review also depicts how studies using iPad application has yielded no significant results. An approach observed in telehealth is the usage of both clinic-based and remote therapy using technological assistance while assessing the gains obtained in the children and parental knowledge and education. Comparing parental groups that were self-directed and the other group that received assistance from therapists supplementally, there were significant differences between the two groups. The assistance from the therapist supplementally was helpful for the group to mediate with their children successfully.

Table 5.2 International Studies Using Telehealth in ASD

Aim of the Study	Citation	Study Design	Sample Size (parents/children)	Age of children (months)	F2F/Online mode of intervention	Type of Technology	No of sessions	Results
To assess the efficacy of tele practice / remote technology to coach parents	Baharav and Reiser, 2010	Single subject time series	2	54 and 62	Speech and language therapy via the clinical model and remote technology-based model	Video conferencing through Skype	Six weeks each of 50 mins sessions per week: control period one 50 min session at the clinic and one 50 min session from home	Gains obtained maintained by both the clinical and home-based remote technology modes
To assess if the use of a self-directed learning program could result in changes in behavior for parents and their children	Nefdt et al., 2010	RCT	27	Under 60	PRT	DVD interactive sessions	14 chapters with each chapter for 1 hour 6 minutes	Significant differences between treatment and control groups
To assess the efficacy using web-based parent training	Kobak et al., 2011	Pre-Post	23	18 to 72	Interactive videotaped multimedia-based tutorials	Enhancing Interaction Program (web-based version)	Three modules	Parent satisfaction and efficiency was proven for this program
To assess the efficacy of an eLearning program in parents	Jang et al., 2012	RCT with waitlist between groups	26	37 to 137	Multimedia interactive web-based training	eLearning program using ABA-based sessions	Nine modules total of 30–40 hours	Significant increase in knowledge in the e-Learning group

Aim of the Study	Citation	Study Design	Sample Size (parents/children)	Age of children (months)	F2F/Online mode of intervention	Type of Technology	No of sessions	Results
To deliver an online intervention curriculum to parents	Vismara et al., 2012	Single case	9	Under 36	ESDM provided online	2-way Video conferencing with DVD learning	12 hourly sessions per week	Significant differences at six weeks with gains maintained across six weeks of follow-up
To assess the proximal effects of a naturalistic language intervention using distance video conferencing	McDuffie et al., 2013	Single case	8	24 to 72	Parent education using AV, Distance coaching using desktops, and F2F coaching	Video-Tele-conferencing for language intervention	Eight sessions on-site, F2F clinical, and 12 distance coaching sessions	Parents increased the use of verbal responses, frequency of prompts, parent strategy improvement for both on-site and distance sessions
To assess the results of tele-delivery of FCT to parents	Wacker et al., 2013	Single case	17	29 to 80	FCT using Tele-consultation left	Tele-consultation left	60 mins per session for 4 to 21 weeks	Significant reduction in problem behavior observed after tele-delivery

Aim of the Study	Citation	Study Design	Sample Size (parents/children)	Age of children (months)	F2F/Online mode of intervention	Type of Technology	No of sessions	Results
To assess online-based parent training	Vismara et al., 2013	Single case	8	20 to 45	ESDM provided online	2-way Video conferencing	12 weekly 1.5 hours & three monthly 1.5 hours as a follow-up	Results indicate parent satisfaction, parent intervention skills & engagement, website usage and child behaviors improvement
To assess online and applied system for intervention skills	Heitzman-Powell et al., 2014	Pre-post test	Seven parents; Four children	Age not reported	Online tutorials and live video conferencing	OASIS	90 to 120 mins on an average of 17 (13–19) sessions	Gains in knowledge, skills, and satisfaction with the training sessions
To assess discrete trial procedures as early interventions	St. Peter et al., 2014	Quasi-random two group	32	Under 60	Discrete trial instruction procedures	Written manual and Video instructions	12 trials	Video group adhered five times more on using the procedures
To assess themes of engagement and improvement of sensory processing issues	Ringland et al., 2014	Single case	4	48 to 144	Daily clinic sessions with weekly interventions online	Sensory Paint System	30 mins daily at clinic total five weeks	A significant difference in sensory processing skills

Aim of the Study	Citation	Study Design	Sample Size (parents/children)	Age of children (months)	F2F/Online mode of intervention	Type of Technology	No of sessions	Results
To assess the fidelity of telehealth coaching on FCT in parents	Suess et al., 2014	Between groups	3	18 to 83	Telehealth versus independent of tele-coaching	Skype	Eight to 12 coached trials once a week for one hour each	Procedural fidelity showed telehealth to be an effective method to deliver treatments
To assess if engagement to telehealth-based parent mediated intervention	Ingersoll and Berger, 2015	RCT	27	24 to 72	Self-directed program and therapist-assisted online program	ImPACT online program	12 lessons per 80 mins and 24 sessions of 30 mins per week online	Parental engagement and satisfaction with online content of intervention high in both the groups
To assess early intervention for social communication skills in preschoolers using technology-based tools	Fletcher-Watson, 2016	RCT	54	Under 72	Online game access with treatment on a one-to-one basis of schooling and speech/occupational therapy	Gameplay activities on iPad	5 mins per day or 10 min every alternate day for two months	No significant effects

Aim of the Study	Citation	Study Design	Sample Size (parents/children)	Age of children (months)	F2F/Online mode of intervention	Type of Technology	No of sessions	Results
To study internet-based parent training	Pickard et al., 2016	RCT	28	19 to 73	Self-directed and therapist-assisted	ImPACT online program	Self-directed group completed 12 online lessons; the therapist-assisted group met 12 online lessons + 30 mins two times per week Skype meetings	Significant differences seen
To assess the efficacy of early intervention program using technology as delivery mode	Whitehouse, 2017	Case-control	80	39 to 40	Therapy versus iPad application	iPad Application	20 mins per day for six months on iPad activities	No difference noted
To investigate developmental skills in children using tablet-based applications	Esposito et al., 2017	Case-Control	30 (15 each)	26 to 70	Clinical therapy for one year and then training for four weeks on e-intervention	Tablet applications	30 mins daily for four weeks	No significant differences
To assess visual-spatial skills	Coutinho et al., 2017	Two group comparative	20	48 to 84	Online and clinical therapy	iPad applications	Two 40 min sessions per week for ten weeks	No significant differences

Aim of the Study	Citation	Study Design	Sample Size (parents / children)	Age of children (months)	F2F/Online mode of intervention	Type of Technology	No of sessions	Results
To find if an internet-based serious game could be used to teach emotions	Fri-denson-Hayo et al., 2017	Case-Control	UK: 15; Israel: 43; Sweden: 40	72 to 108	Internet-based game	Emotiplay online game	8–12 weeks; Two hours per week	Significant differences between all clinical groups and control group
To understand a self-directed, tele-health-based parent-mediated intervention	Ingersoll et al., 2017	Two-group comparative	112 and 50	26 to 150 in open trial; 18 to 72 in Controlled trial	Open trial group and Controlled trialgroup	ImPACT online program	12 self-directed lessons each for 75 minutes	Parents engaged poorly in the Open trial vis-a-vis Controlled trial
To impart social communication skills through parent-mediated telehealth interventions	Simacek et al., 2017	Single case Pre-Post	Three (girls)	36 to 60	Early communication skills using FCT	Two-way video meeting using Google Hangout	Initial coaching was for three sessions: seven sessions lasting three mins each as FCT online	Two children acquired skills in two contexts while one child acquired skills in all three contexts

Aim of the Study	Citation	Study Design	Sample Size (parents / children)	Age of children (months)	F2F/Online mode of intervention	Type of Technology	No of sessions	Results
To assess if challenging behavior are treated using telehealth services in parent training	Lindgren et al., 2020	Single-subject and between-group	107	21 to 84	Group 1: Home-based Group 2: Clinic-based telehealth Group 3: Home-based telehealth	Internet-based video conferencing	One hour for more than or equal to 25 weeks with 10–15 min of daily practice of FCT	Significant reduction of problem behavior in all three groups. The cost of treatment was lower for home-based telehealth groups than others

Note: Demographic profile, methods, and results obtained on the studies using e-interventions for children with Autism Spectrum Disorder and their parents have been outlined. OASIS = Online and applied system for intervention skills, PRT = Pivotal response training, ESDM = Early start Denver model, RIT = Reciprocal initiation training, FCT = Functioning communication training, DVD = Digital video disc, iPad = Interactive personal application device, AV = Audio-video, F2F = Face to face, RCT = Randomized Control Trial.

As a clinician/researcher designs telehealth services, pre and post-coaching of the parents on the modules of training and design, acute pre-design and post-design measurement of outcome variables, strict outline, and adherence of the sessions, assessing knowledge, and skill-wise understanding of the parents who mediate the therapeutic interventions are found to be of utmost importance.

Thus, the international studies on telehealth in ASD seem promising and acceptable to the parent population.

Telehealth in ASD: Indian Studies

A brief review of the Indian studies revealed very sparse results. A Google Scholar search using the terms "Internet-Based Intervention for Autism in India," "Telehealth in Autism Spectrum Disorder on Indian children and parents," or "Web-Based Intervention for Autism in India" yielded 1200 results. Out of this, only two studies on telehealth / e-interventions in ASD were noted. One highlighted the need and development of a web-based training model for Indian children by Kohli and Kohli (2016) and hence had to be discarded. Therefore, one study is given in Table 5.3.

This study was conducted on one child with ASD and their mother. They used behavior skills training via WhatsApp mode of delivery. It was provided for eight weeks, and each session was for eight to 19 minutes. Though the tools used for assessment were not standardized on Indian children, results showed improvement compared to their pretest scores in social-communication skills. They reported positive bonding between the child and parent.

Telehealth for ASD in Our Country: Need Versus Challenges

Technological inputs have been upcoming in India's past three to five years in psychiatry and clinical psychology, albeit incipiently. While the clinicians attempt to assess the efficacy of using technological methods (Pandey et al., 2017), non-clinicians have been contributing to assistive inputs in the same (Wadhera and Kakkar, 2019).

Nevertheless, the comparison between the Western and Indian studies in this domain appears weak and disengaging. The need for many web-based models for e-training / e-intervention is to be noted for attending to the variety of skills training and behavioral problems of the children with ASD. Such attempts to develop e-interventions would reduce time and money for the families while improving their access to interventions immensely (Kohli and Kohli, 2016).

E-health/telehealth is visibly crucial for our country as provided by many e-healthcare facilities initiated by our government and offered online (National Health Portal, 2021). Many reasons could be observed for telehealth is one of the modes of treatment in the present age and era.

i *Internet and gadget usage*: India is the second-largest in the number of internet users in 2019, with 560 million, next only to China (Asher, 2020).

Table 5.3 Indian Studies Using telehealth in ASD

Aim of the Study	Citation	Study Design	Sample Size (parents/ children)	Age group of children (months)	F2F/Online mode of intervention	Type of Technology	No of sessions	Results
To assess the training of a parent via telehealth platforms	Narayan and Sri-kanth, 2020	Single case pre-post test	One child and his mother	Age not reported	Live telecast or video recordings	WhatsApp	8 to 19 mins each session for eight weeks	The improvement observed in social communication and language skills along with parent-child bonding

Note: The demographic profile, design, and method adopted in this study are outlined.

By December 2020, around 639 million have actively used the internet (Kumar and Dwivedi, 2020). The usage of the internet for the alleviation of symptoms by the patients and their caregivers/family members in mental illnesses has been 82.1% and 79.4%, respectively, in India (Singha Deb et al., 2018).

ii *Evidence for e-interventions from the West*: With the studies from the West noted, much more evidence-based use of e-interventions should be encouraged for our Indian population. Telepsychiatry has been regarded as noteworthy for solving problems of reach, offering quality consultations to rural areas, and imparting psychotherapeutic services. It is essential for a vast populous country such as India (Naskar et al., 2017). For interventional purposes, guidelines for tele-psychotherapeutic services have been provided by the National Institute of Mental Health and Neurosciences (2020). It clearly outlines the consent process, confidentiality and privacy issues, and record-keeping governing teleconsultations.

iii *Difficult situations*: Our cases narrative provided at the beginning of the chapter enumerates examples of the conditions in which parents and children with NDD find themselves in today's circumstances. The COVID-19 (World Health Organization, 2020) warranted the nationwide lockdown (Ministry of Home Affairs, 2020). This situation triggered web-based video and audio consultations for many medical illnesses, including psychiatry and clinical psychology. Geographic isolation, lack of transportation, and shortage of trained professionals are some of the situations warranting the use of e-interventions (Wainer and Ingersoll, 2014). These methods, therefore, assist in providing a quicker diagnosis and treatment plan for the families staying in rural or remote areas, reduces costs of travel, and could be used for emergency purposes, too (Alfuraydan et al., 2020).

Many factors might play differently for our Indian scenario and would have to be considered with all these reasons, such as:

i socioeconomic status of the families: urban versus rural children and their parents.
ii parental interest and ability to become co-therapist for undertaking such training online
iii research support and education for the parent
iv security and privacy in home environment vis-a-vis clinical/hospital environment
v insufficient funding towards enabling clinicians/researchers to set up e-interventional units. This would guide our ability to provide computers/ laptops and programs/applications to the child and parents.
vi research network and resources for designing and implementing telehealth programs of intervention modules for our Indian children with ASD.

Conclusion

As technological advancements are burgeoning with long strides, India could be considered as an infant trying to stand. Clarity on the applicability, design, and technology to be used for benefits to be observed in the child via their parents in the diathesis of NDD, in general, is needed. Hence, this chapter focuses on bringing a narrative review of the list of studies in the West, albeit not exhaustive. This could help us to understand how to maneuver our studies, solve our population and setting problems, and navigate towards better results. In conclusion, understanding telehealth's prospects and challenges for children with ASD would be sensible to implore in our country.

References

Alfuraydan, M., Croxall, J., Hurt, L., Kerr, M., and Brophy, S. (2020). Use of telehealth for facilitating the diagnostic assessment of autism spectrum disorder (ASD): A scoping review. *PLoS ONE*, 15(7). doi:10.1371/journal.pone.0236415.

American Psychiatric Association. (2013). "Autism spectrum disorders." In *Diagnostic and statistical manual of mental disorders* (5th ed., pp. 50–59). doi:10.1176/appi.books.9780890425596.dsm01.

Andersson, G. (2016). "Internet-Delivered psychological treatments." *Annual Review of Clinical Psychology*, 12, 157–179. doi:10.1146/annurev-clinpsy-021815-093006.

Arora, N. K. et al. (2018). "Neurodevelopmental disorders in children aged 2–9 years: Population-based burden estimates across five regions in India." *PLOS Medicine*, 15 (7): e1002615. doi:10.1371/journal.pmed.1002615.

Asher, V. (2020). "Smartphone user penetration rate as share of mobile phone users India 2014–2022." Statista. Retrieved from www.statista.com/statistics/257048/smartphone-user-penetration-in-india.

Bada Math, M., Manjunatha, N., Kumar, N. C., Basavarajappa, C., and Gangadhar, B. N. (2020). *Telepsychiatry operational guidelines*. NIMHANS Publication Division.

Baharav, E. and Reiser, C. (2010). "Using tele practice in parent training in early autism." *Telemedicine and E-Health*, 16(6): 727–731. doi:10.1089/tmj.2010.0029.

Barak, A., Klein, B. and Proudfoot, J. G. (2009). "Defining internet-supported therapeutic interventions." *Annals of Behavioral Medicine*, 38(1): 4–17. doi:10.1007/s12160-009-9130-7.

Carr, E. G. and Durand, V. M. (1985). "Reducing behavior problems through functional communication training." *Journal of Applied Behavior Analysis*, 18(2): 111–126. doi:10.1901/jaba.1985.18-111.

Chauhan, A. et al. (2019). "Prevalence of autism spectrum disorder in Indian children: A systematic review and meta-analysis." *Neurology India*, 67(1): 100. doi:10.4103/0028-3886.253970.

Coutinho, F. et al. (2017). "Effectiveness of iPad apps on visual-motor skills among children with special needs between 4y0m–7y11m." *Disability and Rehabilitation: Assistive Technology*, 12(4): 402–410. doi:10.1080/17483107.2016.1185648.

Dean, B. B., Lam, J., Natoli, J. L., Butler, Q., Aguilar, D., and Nordyke, R. J. (2009). "Review: Use of electronic medical records for health outcomes research: a literature review." *Medical Care Research and Review*, 66(6): 611–638. doi:10.1177/1077558709332440.

Dinakaran, D., Basavarajappa, C., Manjunatha, N., Kumar, C. N., and Math, S. B. (2020). "Telemedicine practice guidelines and telepsychiatry operational guidelines, india—a commentary." *Indian Journal of Psychological Medicine*, 42(5): 1–3. doi:10.1177/0253717620958382.

Divan, G., Vajaratkar, V., Desai, M. U., Strik-Lievers, L., and Patel, V. (2012). "Challenges, coping strategies, and unmet needs of families with a child with autism spectrum disorder in Goa, India." *Autism Research*, 5(3): 190–200. doi:10.1002/aur.1225.

Esposito, M. et al. (2017). "Using tablet applications for children with autism to increase their cognitive and social skills." *Journal of Special Education Technology*, 32(4): 199–209. doi:10.1177%2F0162643417719751.

Fletcher-Watson, S. et al. (2016). "A trial of an iPad™ intervention targeting social communication skills in children with autism." *Autism*, 20(7): 771–782. doi:10.1177/1362361315605624.

Fridenson-Hayo, S. et al. (2017). "'Emotiplay': A serious game for learning about emotions in children with autism: results of a cross-cultural evaluation." *European Child & Adolescent Psychiatry*, 26(8): 979–992. doi:10.1007/s00787-017-0968-0.

Grantham-McGregor, S. et al. (2007). "Developmental potential in the first 5 years for children in developing countries." *Lancet*, 369(9555): 60–70. doi:10.1016/S0140-6736(07)60032–60034.

Heitzman-Powell, L. S., Buzhardt, J., Rusinko, L. C., and Miller, T. M. (2014). "Formative evaluation of an ABA outreach training program for parents of children with autism in remote areas." *Focus on Autism and Other Developmental Disabilities*, 29(1): 23–38. doi:10.1177/1088357613504992.

Ingersoll, B. and Berger, N. I. (2015). Parent engagement with a telehealth-based parent-mediated intervention program for children with autism spectrum disorders: predictors of program use and parent outcomes. *Journal of Medical Internet Research*, 17 (10). doi:10.2196/jmir.4913.

Ingersoll, B. and Dvortcsak, A. (2009). *Teaching Social Communication to Children with Autism: A Practitioner's Guide to Parent Training and a Manual for Parents*. Guilford Press.

Ingersoll, B., Shannon, K., Berger, N., Pickard, K., and Holtz, B. (2017). Self-Directed telehealth parent-mediated intervention for children with autism spectrum disorder: Examination of the potential reach and utilization in community settings. *Journal of Medical Internet Research*, 19(7). doi:10.2196/jmir.7484.

Jang, J. et al. (2012). "Randomized trial of an eLearning program for training family members of children with autism in the principles and procedures of applied behavior analysis." *Research in Autism Spectrum Disorders*, 6(2): 852–856. https://psycnet.apa.org/doi/10.1016/j.rasd.2011.11.004.

Knutsen, J.et al. (2016). "A systematic review of telemedicine in autism spectrum disorders." *Review Journal of Autism and Developmental Disorders*, 3(4): 330–344.

Kobak, K. A. et al. (2011). "A web-based tutorial for parents of young children with autism: Results from a pilot study." *Telemedicine Journal and E-Health*, 17(10): 804. doi:10.1089/tmj.2011.0060.

Koegal, R. L. and Koegal, L. K. (2006). *Pivotal response treatments for Autism: Communication, social and academic development* (1st ed.). Paul H. Brookes Publishing Co.

Kohli, M. and Kohli, S. (2016). "Electronic assessment and training curriculum based on applied behavior analysis procedures to train family members of children diagnosed with autism." *2016 IEEE Region 10 Humanitarian Technology Conference (R10-HTC)*, 1–6. doi:10.1109/R10-HTC.2016.7906785.

Kumar, M. and Dwivedi, S. (2020). "Impact of coronavirus-imposed lockdown on Indian population and their habits." *International Journal of Science and Healthcare Research*, 5(2): 88–97.

Lindgren, S. et al. (2020). "A randomized controlled trial of functional communication training via telehealth for young children with autism spectrum disorder." *Journal of Autism and Developmental Disorders*, 50(12): 4449–4462. doi:10.1007/s10803-020-04451-1.

McCoy, D. C. et al. (2016). "Early childhood developmental status in low- and middle-income countries: national, regional, and global prevalence estimates using predictive modeling." *PLoS Medicine*, 13(6). doi:10.1371/journal.pmed.1002034.

McDuffie, A. et al. (2013). "Distance video-teleconferencing in early intervention: pilot study of a naturalistic parent-implemented language intervention." *Topics in Early Childhood Special Education*, 33(3): 172–185. doi:10.1177/0271121413476348.

Ministry of Health and Family Welfare. (2020a). *Telemedicine practice guidelines*. Retrieved from www.mohfw.gov.in/pdf/Telemedicine.pdf.

Ministry of Health and Family Welfare. (2020b*). Guidelines on managing mental illness in hospital settings during COVID 19*. National Institute of Mental Health and Neurosciences. Retrieved from www.mohfw.gov.in/pdf/GuidelinesforDeliveryofMentalMentalHealthcareServicesduringtheCOVID19.pdf.

Ministry of Home Affairs. (2020). "MHA requests states/U.T.s to implement lockdown measures in letter and spirit to fight COVID-19." Retrieved from www.mha.gov.in/sites/default/files/PR_MHArequestsStatesUTstoimplementLockdown_01042020%20_0.pdf.

Moher, D., Liberati, A., Tetzlaff, J., and Altman, D. (2009). "Preferred reporting items for systematic reviews and meta- analyses: The PRISMA statement." *PLOS Medicine*, 6(7). doi:10.1371/journal.pmed1000097.

Narayan, S. and Srikanth, G. (2020). "Telehealth as a parent training platform: a behavioral development approach to autism intervention." *IOSR Journal of Research & Method in Education*, 10(4): 48–54. doi:10.9790/7388–1004044854.

Naskar, S., Victor, R., Das, H., and Nath, K. (2017). "Telepsychiatry in India - Where do we stand? a comparative review between global and Indian telepsychiatry programs." *Indian Journal of Psychological Medicine*, 39(3): 223–242. doi:10.4103/0253-7176.207329.

National Health Portal. (2021). National teleconsultation service. Ministry of Health and Family Welfare, Government of India. Retrieved from www.esanjeevaniopd.in/Home.

National Institute of Mental Health and Neurosciences. (2020). *Guidelines for tele-psychotherapy services*. Retrieved from https://nimhans.ac.in/wp-content/uploads/2020/04/Guidelines-for-Telepsychotherapy-Services-17.4.2020.pdf.

Nefdt, N., Koegel, R., Singer, G., and Gerber, M. (2010). "The use of a self-directed learning program to provide introductory training in pivotal response treatment to parents of children with autism." *Journal of Positive Behavior Interventions*, 12(1): 23–32.

Pandey, J. M., Garg, S., Mishra, P., and Mishra, B. P. (2017). "Computer based psychological interventions: subject to the efficacy of psychological services." *International Journal of Computers in Clinical Practice (IJCCP)*, 2(1): 25–33. doi:10.4018/IJCCP.2017010102.

Pickard, K. E., Wainer, A. L., Bailey, K. M., and Ingersoll, B. R. (2016). "A mixed-method evaluation of the feasibility and acceptability of a telehealth-based parent-mediated intervention for children with autism spectrum disorder." *Autism*, 20(7): 845–855. doi:10.1177/1362361315614496.

Ringland, K. E. et al. (2014). SensoryPaint: A multimodal sensory intervention for children with neurodevelopmental disorders. Proceedings of the 2014 ACM International Joint Conference on Pervasive and Ubiquitous Computing, 873–884.

Rogers, S. J. and Dawson, G. (2010). *Early Start Denver Model for Young Children with Autism: Promoting Language, Learning, and Engagement.* Guilford Press.

Simacek, J., Dimian, A. F., and McComas, J. J. (2017). "Communication intervention for young children with severe neurodevelopmental disabilities via telehealth." *Journal of Autism and Developmental Disorders*, 47(3): 744–767. doi:10.1007/s10803-016-3006-z.

Singh, P., Ghosh, S., and Nandi, S. (2017). "Subjective burden and depression in mothers of children with autism spectrum disorder in India: Moderating effect of social support." *Journal of Autism and Developmental Disorders*, 47(10): 3097–3111.

Sinha Deb, K.et al. (2018). "Is India ready for mental health apps (MHApps)? A quantitative-qualitative exploration of caregivers' perspective on smartphone-based solutions for managing severe mental illnesses in low resource settings." *PLoS ONE*, 13(9). doi:10.1371/journal.pone.0203353.

St. Peter, C. C. et al. (2014). "Adherence to discrete-trial instruction procedures by rural parents of children with autism: Adherence to DTI." *Behavioral Interventions*, 29, 200–212. doi:10.1002/bin.1386.

Suess, A. N. et al. (2014). "Evaluating the treatment fidelity of parents who conduct in-home functional communication training with coaching via telehealth." *Journal of Behavioral Education*, 23(1): 34–59. doi:10.1007/s10864-013-9183-3.

Sutherland, R., Trembath, D., and Roberts, J. (2018). "Telehealth and autism: A systematic search and review of the literature." *International Journal of Speech-Language Pathology*, 20(3): 324–336. doi:10.1080/17549507.2018.1465123.

Vismara, L. A., McCormick, C., Young, G. S., Nadhan, A., and Monlux, K. (2013). "Preliminary findings of a telehealth approach to parent training in autism." *Journal of Autism and Developmental Disorders*, 43(12): 2953–2969. doi:10.1007/s10803-013-1841-8.

Vismara, L. A., Young, G. S., and Rogers, S. J. (2012). "Telehealth for expanding the reach of early autism training to parents." *Autism Research and Treatment*, 2012, 1–12. doi:10.1155/2012/121878.

Wacker, D. P. et al. (2013). "Conducting functional communication training via telehealth to reduce the problem behavior of young children with autism." *Journal of Developmental and Physical Disabilities*, 25(1): 35–48. doi:10.1007/s10882-012-9314-0.

Wadhera, T. and Kakkar, D. (2019). "Eye tracker: An assistive tool in diagnosis of autism spectrum disorder." In: S. K. Gupta, S. Venkatesan, S. P. Goswami and R. Kumar (Eds), *Emerging Trends in the Diagnosis and Intervention of Neurodevelopmental Disorders*. IGI Global. doi:10.4018/978-1-5225-7004-2.ch007.

Wainer, A. and Ingersoll, B. (2014). "Increasing access to an ASD imitation intervention via a telehealth parent training program." *Journal of Autism and Developmental Disorders*, 45. doi:10.1007/s10803-014-2186-7.

Whitehouse, A. J. et al. (2017). "A randomized controlled trial of an iPad-based application to complement early behavioral intervention in Autism Spectrum Disorder." *Journal of Child Psychology and Psychiatry*, 58(9): 1042–1052.

Walker, S. P. et al. (2011). "Inequality in early childhood: Risk and protective factors for early child development." *The Lancet*, 378(9799): 1325–1338.

World Health Organization. (2010). *Telemedicine: Opportunities and developments in member states: report on the second global survey on eHealth 2009*. Retrieved from www.who.int/goe/publications/goe_telemedicine_2010.pdf.

World Health Organization. (2011). *World report on disability*. Retrieved from www. who.int/teams/noncommunicable-diseases/disability-and-rehabilitation/world-report-on-disability.

World Health Organization. (2016). *Telehealth*. Global Health Observatory Data. Retrieved 16 December 2020 from who.int/gho/goe/telehealth/en.

World Health Organization. (2020). "WHO Director-General's remarks at the media briefing on 2019-nCoV on 10 February 2020." Retrieved from www.who.int/direc tor-general/speeches/detail/who-director-general-s-remarks-at-the-media-briefing-on-2019-ncov-on-10-february-2020.

6 Advances in Innovative Technologies for overcoming Adversial External Factors Affecting Individuals with Neurodevelopmental Disorders

Current and future concerns

Sana Nafees, Md Asad Khan and Moshahid A. Rizvi

1 Introduction

1.1 Neurodevelopmental disorders

Neurodevelopmental disorders (NDD) cover a range of conditions which have as their starting points the beginning phases of a child's growth. NDDs are defined by formative deficits that hinders individual's social performance, and world-related interactions. The most widely recognized NDDs incorporate attention–deficit/hyperactivity disorder (ADHD) (Althea et. al., 2020), explicit language disorders, disability influencing discourse, correspondence, mental imbalance range disorder, and autism spectrum disorder (ASD). NDDs regularly co-exist with each other (Kalyva et al., 2016), making an appraisal, determination, and choosing effective interventions a perplexing, protracted, and often exorbitantly expensive cycle. Moreover, the existence of these conditions demands huge wellbeing and economically for communities and societies. An evaluation for ASD in the UK costs about £32bn every year (Buescher et al., 2014; Althea et. al., 2020). In addition, the total expenditure on ADHD has been reported as US $143–266 billion every year in the USA which leads to economic effective loss in medical healthcare (Doshi et al., 2012; Althea et. al., 2020). Patients for a NDD evaluation frequently experience significant deferrals in getting an analysis; for instance, a new randomized controlled preliminary test (RCT) indicated that 40% of patients put forward for an ADHD appraisal were still waiting for a result a half year after beginning the appraisal (Hollis et al., 2018a; Althea et. al., 2020).

1.2 Technology in Observation and Screening of NDDs

Once analyzed, families report critical postponements in treatment commencement and inadmissible degrees of treatment monitoring (Hall et al., 2016). Just

DOI: 10.4324/9781003165569-6

one of every five persons with Tourette Syndrome can get to receive treatment for spasms, and the individuals who do get treatment normally do not receive a large number of the recommended consultations (Cuenca et al., 2015; Althea et. al., 2020). Because of these time deferrals and restricted admittance to treatment, adults cannot benefit ultimately from the mediation, which might have an adverse result on their socioeconomic and scholastic performance (Althea et. al., 2020). Explanations behind poor treatment for NDDs include the absence of admittance to specialists (Hall et al., 2017), especially in geographically remote areas, and lacking clinical opportunities (Hall, et al., 2016). It is a requirement to recognize simple practical techniques for showing and checking of NDDs. Innovation has led to improved computerized and self-coordinated interventions, enhanced admittance for treatment over a distance (Hall, et al., 2019), facilitation of the in-person consultations (Hall, et al., 2016), and improved customized treatment approaches (Hall et al., 2017; Althea et. al., 2020). As anyone might expect, the pace of mechanical interventions focused on emotional wellbeing is developing dramatically; for instance, in 2017, there were more than 10,000 individuals identified with psychological wellness, with the number expanding day by day (Torous and Roberts, 2017). With a large number of cases improved through medical healthcare administrations,it is significant that these innovations are ,objectively, and precisely assessed. In the UK, the National Health Service (NHS) Five-Year Plan for Personalized Health and Care 2020 (Department of Health, 2014) portrays the extraordinary capability of innovation to drive efficiencies, improve results, and enlarge access in medical healthcare conveyance. Innovation incorporates a wide scope of gadgets, modalities, and strategies. Augmented treatment, computerized advances, telehealth, PC-based treatments, constant observing and wearable gadgets, cell phone applications, and sensors that can improve results and health administration efficiencies are achieved.

Innovations that can identify NDD using with Ineterent-of-things based neuroimaging, biomarker tests/gadgets, and neuro–input techniques without demanding NDD individuals in direct-contact (i.e., telehealth) need to be developed to promote early diagnosis for individuals reported with atypicality (Van Doren et al., 2019) Ongoing precise research reports have summed up the accessible evidence base for explicit innovations in disorder detection, for example, the utilization of consistent behaviour tests in ADHD (Hall et al., 2016), advances used to encourage the self-administration of ADHD (Powell et al., 2018; Althea et. al., 2020), telepsychiatry with kids to teenagers as per the American Academy of Child and Adolescent Psychiatry, and games for individuals with learning disabilities (Terras et al., 2018; Althea et. al., 2020).

= The biggest assortment of evidence is in the field of mental imbalances, where various innovations, for example, applications, telehealth, robots, and video demonstrations, has been utilized (Qi et al., 2017; Althea et. al., 2020). Different investigations have focussed comprehensively over advancementsin detection of disorders; for example Hall et al. (2017) looked at the viability of advanced wellbeing interventions to detect emotional wellness condition in kids and youngsters and (Free et al. 2013) summarized evidence for portable innovation for wellbeing administrations. Aggregately research reports researching adequacy have discovered that natural methodological short-comings, such as low-quality examination plans, absence of control gatherings, and a small sample set of affected individuals, hinders any complete conclusions about viability.

Although viability (as decided by a meta-examination) is significant in assessing the legitimacy of tech innovation, given the absence of any direct test that can cover the entire spectrum of disorder, it is imperative to incorporate more exten-sive researchto comprehend the current percentage of disordered individuals (Murray et al., 2016). Moreover, the exisiting methods have focussed exclusively on youngsters with NDDs, and significant evidence is also foundfor disorder detection among grown-up populaces (Table 6.1). The tabular summary features which innovations might be reasonably efficient or inefficient in detecting NDD (Althea et. al., 2020). We arranged existing estimation and subjective examination to provide evidence for the future utilization of innovations inside wellbeing administrations. In particular, the audit reports discoveries on clinical/administra-tion viability, monetary effect, and client sway (possibility/adequacy) for accessible innovations to help evaluate, analyse, observe, and treat NDDs. We incorporate investigations from administration clients (youngsters/families and grown-ups) such as medical care experts (Table 6.2). We assess the nature of the evidence and feature gaps in the current scenarios for future advancements.

1.3 Technology in NDD Rehabilitation

Assistive innovation is progressively becomingthe mainstream inside various instruction, rehabilitation, and care settings. It incorporates a mixture of inno-vation arrangements (Puanhvuan et al. 2017; Schlosser et al. 2017) due to usage among various people of different destinations. This demonstrates that a wide range of people with various disability narratives, necessities, and instructive care objectives (e.g., people with numerous incapacities because of pre-birth causes, people with neurodisorder sickness, and people with gained cerebrum harm) might profit by the utilization of innovation-aided systems (Boyd et al., 2017; Lancioni and Singh, 2014). The innovation-supported program needed to assist these peopleincludes (a) microswitch (sensor) that gets actuated with a little touch or contact (e.g., a little head, finger, lip, or retina contact) and (b) a PC or electronic gadget that reacts to microswitch initiations by conveying explicit incitement. The utilization of such innovation programs can give fun-damental help to people to access and control the external noise factors that can amplify the problems/suffering of individuals with NDDs (Lancioni and Singh, 2014). An innovation-supported program to assist the external noise-generating devices could depend on the use of (a) sound boxes put in different zones/ direction and (b) controlling PC/other framing tools (pause/mute and actuate) (Lancioni et al., 2018c). People affected by these disabilities face a cycle of crumbling until they can bear, with no chance of preventing this. A feasible

Table 6.1 Summary of Physiological measurements via smartphone apps to detect NDDs

Number	App	Smartphone	Applicants	Outcome	Reference of study
Blood pressure	Instant Blood Pressure	iPhone 5 and 6. 85	85 patients and staff; 53% with hypertension.	Trials "were highly imprecise"	Patel et al. (2016)
Heart frequency	Instant Heart Rate Heart Fitness Whats My Heart Rate Cardio Version	iPhone 4 and 5.	108 patients, without those in dangerous disorder.	Significant performance differences" between the four apps	Coppetti et al. (2017)
Step numeration	Argus: calorie counter and step	Android phones: Sam-sung, One-Plus, Moto, Oppo, Galazy, Huawei, LG, Google, Sony and Agora running Android 4.4 to 8.1 Apple: iPhone 6, 6S, 7, 8, running iOS10.3–11.4.	48 healthy Applicants	Very large error ranges for both. phones" "appear inappropriate to perceive steps in short, slow, or non-stereo-typical gait patterns"	Brodie et al. (2018)
Sleep	Sleep time	iPhone 4 s and 5	20 Applicants with no sleep disorder	Absolute parameters and sleep staging.... correlate poorly with polysomnography"	Bhat et al. (2015)

Table 6.2 Recent Trends in App-based Studies.

Measure	App	Year of search	Country of search	Number of apps	Reference of study
Depression	Google Play, Apple iTunes store	2017	**US**	**116**	O'Loughlin et al. (2019)
Depression	Google Play, Apple App store	2018	UK	353	Bowie-Da Breo et al. (2019)
Dementia	Apple iTunes store Apr–	2016	US	72	Rosenfeld et al. (2017)
Migraine	Google Play, Apple App store, health- line.com	2017	US	29	Minen et al. (2018)
Depression and smoking cessation	"official Android and iOS marketplaces"	2018	US and Australia	36	Huckvale et al. (2019)

method of helping the NDD people from such external noise pollution is to give them ideal innovation arrangements that can reduce such noise and lighten the effect of such factors on amplification of the disability. For instance, people with mild symptoms might have problems recalling the various exercises they need to do during the day and external noise factors generated from electronic gadgets (mixers, grinder) or cell phones can make it more difficult for them to focus on excercise. In such cases, the utilization of a business gadget, for example, a laptop/cell phone, could be customized to alert the patient about the exercises (suitable occasions) and verbal guidelines/prompts that they need to complete. People can get all necessary sources or information using a remote Bluetooth earpiece connected to a tablet or cell phone (Lancioni et al. 2017). The people in serious or moderate phases of NDD severity represent broad disabilities that reduce their work-related chances. Indeed, a considerable number of these people are not able to walk without support and lose energy on wheelchairs. People endeavor to examine them depending on the utilization of walker gadgets. The issue might be because of wheelchair rugged engine which is a shortcoming as it do not inspire the people to walk. One approach to manage the issue to join the utilization of a gadget with (a) touch-screen and (b) an electronic gadget to record and follow the person's walk.. People might get 3–5 seconds of favoured alarm at each progression that can motivate them to walk more (Lancioni et al. 2018d). People with brain damage are insignificantly cognizant, along with unavoidable engine disability become an exceptionally extreme testcase for any expert in the field. These people could benefit from an innovative program that permits their reacting (although restricted) and get the attention of staff/guardians. The innovation might be required to create a gadget (SGD) and a switch touch associated with a PC framework (Lancioni and Singh, 2014). The switch touch should permit them autonomous admittance to favored ecological incitement. The SGD should help patients to ask for (regardless of the absence of local abilities) the focus of the parental figure/staff individuals. The SGD should transmit a local solicitation for such observation comparable to a straightforward engine reaction of the person. However, people who have risen out of a negligibly cognizant state present engine and correspondence hindrances might utilize a further developed innovation helped program. Such a program could depend on a PC framework introducing relaxation and correspondence choices (e.g., alarm, calls, messages, and recordings) and a switch touch. The switch touch would permit people to choose anyone introduced by the PC framework. When a choice is determined, the individual is allowed to settle on decisions inside that alternative (pick anyone in various tunes, calls, or instant messages) (Lancioni and Singh, 2014).

1.4 Case Study on NDD Rehabilitation using Technology

The adequacy of innovation in telemedicine is evaluated to prepare guardians of thirty-two teenagersgrown-ups on a care-based wellbeing health (MBHW) program (Myers et al. 2018). The thirty-two kids (i.e., youths/ youthful grown-ups) with huge body weight can gave a gentle degree of scholarly inability among individuals.Theimpact of the electronic programs on the youngsters' body weight were evaluated inside a measure changing in the body. The mediation included local exercise, regular dieting and sustenance, careful reaction for appetite, and practice to control the inclination for eating. The thirty kids who experienced the design program effectively decreased weight of 38.27 lb. before the mediation and kept up their new weight for a continuous 4years. Inside a social legitimacy, youngsters likewise revealed extraordinary fulfillment with the program impacts. Davies et al. 2018 evaluated an innovation arrangement (GeoTalk) comprising of a hand set gadget that incorporates worldwide situating framework (GPS) and other electronic wave advancements to consequently switch between speech sets when the client enters an assigned geographic zone for example, a college, university, school, bank, and market places. When client enters a GPS correspondence zone, the client was provided with the comparing speech set to solicitations relating to that zone.. A change should happen when the client naturally move to another zone. The new zone gets declared and the client naturally get to another speech set relating to the new zone. The members could work the GPS-empowered Geo Talk gadget with fewer blunders and prompts and more prominent speed than two economically accessible examination AAC gadgets. Damianidou et al. 2018 broadened an as-of-late distributed meta-investigation on the effect of innovation to help business-related results of individuals with scholarly and formative inabilities by dissecting the sorts of invention and work settings.. As to kinds of innovation, noticeable impact contrasts were found between figure prompts (least viable) and choices, for example, hearable inciting gadgets, work area, and PCs, palmtops. As to setting, discoveries demonstrated that the interventions occurring in genuine work settings had an essentially below result than those occurring in reproduced work settings. Massive connections were likewise found between the presence of all-inclusive plan highlights and sorts of innovation. Palmtops, and work area and PCs, model, incorporated the all-inclusive plan that includes more time than pictorial prompts. The consequences of those discoveries for new exploration in the zone were also examined. Desideri et al. 2018 did a starter assessment of a socioeconomic robot inside a public kid and young adult emotional wellness administration. Their objective was to decide if the robot could build commitment and language accomplishment in 2-9 old kids. They had chemical imbalance range disorder (ASD) joined with scholarly incapacity, learning-correspondence impedances, and diminished versatile aptitudes. The observation depended on an ABA1 (i.e., pattern, mediation, and post-intercession) plan. The kids took an interest in informational meetings focusing on formative and social aptitudes (e.g., engine impersonation, expressive/responsive language, unconstrained solicitations). The outcomes demonstrated that connecting with a social robot expanded commitment and objective accomplishment in any youngsters and just objective achievement in the other. This outcome was challenging to help the usage of more strong examination conventions in the territory.

Discourse language pathologist (SLPs) should have the option to convey without hands visual backings using the Echo Show^{TM}, a voice-actuated smart individual like a touch screen showing realistic substance (photos, recordings) as discussed by the studies (Yu, et al. 2018). The examination included five members, that is, 5 SLPs utilized in an OPD pediatric emergency clinic, and researched three inquiries concerning (a) capacity of the SLPs to dependably utilize a particular (transporter) expression to recover visual backings on the Echo Show^{TM}, (b) capacity of the Echo Show^{TM} to dependably recover customized visual backings, and (c) perspective on the SLPs about the convenience and expected effect of the Echo Show^{TM} inside a medical setting. The outcomes of each of the three inquiries were empowering. The creators discussed the expected ramifications of these outcomes for clinical work with people with ASD. They focused on the requirement for research testing the innovation straightforwardly with people with ASD. Lancioni et al. 2018a assessed on cellphone-based program to empower 5 members with direct, intelligent incapacity, visual or potentially engine disabilities, and helpless discourse to freely get to recreation and correspondence exercises. The Samsung smart cell phone gadgets were utilized for the plan. The members could make their action demands by setting small items or photos (spoke to these exercises and fitted with recurrence code marks) on one of the two cell phones. This cell phone read the bar code and expressed the connected movement on demands. Solicitation verbalizations enacted S-voice of the second cell phone, which opened the coordinating recreation movement documents or phone contacts for the members. All members utilized the program effectively and invested a large portion of the meeting energy occupied with freely got to recreation and correspondence exercises. It was sought after two explicit destinations. The principal aim was to inspect the viability of an eye stare inclination evaluation utilizing eye stare innovation to distinguish exceptionally alluring (i.e., conceivably strengthening) boosts for three young people with extreme scholarly and actual handicaps (Cannella-Malone, et al. 2018). The next target was to decide the dependability of the eye stare evaluation results. An objective was sought after by utilizing an "ABCACB" plan, in which A spoke to pattern stages while B and C spoke to mediation stages. During the B and C, the boosts distinguished (eye stare innovation) with high and low inclination was utilized dependent upon members reacting, separately (Giulio, 2018). Information indicated that during the pattern, the members' reacting zero or almost zero. At the B stages, the members were reacting consistently higher than that seen during the C stages, in this manner demonstrating that the eye stare's segregation among up-and low-inclination improvements was dependable. The initial segment of this book chapter is to look at the basic sequelae of awful mind injury (TBI), which is the main wellspring of inability and demise among kids (Martinez et al., 2018). Surely, the depicted debilitating effect that TBI has on (a) psychological measurements, for example, attention, language, and lead work, (b) passionate measurements, for example, tension and discouragement, (c) college/school accomplishment. In this book chapter, the authors focused on that ideal innovation on secret tools for youngsters with awful mind blowing and help them fabricate compensatory procedures and improve the probability of carrying on free lives. By the above mentioned, the creators gave a rundown of different assistive innovation assets for every one of the principal trouble spots portraying those youngsters. For instance, innovation assets, for example, voice recorders, voice recorder programming for iPod screen touch or windows operating mobile, just sign and shaded list cards were recorded as apparatuses to check the handicapping impacts of TBI on memory. The main examination broadened the appraisal of a switch tough-based mediation program for aiding MCS people to increment utilitarian reacting as an approach to control ecological incitement (Giulio, 2018). Ten members were incorporated and subsequent examination done to look at the impacts of the microswitch-supported mediation program with those of ordinary natural incitement methodologies regarding members' readiness and inclusion. Eight of the 10 members associated with the principal study were additionally selected for the subsequent examination. The consequences of the main examination affirmed the propriety of a microswitch-helped mediation program for supporting versatile reacting and incitement command on MCS people. The subsequent examination demonstrated that a switch tough-supported intercession program might be more compelling than essential and expand incitement methodologies in advancing members' sharpness and association.

All in all, the articles remembered for this extraordinary issue concern an assortment of destinations, include various sorts of members, centre around various handicaps, and cover diverse innovation arrangements significant for training, rehabilitation, and care settings. This book chapter can be viewed as supportive to the particular proposals and justification to the per user and their overall commitment and discussion on assistive innovation. These discussions are basic to (a) advance our insight in the zone, (b) investigate the chance for utilizing explicitly masterminded standard innovation gadgets to help people with various inabilities and necessities, and (c) build up another scope of mediation programs that utilize the innovation all the more productively and seek after the accomplishment of more major goals.

The absolute generally fundamental and effectively perceived assistive innovation gadgets to improve working people groups' through listening devices and video magnifiers devices (Puanhvuan et al., 2017). In addition, another gathering of exceptionally esteemed innovation devices incorporates; touch switches, discourse creating gadgets, memory card, robots and video devices (Lancioni and Singh, 2014). Touch switches are also used devices to permit people to inescapable engine/numerous inabilities for associate with their setting through exceptionally basic reactions (developments of their hands/fingers, lips, or retina). The basic reactions, influenced individuals can (a) entrance a PC framework and pick and initiate distinctive program alternatives or (b) enact basic ecological incitement (for example contingent upon their degrees of scholarly working and commitment interests). Discourse producing gadgets serve to empower people without discourse capacities to utilize local sentences for giving responses. People might enact these gadgets by contacting viewable signs (pictures) of the gadgets' by setting off sensors/touch switches associated with gadgets. Memory card can help different types of innovation (cell phones and PC gadgets) and are for the most part pointed toward giving individuals memory issues updates about explicit exercises/reactions to complete at explicit times (Baldwin and Powell, 2015). Video gadgets are film clasps of various activities (steps engaged with an unpredictable action) and are utilized to represent those activities to the people who require doing them. The gadgets are typically appeared on a screen of PC for a couple of moments (Wu, et al., 2016). Robots might need to be used for various shapes and utilized for helping people with various incapacities during their ambulation and help the people to read the correct objections (hence guaranteeing direction and portability) (Lancioni, et al., 2017). Robots can also utilize the management of people under neurodegenerative illness or post-stroke rehabilitation at the work area adjusted gadgets to serve people's help through a progression of practical developments (Masiero, et al., 2014). Robots also utilized for advancing social works with kids during mental imbalance disorders and fitted with human highlights point toward rearranging their collaboration work (Cabibihan, et al., 2013). Considering the over, one could undoubtedly contend that different innovative arrangements are accessible and they might be chosen based on the particular attributes and needs of the people remembered for the mediation cycle. While the present circumstance might be taken as empowering and new improvements in the zone can be normal, one ought to likewise stretch that the accessibility of innovation helps as such cannot be adequate the advancing for ideal result. The accomplishment a significant result is more likely or just conceivable when a deliberately planned mediation system- (a) show members to utilize the innovation additionally (b) guarantee the utilization of the innovation could prompt significant outcomes accordingly propelling the members to be dependably dynamic with it. The ramifications of this endeavor are to build an innovation and expand its utilization inside the applied settings with accomplishment members who are particularly involved in the innovation of powerful intercession programs. This connection among innovation and mediation programs (a) might be viewed as a significant variable in deciding the convenience of the innovation arrangements and achievement, and (b) flag the rise of another strength zone coordinating crafted by rehabilitation designing from one viewpoint with crafted by rehabilitation brain science, conduct investigation and custom curriculum on different (Lancioni, et al., 2013; Lancioni and Singh, 2014). The union of territory could guarantee the improvement of innovation arrangements dynamically fit members' qualities and instruction/rehabilitation prerequisites and advancement of progressively more compelling mediation system (cultivating the proper utilization of arrangements and expanding the member's inspiration). This extraordinary issue incorporates eight articles that speak to noble endeavours to assess the capability of ideal innovation for people with neurological disorders (for example scholarly inability, mental imbalance range disorder, and mixes of scholarly handicap with mental imbalance range disorders or with tactile or tangible engine weaknesses). For different youngsters who show more dis-orders, nonetheless, the chance of getting a precise determination would require deliberately arranged, direct assessment. Evaluation of telemedicine innovation might be involved to encourage instructors in college/school area to utilize a straight forward care-based technique, estimated constancy of the educators to showing the methodology for their understudies, and decided the effect of utilization of these studies on the strategy of their physical and local hostility. Information indicated that the telemedicine innovation could be applied adequately to empower the instructors to utilize the method and give it to their followers dependably. The understudies, thusly, profited by utilizing the technique with a decrease of their hostility conduct to zero or approach zero levels.

   This book chapter assessed a PC helped framework that was set up to control grown-up member's inability through an examination circumstance (Davies, et al., 2018). The framework (a) locally introduced the inquiries that the members said to reply (b) permitted members have to inquiries rehashed (c) expressed answers of the members investigated and (c) permitted members to continue the following inquiry after they had given a response from the past. The investigator can be utilized a standard subject's plan utilized by the mem-bers from both traditional composed and PC examination. Information showed that the PC helped variant was presented through a short practice period, per-mitted by the members to finish the examination with more noteworthy exactness, expanded freedom, and predominant proficiency. The accompany-ing authors of this chapter evaluated the effect of innovation helped viewable prompts on members exhibition (Cannella-Malone, et al., 2018; Schlosser, et al., 2017). In particular, the impacts of evaluated self-coordinated video provoked through iPod securing the professional abilities by grown-ups with a moderate scholarly handicap (Cannella-Malone, et al., 2018). The members were educated to utilize the video inciting with one assignment and a least-to-most provoking methodology with another errand. We showed the instructional procedures successfully showed the abilities and understudies summed up their utilization for the innovation to get familiar with another aptitude with no extra guidance (Giulio, et. al., 2013). Utilizing an Apple watch, give the nick of time (JIT) viewable prompts (pertinent photographs or video cuts) to enhance the verbal mandates accessible for five kids with a double determination of scholarly inability and mental disparity (Schlosser et al., 2017). The inquiry was whether the accessibility of JIT-conveyed obvious signals expanded the kid's capacity to follow the orders. Information indicated that the youngsters effectively followed twenty one of the fifty mandates accessible through local information alone. The figured out how to react to (a) twenty static signals were added and (b) three of the leftover nine orders with dynamic prompts were presented. The utilization showed through iPod-contact or introduction of improves plan video with scholarly incapacity and chemical imbalance variety disorder. This improved video was viable in showing the members to autonomously finish an assortment of scholastic undertakings. Assumption and support impacts were likewise noticed. This connection among innovation and mediation programs might be viewed as the absolute most significant variable in deciding the convenience of the innovation arrangements and their last achievement, and might ensign the rise of another claim to fame territory coordinating crafted by rehabilitation designing from one perspective with crafted by rehabilitation brain research, conduct examination and custom curriculum on different (Lancioni, et al. 2013; Lancioni and Singh, 2014). The guarantee of dynamically improved innovation arrangements is fit for attributes members and rehabilitation instructor's necessities and advancement of progressively more successful mediation system (cultivating the fitting utilization of the arrangements and expanding the members' inspiration). This unique issue incorporates in this chapter that speak to endeavours for assess capability of ideal innovation for people with neurological disorders (scholarly handicap, mental imbalance range disorder, and mixes of scholarly incapacity with mental imbalance range disorders or with tangible or tactile engine debilitations). The significant writing and direct involvement in a telehealth project drove them to stay mindful with respect to the convenience of this methodology for demonstrative purposes. Their decision was that for various kids, especially for those with the most exemplary indications, a solid analysis is conceivable using telehealth innovation. For different youngsters who show more disorders, nonetheless, the chance of getting an exact determination would require deliberately arranged, direct assessment. The evaluation of telemedicine innovation might be applied to train the instructors in college/ school area for utilization of straightforward care-based system, estimated constancy of the educators in showing the technique for their understudies, and decided the effect of these studies utilization for the strategy on their physical appearance and local hostility. Information demonstrated that the telehealth innovation could be applied successfully to empower the educators to utilize the system and give it to their understudies dependably.

Thus, these examinations were profited by utilizing the technique to decrease their animosity conduct to zero approach levels. This book chapter assessed a PC helped framework that was set up to direct grown-up members with scholarly inability *via* examination circumstance (Davies, et al. 2018). These frameworks locally introduced the inquiries that members were to reply, permitted members have received inquiries express answer by the members investigated and continue the permitted members to following inquiry exclusively after they have given response from past. Information demonstrated that the PC supported form presented *via* a concise acquaintance. The permitted members were finished examination through noteworthy accuracy, expanded autonomy and predominant proficiency. The impact showed on self-coordinated video provoking through iPod, the procurement of professional aptitudes by two grown-ups with moderate scholarly inability (Cannella-Malone, et al., 2018).The members were instructed to utilize the video inciting with one assignment and a least-to-most provoking technique with another task. Both instructional procedures were viable in showing the abilities, and understudies summed up their utilization of the innovation to become familiar with another aptitude with no extra guidance. The chance of evaluation for utilizing an Apple gadget to give without a moment to spare (JIT) viewable signs (for example important photographs or video cuts) to enhance the verbal mandates accessible for five kids with a double conclusion of scholarly incapacity and chemical imbalance. The inquiry was whether the accessibility of JIT-conveyed viewable signs expanded the youngsters' capacity to follow the orders. Information demonstrated that the kids effectively followed twenty of the fifty mandates accessible by means of verbal information alone. They figured out how to react to twenty extra orders when static obvious signals were included, 3 of the leftover 9 orders for dynamic prompts were presented. In particular, for each stage of visual picture and video clasp for model playing out particularly advance versions were incorporated. The introduction of upgraded video mode was viable in showing the two members to freely finish an assortment of scholastic undertakings. Speculation and upkeep impacts were likewise noticed. Information indicated that the program was powerful and the members had an expansion in practical correspondence. However, the increases were kept up just for a portion of the members. The new gadget incorporated a cell phone and a progression of small-scale articles or fitted pictures chips with explicit codes. When the members set one of the small-scale chips with pictures for the cell phone, these discharged a local solicitation engaging the movement showed by the chips.

2.1 Strengthen Patient Conclusion of Technology

The focal point of innovation in psychiatry ought to be on robotizing capacities that will permit understanding information or contact utilizing numerous sorts of buyer advances, regarding the patient's way of life, financial plan and range of abilities. For instance, the individuals who can just bear the cost of discontinuous cell phone administration might like to get messages instead of instant messages (Alcaraz et al., 2018). It is additionally essential to think about that individuals of any age with inabilities, including visual or engine disabilities, might like to utilize innovation other than a cell phone (Bauer et al., 2018a).

Silent innovations for medication, including psychological instability, ought not bar those with actual handicaps (Wolbring and Lashewicz, 2014). A drug update framework could send instant messages to a cell phone or highlight telephone, email to a PC, call a standard phone, or associate with a voice collaborator. In a US public example, the most usually utilized wellbeing innovation in 2018 (by 59%) was to reorder remedies (Abrams and Korba 2018), which would not need a cell phone. Because of the numerous limits talked about above, investigations dependent on patient information should uphold numerous kinds of advances, instead of zeroing in on unregulated, sensor-based estimations. A modest quantity of information could be entered from all generally utilized buyer innovations, at a recurrence, for example, day by day or week by week. Help to improve advanced abilities. An optional advantage of prescribing the utilization of innovation to those with dysfunctional behaviour is to increment computerized abilities, and the utilization of numerous shopper advances ought to be energized and upheld. A few analysts feel that cell phone just admittance to the Internet is making another kind of "portable underclass" with less computerized abilities and more uninvolved online contribution (Napoli and Obar, 2014). Studies from different nations including The Netherlands and Chile report less data chasing, dynamic support and assortment of Internet use when access is exclusively by cell phone (van Deursen and van Dijk, 2019). In a US investigation of cell phone clients more than age 18, 87% of cell phone time was spent on applications and just 13% on the Internet (ComScore, 2017b). Projects to help local area mix of those with genuine psychological maladjustment could remember preparing for the protected utilization of innovation.

2.2 Recommendations for the Future

Expanded comprehension of the unpredictable issues encompassing customer advances is expected to effectively incorporate applications into the act of psychiatry. New approaches should be characterized and normalized to assess the adequacy of applications utilized for screening or treatment. Notwithstanding the innovation stage, just a few patients will utilize the application. Given the real factors of application precision, viability, protection, security, and the administrative climate, and to amplify interest, an assortment of innovation stages ought to be utilized for information assortment instead of zeroing in on cell phones. Advancement ought to likewise incorporate regulatory applications that might expand care interest, and applications that instruct about psychological sickness. Application improvement requires multidisciplinary mastery in clinical, legitimate, customer, and specialized territories, with doctors and patients vigorously engaged with all stages, and huge scope testing in clinical settings. Complete security data ought to be given to patients prior to suggesting any applications on any innovation stage. Preparing and continuous help from people ought to be accessible for all suggested applications. Patients ought to be permitted to pick on the off chance that they need their application information remembered for their EMR, imparted to anybody other than their specialist, or utilized in exploration. Understanding information from applications ought not be moved into EMR if inadequate IT assets are accessible to deal with safely, or if incapable to oblige persistent decision as to access and utilize.

2.3 Advantages

Mental health in neurodevelopmental disorders has been considered to contain a grouping of basic periods, and irregularities happening during early advancement viewed as irreversible in adulthood. Nonetheless, discoveries in mouse models of neurodevelopmental condition, including delicate X, Rett Syndrome, Down Syndrome, and neurofibromatosis type I recommend that it is conceivable to turn around certain molecules, electrophysiological, and social deficiencies related with these issues in grown-ups by hereditary or pharmacological controls. Individuals with serious neurological weaknesses face numerous difficulties in sensorimotor capacities and correspondence with the climate; in this manner, they have expanded interest for cutting-edge, versatile, and customized restoration.

The advantages are valuable in recognizing the needs at worldwide, regional and public consideration level. Some type of need setting is vital as there are a greater number of cases on assets than there are properties accessible. Generally, the assignment of assets in wellbeing associations will in general be directed based on recorded examples, which frequently do not consider ongoing changes in the study of disease transmission and relative weight just as late data on the adequacy of mediations. This can prompt imperfect utilization of the restricted assets. Financial assessments consider minimal expenses and advantages and use result estimates, for example, DALYs to educate choices. For instance, phenobarbital, by a wide margin, is the most practical intercession for overseeing epilepsy and hence should be suggested for inescapable use in general wellbeing efforts against epilepsy in low-and centre pay nations. This section reinforces the evidence suggested before revealing that expanded assets are expected to improve administrations for individuals with neurological issues.

Acknowledgment: The authors would like to thank the Department of Biochemistry, Faculty of Dentistry Jamia Millia Islamia, New Delhi for providing assistance with this chapter.

References

Abrams, K. and Korba, C. 2018. *"Consumers are on board with virtual health options."* *Deloitte Insights.* Retrieved from www2.deloitte.com/insights/us/en/industry/health-care/virtual-health-care-consumer-experience-surve y.html.

Alcaraz, K. I., Riehman, K., Vereen, R., Bontemps-Jones, J., and Westmaas, J. L. 2018. "To text or not to text? Technology-based cessation communication preferences among urban, socioeconomically disadvantaged smokers." *Ethnicity & Disease*, 28: 161–168.

Althea, Z. V., Beverley, J. B., Madeleine, J. G., Emma, Y., Chris, H., and Charlotte, L. H. 2020. "A systematic review evaluating the implementation of technologies to assess, monitor and treat neurodevelopmental disorders: A map of the current evidence." *Clinical Psychology Review*, 80(10): 1870. doi:10.1016/j.cpr.2020.101870.

Baldwin, V. N. and Powell, T. 2015. "Google calendar: A single case experimental design study of a man with severe memory problems." *Neuropsychological Rehabilitation*, 25(4): 617–636. doi:10.1080/09602011.2014.956764.

Bauer, R., Glenn, T., Strejilevich, S., Conell, J., Alda, M., and Ardau, R., et al. 2018a. "Internet use by older adults with bipolar disorder: international survey results." *International Journal of Bipolar Disorders*, 6: 20.

Bhat, S., Ferraris, A., Gupta, D., Mozafarian, M., De Bari, V.A., and Gushway-Henry, N., et al. 2015. "Is there a clinical role for smartphone sleep apps? Comparison of sleep cycle detection by a smartphone application to polysomnography." *Journal of Clinical Sleep Medicine*. 11: 709–715.

Bowie-Da Breo, D., Sunram-Lea, S.I., Sas, C., and Iles-Smith, H. 2019. "A content analysis and ethical review of mobile applications for depression: exploring the app market place." Retrieved from http://eprints.lancs.ac.uk/132009/1/CMH,2019.

Boyd, H. C., Evans, N. M., Orpwood, R. D., and Harris, N. D. 2017. "Using simple technology to prompt multistep tasks in the home for people with dementia: An exploratory study comparing prompting formats." *Dementia*, 16(4): 424–442. doi:10.1177/1471301215602417.

Brodie, M.A. et al. 2018. "Big data vs accurate data in health research: large-scale physical activity monitoring, smartphones, wearable devices and risk of unconscious bias." *Medical Hypotheses*. 119: 32–36.

Buescher, A. V., Cidav, Z., Knapp, M., and Mandell, D. S. 2014. "Costs of autism spectrum disorders in the United Kingdom and the United States." *JAMA Pediatrics*, 168(8): 721–728. doi:10.1001/jamapediatrics.210.

Cabibihan, J. J., Javed, H., Ang, M., and Aljunied, S. M. 2013. "Why robots? A showed of the roles and benefits of social robots in therapy of children with autism." *International Journal of Social Robotics*, 5(4): 593–618. doi:10.1007/s12369-013-0202-2.

Cannella-Malone, H. I., Schmidt, E. K., and Bumpus, E. C. 2018. "Assessing preference using eye gaze technology for individuals with significant intellectual and physical disabilities." *Advances in Neurodevelopmental Disorders*, 2(3): 300–309. doi:10.1007/s41252-018-0072-6.

Collishaw, S. 2015. "Annual research review: Secular trends in child and adolescent mental health." *Journal of Child Psychology and Psychiatry, and Allied Disciplines*, 56(3): 370–393. doi:10.1111/jcpp.12372.

ComScore. 2017b. *The 2017 US mobile app report*. Retrieved from www.comscore.com/Insights/Presentations-and-Whitepapers/2017/The-2017-USMobile-App-report.

Coppetti, T., Brauchlin, A., Muggler, S., Attinger, Toller, A., Templin, C., and Schonrath, F. et al. 2017. "Accuracy of smartphone apps for heart rate measurement." *European Journal of Preventive Cardiology*, 24 : 1287–1293.

Cuenca, J.et al. 2015. "Perceptions of treatment for tics among young people with Tourette syndrome and their parents: A mixed methods study." *BMC Psychiatry*, 15 (1): 46. doi:10.1186/s12888-015-0430-0.

Damianidou, D., Foggett, J., Arthur-Kelly, M., Lyons, G., and Wehmeyer, M. L. 2018. *"Effectiveness of technology types in employment-related outcomes for people with intellectual and developmental disabilities: An extension meta-analysis." Advances in Neurodevelopmental Disorders*, 2(3): 262–272. doi:10.1007/s41252-018-0070-8.

Davies, D. K., Stock, S. E., Herold, R. G., and Wehmeyer, M. L. 2018. "GeoTalk: A GPS-enabled portable speech output device for people with intellectual disability." *Advances in Neurodevelopmental Disorders*, 2(3): 253–261. doi:10.1007/s41252-018-0068-2.

Desideri, L.et al. 2018. "Using a humanoid robot as a complement to interventions for children with autism spectrum disorder: A pilot study." *Advances in Neurodevelopmental Disorders*, 2(3): 273–285. doi:10.1007/s41252-018-0066-4.

Doshi, J.A. et al. 2012. "Economic impact of childhood and adult attention-deficit/hyperactivity disorder in the United States." *Journal of the American Academy of Child and Adolescent Psychiatry*, 51(10): 990–100. doi:10.1016/j.jaac.2012.07.008.

Free, C.et al. 2013. "The effectiveness of mobile-health technology-based health behaviour change or disease management interventions for health care consumers: A systematic review." *PLOS Medicine*, 10(1): 1001362. doi:10.1371/journal.pmed.1001362.

Giulio, E. L. 2018. "Assistive Technology Programs to Support Persons with Neuro-developmental Disorders." *Ad. Neurodevelop Disorders*, 2: 225–229. doi:10.1007/s41252–41018–0074–0074.

Giulio, E. L., Jeff, S., and Mark, F. 2013. *O'Reilly*, Nirbhay N. Singh. "Assistive Technology", Springer Science and Business Media LLC.

Kalyva, E., Kyriazi, M., Vargiami, E., Dimitrios, I, and Zafeirioub, D. 2016. "A review of co-occurrence of autism spectrum disorder and Tourette syndrome." *Research in Autism Spectrum Disorders*, 39–51.

Hall, C. L. et al. (2019). "Investigating a therapist-guided, parent-assisted remote digital behavioural intervention for tics in children and adolescents—'Online Remote Behavioural Intervention for Tics'(ORBIT) trial: Protocol of an internal pilot study and singleblind zrandomized controlled trial". *BMJ Open*, 9(1): 027583. doi:10.1136/bmjopen-2018-027583.

Hall, C.L. et al. 2016. "Innovations in practice: An objective measure of attention, impulsivity and activity reduces time to confirm attention deficit/hyperactivity disorder diagnosis in children—A completed audit cycle." *Child and Adolescent Mental Health*, 21(3): 175–178. doi:10.1111/camh.12140.

Hall, C. L., et al. 2017. "Study of user experience of an objective test (QbTest) to aid ADHD assessment and medication management: A multi-methods approach." *BMC Psychiatry*, 17(1): 66. doi:10.1186/s12888-017-1222-5.

Hollis, C. et al. 2018a. "The impact of a zcomputerized test of attention and activity (QbTest) on diagnosticdecision-making in children and young people with suspected attention deficit hyperactivity disorder: Single-blind zrandomized controlled trial." *Journal of Child Psychology and Psychiatry*, 59(12): 1298–1308.

Huckvale, K., Torous, J., and Larsen, M. E. 2019. "Assessment of the data sharing and privacy practices of smartphone apps for depression and smoking cessation." *JAMA Network Open*, 2: 192542.

Lancioni, G. E., Sigafoos, J., O'Reilly, M. F., and Singh, N. N. 2013. *Assistive technology: Interventions for individuals with severe/profound and multiple disabilities.* New York, NY: Springer.

Lancioni, G. E. and Singh, N. N. 2014. *Assistive technologies for people with diverse abilities.* New York, NY: Springer.

Lancioni, G.E. et al. 2017. "Supporting ambulation in persons with intellectual and multiple disabilities: An overview of technology-aided intervention programs." *International Journal of Sport Psychology*, 48: 55–70.

Lancioni, G.E. et al. 2018a. "A modified smartphone-based program to support leisure and communication activities in people with multiple disabilities." *Advances in Neurodevelopmental Disabilities*, 2.

Lancioni, G.E.et al. 2018b. "A smartphone-based technology package to support independent activity in people with intellectual disability and blindness." *Internet Technology Letters*, 1(5): 34. doi:10.1002/itl2.34.

Lancioni, G.E. et al. 2018c. "Promoting supported ambulation in persons with advanced Alzheimer's disease: A pilot study." *Disability and Rehabilitation. Assistive Technology*, 13 (1): 101–106. doi:10.1080/17483107.2017.1297856.

Martinez, A. P., Scherer, M., and Tozser, T. 2018. "Traumatic brain injury (TBI) in school based populations: Common sequelae and assistive technology interventions." *Advances in Neurodevelopmental Disabilities*, 2

Masiero, S. et al. 2014. "The value of robotic systems in stroke rehabilitation." *Expert Review of Medical Devices*, 11(2), 187–198. doi:10.1586/17434440.2014.882766.

Minen, M. T., Stieglitz, E. J., Sciortino, R., and Torous, J. 2018. "Privacy issues in smartphone applications: an analysis of headache/migraine applications." *Headache*, 58: 1014–1027.

Murray, E. et al. 2016. "Evaluating digital health interventions: Key questions and approaches." *American Journal of Preventive Medicine*, 51(5): 843–851.

Myers, R. E.et al. 2018. "A telehealth parent-mediated mindfulness-based health wellness intervention for adolescents and young adults with intellectual and developmental disabilities." *Advances in Neurodevelopmental Disabilities*, 2.

Napoli, P. M. and Obar, J. A. 2014. "The emerging mobile internet underclass: a critique of mobile internet access." *Journal of Information Science*, 30: 323–334.

O'Loughlin, K., Neary, M., Adkins, E.C., and Schueller, S.M. 2019. "Reviewing the data security and privacy policies of mobile apps for depression." *Internet Interventions*, 15: 110–115.

Patel, V., Hughes, P., Barker, W., and Moon, L. 2016. "Trends in individuals' perceptions regarding privacy and security of medical records and exchange of health information: 2012–2014." *ONC Data Brief*, no. 33. Washington, DC: Office of the National Coordinator for Health Information Technology.

Powell, L., Parker, J., and Harpin, V. 2018. "What is the level of evidence for the use of currently available technologies in facilitating the self-management of difficulties associated with ADHD in children and young people? A systematic review." *European Child and Adolescent Psychiatry*, 27(11): 1391–1412. doi:10.1007/s00787-017-1092-x.

Puanhvuan, D., Khemmachotikun, S., Wechakarn, P., Wijarn, B., and Wongsawat, Y. 2017. "Navigation-synchronized multimodal control wheelchair from brainto alternative assistive technologies for persons with severe disabilities." *Cognitive Neurodynamics*, 11(2): 117–134. doi:10.1007/s11571-017-9424-6.

Qi, C. H., Barton, E. E., Collier, M., and Lin, Y. L. 2018. "A systematic review of single-case research studies on using video modeling interventions to improve social communication skills for individuals with autism Spectrum disorder." *Focus on Autism and Other Developmental Disabilities*, 33(4): 249–257. doi:10.1177/1088357617741282.

Rosenfeld, L., Torous, J., and Vahia, I.V 2017. "Data security and privacy in apps for dementia: an analysis of existing privacy policies." *American Journal of Geriatric Psychiatry*, 25: 873–877.

Schlosser, R. W. et al. 2017. "Repurposing everyday technologies to provide just-in-time visual supports to children with intellectual disability and autism: A pilot feasibility study with the Apple Watch®." *International Journal of Developmental Disabilities*, 63(4): 221–227. doi:10.1080/20473869.2017.1305138.

Terras, M. M., Boyle, E.A., Ramsay, J., and Jarrett, D. 2018. "The opportunities and challenges of serious games for people with an intellectual disability." *British Journal of Educational Technology*, 49(4): 690–700. doi:10.1111/bjet.12638.

Torous, J. and Roberts, L. W. 2017. "Needed innovation in digital health and smartphone applications for mental health: Transparency and trust." *JAMA Psychiatry*, 74(5): 437–438. doi:10.1001/jamapsychiatry.2017.0262.

Van Doren, J. et al. 2019. "Sustained effects of neurofeedback in ADHD: A systematic review and meta-analysis." *European Child and Adolescent Psychiatry*, 28(3): 293–305. doi:10.1007/s00787-018-1121-4.

van Deursen, A.J. and van Dijk, J.A. 2019. "The first-level digital divide shifts from inequalities in physical access to inequalities in material access." *New Media & Society*, 21(2): 354–357.

Wolbring, G. and Lashewicz, B. 2014. "Home care technology through an ability expectation lens." *Journal of Medical Internet Research*, 16(6): 155.

Wu, P. F., Wheaton, J. E., and Cannella-Malone, H. I. 2016. "Effects of video prompting and activity schedules on the acquisition of independent living skills of students who are deaf and have developmental." *Education and Training in Autism and Developmental Disabilities*, 51: 366–378.

Yu, C.et al. 2018. "An exploratory study of speech-language pathologists using the Echo ShowTM to deliver visual supports." *Advances in Neurodevelopmental Disorders*, 2 (3): 286–292. doi:10.1007/s41252-018-0075-3.

7 Assistive Technology for Promoting Inclusive Education of Children with Neurodevelopmental Disorders

Dr G. Malar and Prof. S. P. Goswami

Introduction

Neurodevelopmental disorders (NDD) are any delay, deficiency, or deviance in the typical course of child development, owing to maldevelopment or malfunction in the central nervous system. They could occur anytime from the early stages of gestation to early childhood, and result in impairment of affective, behavioral, cognitive and/or motor functioning in children (American Psychiatric Association, 2014). Remedial rehabilitation could include neurobiological treatment, clinical therapies, special education, vocational training, and socio-familial assimilation to promote independent, productive, and integrated living skills (Ahn and Hwang, 2017; Hamilton, 2015; Thapar et al., 2017). Among these, educational habilitation for children with NDDs focuses on initiating them into a life-long process of developing awareness and adeptness necessary to lead a self-sustained and socially integrated life. Such efforts are found to result in enhanced outcomes in the mainstreams of education while these children learn and grow along with their typically developing peers. But it is a task easier said than done amid manifold constraints like inadequate awareness, incompatible mind-sets and insufficient means (Alberta Learning, 2003; Reagan, 2012). But technology comes as relief and rescue for many of the deprivations to be dealt with in inclusive educational habilitation. Assistive technology includes both devices as well as services used to maintain, increase the quantity, and/or improve the quality of functional capabilities of individuals with disabilities. From the educational perspective it is any manoeuvring made to alleviate the difficulties caused by a disabling condition, ensuring secure existence overcoming the constraints caused by it, while also enabling functioning with increased efficiency in the learning environment (Assistive Technology Act, 2004; Dell et al., 2012).

Nevertheless, not all children with NDDs in the learning environment require assistive technology, and again those children who need might not require all available types of technology. Provision of supports that are unnecessary, inappropriate or in excess will rather harm the children with regression of abilities and/or complications. Decisive indicators represented in Figure 7.1, such as independent and interactive functioning being obstructed, inability to convert competence into productive performance, and/or performances lagging considerably behind their peers without

DOI: 10.4324/9781003165569-7

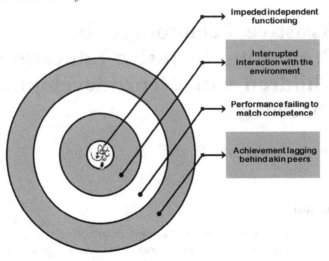

Figure 7.1

valid reasons might imply need for assistive technology (Ahmad, 2015; Cook, 2020; Dikusar, 2019; Donovan et al., 2010).

Mundane applications of assistive technology cater to personal care, communication, mobility, education, employment, social interaction and recreation needs of individuals with disabilities. In the educational context they are expected to promote advantageous ambience, communication, instruction and performances in children with disabilities such as NDD as illustrated in Figure 7.2. Assistive aids and devices, special resource materials, and modifications in routines and methods are instrumental in attaining these targets and have been deliberated further in this chapter (Blackhurst, 2005; Watson et al., 2010).

Supportive Surroundings

Children with NDDs initially on entering mainstream learning environment feel threatened with unfamiliar exposures and unanticipated encounters in the form of strange persons, things, and happenings around. The new sights and sounds might be disquieting to many of them in whom sensory processing dysfunction is a common complaint (Understood Team, 2017). Milder reactions might take the form of anxiety, irritability, fatigue, and consequent inability to attend or respond to instructions and interactions optimally. In severe conditions they could lead to somatic maladies such as dizziness, drowsiness, nausea, sore eyes, and severe headaches among others (Ford-Lanza, 2019). Creating an agreeable learning ambience could help in tiding over these difficulties so as to feel and function well.

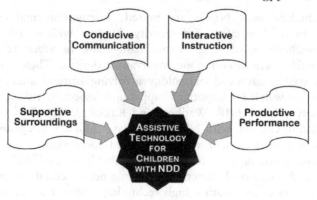

Figure 7.2

Assistive Aids and Devices

Management of environmental lighting depends on several factors such as the nature of the task at hand, which could be visually demanding like copywriting or less-taxing like while listening to a discourse; and more importantly the severity of consequent discomfort experienced by children with NDDs. Severe sensory issues could require alterations in the types of light bulbs (fluorescent, LED, or full-spectrum bulbs), their placement (ceiling, desktop, table, or even floor), and use of accessories such as shades or reflectors to decrease or increase brightness according to need. A few might also need artificial lighting with colored tints which will render the work materials in stark contrast from background objects. In all, portable lamps with auxiliary color-filters, reflectors and shades are handy tools in classrooms with children with NDDs. There might also be need for device-specific arrangements such as colored overlays for printed materials or screen-color inverters for digital displays; and optical/digital/electronic magnifiers for printed/written information/illustrations or digital displays. These facilitate favorable alteration of magnitude and figure-ground contrast of the visual information (Fitzell, 2018; Ford-Lanza, 2019; Howard, 2016; Winterbottom and Wilkins, 2009).

Children with NDDs are either distressed by noise or distracted by them from instruction. Listening devices enhanced with assistive technologies such as frequency-modulation, infrared or sound field induction render instructional information clearer and louder over unimportant sounds. For some children with lowered tolerance, loud, or high-pitched sounds could lead to sensory overload and meltdown. A range of aids from simple earplugs/muffs to specialist ear-defenders or noise-cancelling headphones come handy in such situations. In case of insurmountable difficulty in receiving verbal information/instruction, alternate modes such as live captioning over closed-circuit televised displays can be useful (Griffin, 2018; Neese, 2021; Understood Team, 2017).

Many children with NDDs are inured to environmental events and vulnerable to risks of safety and security. Devices with sound, visual, or tactile-kinaesthetic signals, like alarms, flash-bulbs, or vibrators alert such children with severe attention or observation deficits. These rudimentary devices, as well as advanced technology involving artificial intelligence help them to be on watch for important happenings, especially risks and respond appriopriately (Bigby, 2018; Wadhera and Kakkar, 2018). Technology also comes to aid of children with NDDs who have difficulty integrating socially in the learning environment with videotaped social skills. These promote development of coping skills to overcome difficulties in self-help, linguistic, academic and emotional functioning in general school setting. Facial recognition devices are another high technology support available for these children. These assist children who have difficulty in interpreting others' emotions in the process of social interactions in the mainstream milieu (Gonzalez, 2019; Rice, 2019).

Special Supportive Materials

Social stories describing the learning environment are good means for inculcating desirable behaviors and preparing children for expected roles necessary for better integration. Distinctive demarcation of places and materials in the environment with representative images, symbols or color-codes, as well as physical blocking of forbidden objects and spaces will help hassle-free function and movement of children with NDDs (Arky, 2021; Loring and Hamilton, 2011).

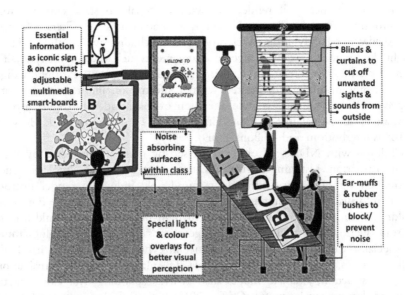

Figure 7.3

In general, evenly spread natural lighting avoiding glares or shadows should be maintained. According to specific needs of children with NDDs, natural sources of lights through doors and windows can be augmented with artificial lights or regulated with blinds/curtains to make them bright or dim according to their level of sensitivity. Simple aids like shades over lamps, blinds across windows help modify the brightness of light or cut-off unwanted scenes, thus controlling overwhelming lights and sights. Other commonplace materials such as beading for doors and shutters, curtains for windows, rubber-footing for furniture, sound-absorbent pin-up boards covering sound-reflecting hard polished wall spaces help in minimizing unwanted noise from inside as well outside the classroom. Soothing music in the background is another useful resource promoting calm and cooperative tendencies among all children, especially those with autistic and hyperactive features (Arky, 2021; Ford-Lanza, 2019; Lonkar, 2014).

Modified Modes of Operation

Simple floor planning that are undisturbed without frequent changes or prior preparation of children with NDDs will minimize factors that upset their routine functioning. Verbal directions that are concrete, clear and crisp supported by iconic visual clues like illustrations, gestures and/or model demonstrations will aid in complying with the demands from the learning environment. Along with these, general maintenance of a disciplined environment with regulated speech, movement and other actions that minimize sudden or severe sights and sounds will render it further amenable (Lonkar, 2014; Wise, 2017).

Conducive Communication

Fluent communication is a fundamental necessity for interacting in the instructional process as well as integrating in the learning environment. However, in many children with NDDs socio-emotional divergences prevent them from indulging in meaningful communication. In certain others, sensory processing disorders as well co-morbid sensory and/or motor impairments hinder the crucial channels of communication and interaction with the environment (Sanz-Cervera et al., 2017). These inherent difficulties are further complicated by the use of abstract academic language, thus impeding the assimilation and achievement of children with NDDs. However, a wide range of unaided, low and high technology systems are available at their disposal to help to tide over these impediments (Arthur-Kelly et al., 2018).

Assistive Aids and Devices

High technology, that is, aids using sophisticated electronic technology along with auxiliary electrical devices for children with NDDs with affected hearing perception or processing might include listening aids with enhancing assistive accessories or alternate devices enabling text or video messaging. For children with visual impairment or processing disorder magnification devices or optical character recognizing software augmented with alternate auditory and tactile output might be necessary (Lonkar, 2014; Neese, 2021). For those with problems in expressive communication due either to motor execution or psycho-social issues, assistive aids such as digital communication boards, or devices utilizing voice/speech-recognition and speech-generating/synthesizing software like 'Apple's Speak Selection, Dragon Dictation, Dragon Naturally Speaking, Good Reader, Intel Reader, Jaws, Kurzweil 3000, Microsoft Narrator, Seeing AI, XpressLab, etc.' will be helpful. These applications enable children with NDDs communicate alternately through the oral or textual mode whichever is convenient. In case of difficulty in speaking, but intact writing or typing skills; the digitized textual information are spoken aloud by the speech-generating/synthesizing devices. Conversely, if the difficulty is in writing or typing, these applications recognize the information conveyed by verbal speech and convert it into textual format (Allen et al., 2018; Dimian et al., 2018; Izzo et al., 2009).

In some of these children both oral as well as fine motor movements are affected, subsequently hindering both oral and written communication skills. For such children, touch screen facilities where letters, words or pictures can be chosen with minimal movements of hands/fingers or head pointers to form/represent words and phrases to communicate their intentions/ideas. If even such rudimentary movements are affected, computers with cameras to track eye movements like eyeball shift or blinking at any particular display on the monitor will recognize the content of their communication (Dell et al., 2012; Simacek et al., 2018; Wadhera and Kakkar, 2019). Many of these software applications serve the dual purpose of enabling use and practice of the secondary mode of verbal communication, that is, reading and writing, which are inevitable for subsistence and success in conventional classrooms. They function on a two-pronged basis – sidestepping difficulties posed by the disabling condition, while providing training to overcome them. For example, audio-book that highlights the text being read out helps evade reading-difficulties, while also working on sight-reading ability (Batorowicz et al., 2012; Strangman and Dalton, 2005; Zhang, 2000).

Special Supportive Materials

In the absence of need or means for high technology communication devices, manual aids generally categorized as low-technology systems might be used. Locally available objects and indigenous materials, printed/drawn images, printed/written words/letters related to learning and other occupations can be used to overcome impediments in verbal transactions. These could be organized in the form of cards, communication boards, or communication/experience books which are either laid out or suspended in front of them. These objects, images, words or letters can be picked up or pointed to manually with fingers/hands, or pointers attached to the head. In case of all these movements being restricted, then human aides can track their eye-gaze directed towards boards or cards with letters, words and/or pictures to make out their communicational intent (Illinois University Library, 2020; Young and MacCormack, 2014).

Modified Modes of Operation

Adoption of helpful communication strategies other than use of aids and materials are considered as unaided technology. These strategies are to be custom-decided according to need of each child. One useful suggestion to overcome drawbacks in verbal communication is to combine verbal information along with multisensory cues in the form of vivid facial expressions, symbolic hand gestures, and expressive body language. Some children might benefit from concurrent use of all these different modes of communication simultaneously. But for certain others they have to be detached without overlap when presenting. Pacing the delivery of information according the receptive ability of the child, while also providing reasonable time to respond is another vital tip for effective instructional communication. In case of severe problems in both receptive and expressive communication, then use of augmentative techniques and/or alternate modes of communication have to be contemplated. Supplementing speech with another assistive means like pictures is described as augmentative communication as in picture-elicited/exchange communication systems. Whereas, alternate communication modes involve altogether supplanting verbal or written mode of communication with other non-verbal means. Examples are sign language which is a manual mode of communication and 'Blissymbols' which makes use of ideographic writing. It is prudent to consult professional speech-language pathologists when making crucial decisions about communication modes. As actual difficulties faced by children with NDDs could lie discreetly under externally deceptive behaviors. Impromptu decisions might not comply with needs, and even lead to further complications (Bigby, 2018; Chmiliar, 2007; Howlin et al., 2007).

Interactive Instruction

As children with NDDs get accustomed and begin relating with the learning environment, the next concern is engaging them in gainful learning. This is accomplished by adapting instruction according to learner-characteristics employing a range of modes for representation, engagement and responses. Such adoption of multiple options to collectively meet educational needs characterized by unique learning abilities and styles in children is pedagogically termed as 'Universal Design for Learning'. It provides for educational intervention catering not only to challenges stemming from disabilities like NDD, but also to other learner-variability in the mainstream classrooms (Rao and Meo, 2016; Watson et al., 2010).

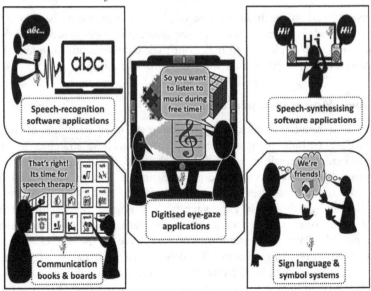

Figure 7.4

The process of adaptation commences with cognizing children's ability and style of learning. Ability for learning is gauged by the capacity for acquiring knowledge and skill for applying it. Regarding learning style generally children can be – auditory learners who understand information or instruction provided in the form of spoken words better; visual learners who are able to grasp easily information or instruction that is rendered with visual images and/or in the written form; and tactile-kinaesthetic children in whom learning is enhanced through hands-on experiences than through other modes (Özdemir et al., 2006). Especially children with NDDs tend to gravitate towards the latter modes of learning (Kemp et al., 2020; Loring and Hamilton, 2011; Reagan, 2012). Apart from these learning qualities, nature of special needs, residual abilities and prior experience with technology are to be considered in choosing appropriate assistive technology for promoting interactive instruction characterized by active and expressive learning (Dikusar, 2019; Pappas, 2012).

Assistive Aids and Devices

Irrelevant instructional purposes and procedures need to be rectified with diversified multilevel targets and multifaceted strategies for inclusive instruction. These provisos are viable in the form of digitized programmed instruction, which entail hardware equipment and software applications essential for computer-assisted instruction. Authentic computer-assisted instruction involves tailor-making lessons to suit extensively variant and exclusively unique learner-characteristics among children with NDDs. Adapted lessons with multimedia components provide scope for dynamic instruction integrating auditory-verbal and textual information complemented with visual graphics, animation, and videos. Ensuing practice usually in the form of simulated games provide for kinaesthetic manoeuvring in the process of exercising learnt knowledge and skills. Specialized software such as 'StoryOnline' offer provisos for creating and operating multimedia lessons and exercises described as augmented virtual reality, which is effective in catering to all three types of auditory, visual and tactile-kinaesthetic learners (Stetter and Hughes, 2010; Taylor, 2016; Wallace, 2018).

Such exercises along with prompt, positive and constructive feedback on the child's participation and performance result in improving learning outcomes as proved by vast evidences generated through numerous pedagogical experiments. The added impetus is that instruction can be rendered over desktop, laptop, or even hand-held devices like iPads and mobile handsets so that it is individualized even among peers in the classroom. Children can continue learning and practising in their convenient pace and place out of classroom bounds until they attain mastery, while concurrently interacting and collaborating with their cohorts via internet connectivity. Such individualized, interesting instruction is found to supplant aversion and fears towards instruction and learning environment with eagerness and enthusiasm in children with NDDs (Bouck et al., 2012; Chiang and Jacobs, 2009; Ferry, 1993; Peterson-Karlan, 2011; Watkins, 1989).

In the course of interactive instruction; children with NDDs might have difficulty organizing scraps of instructional information accrued over several sessions into a meaningful whole and retain them for easy retrieval and effective application later. Variable-speed audio recorders, video recorders–cum-players with automated closed captions, and portable note-takers in the form of pen-top computers with applications such as 'LiveScribe Smartpen and Portronics Electropen' help children with NDDs record verbal and textual information as well as practical demonstrations in the classroom for later retrieval and review at their convenience. Further, digital graphic organizers such as 'Inspiration and Prez' help to categorize information randomly fed during classes and orderly organize them associating related bits and pieces together (Bouck et al., 2009; Rice, 2019; Schmitt et al., 2012).

Alternately, children with NDDs can also visually organize information in the form of concept/mind maps, or create simple outlines of information with software like 'SimpleMind+ and Spark Space'. Digital note-takers like 'Rocket Book' are useful accessories for creating graphically organized information. They help children with NDDs deficient in verbal language skills to jot down large quantities of better quality information with fewer mistakes. These applications have facilities for highlighting and/or adding supplementary information in the form of digital sticky notes. Auxiliary informational data managers such as 'Abbreviation Expanders, Free Books and Tech Matrix' extend access to further, detailed and/or illustrated explanations for difficult data or vocabulary in the notes taken. For children who find noting down information during class difficult, software applications like 'Screen Chomp and Show Me' facilitate video-recording of classroom lectures along with board displays/writings if interactive jam/white-boards or smart-boards are used in the process of instruction (Hetzroni and Shrieber, 2004; Institute for the Advancement of Research Education, 2003; Sturm and Rankin-Erickson, 2002).

Special Supportive Materials

Inaccessible high-technology facilities, as in many remote rural settings with limited resources, are no reason for giving up on multimedia instruction. They could be substituted with tangible multisensory instructional information in the classroom, by ensuring that core verbal instruction is accompanied by visual information and interspersed with ample hands-on learning activities. Visual learners among children with NDDs could be helped with visualized and/or visually emphasized textual information as in illustrated books and color-coded/highlighted notes. Visual aids like cue-cards for discourses/lectures, charts, diagrams, flashcards with printed or pictured information, maps, etc. will also be helpful. However, auditory learners will find recorded lessons/lectures and other useful audio-recorded information commonly called as audio/talking-books useful. Whereas for tactile-kinaesthetic learners, ideas and tools for activity-based learning as in exploratory field-visits, hands-on experiments, model-making and other projects, role-playing, games and play activities among others should be at hand. There are substantial pedagogic evidence suggesting that children with NDDs

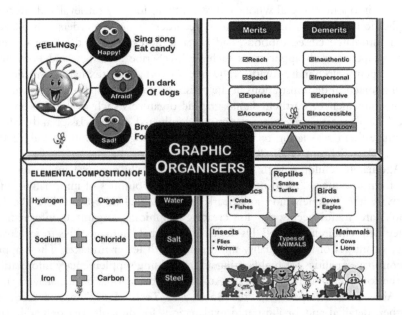

Figure 7.5

learn relatively well from concrete, tangible learning experiences as from alluring virtual exposure. The erstwhile visual organizers and concept maps provided as hand-outs, which were forerunners of the modern digital graphic organizers and mind maps, may resume their due use. And so could picture-dictionaries, real sticky notes and translucent highlighters for enhancing or highlighting textual information presented in writing or print (Bouck et al., 2014; Kemp et al., 2020; Neese, 2021; Sturm and Rankin-Erickson, 2002).

Modified Modes of Operation

As an age-old Chinese adage suggests many children with NDDs hardly respond to oral instruction except for meaningless echolalia. Visual information might be helpful in drawing their attention, but it is practical hands-on activities that ensure meaningful participation in the learning activity. This implies the need for employment of realistic or simulated exposure and experimentation where children handle and manipulate didactic materials both to activate and bolster learning. Such exercises with real objects and realistic experiences have been reported to result in better functional learning. In addition, if these practical aids and activities involve fun components in the form of games and playway learning, they turn out to be strong stimulators of curiosity, facilitators of learning, and perpetrators of its practice in children with NDDs (Alberta Learning, 2003; Bassette et al., 2019; Manitoba Education and Training, 1996; Reagan, 2012).

Furthermore, it is recommended that teachers with the involvement of caregivers get prepared for two alternate levels of input alongside the standard

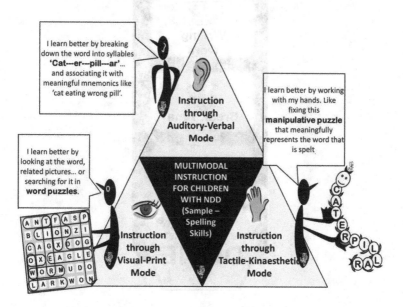

Figure 7.6

instructional content. One of shortened and simplified information for children whose ability to learn is limited. Another of enriched information, as several children with NDDs are reported to have savant abilities for scattered aspects of academic learning (Manitoba Education and Training, 2003; Vaughn and Bos, 2009).

For most types of NDD found in children, structured teaching is found to be effective in directing their attention and efforts towards systematic, distraction-controlled, comprehensive learning. This involves organizing the instructional targets, activities, and environment to include concrete steps and objects positioned and/or sequenced in a particular logical order. Visual scheduling of activities is an essential constituent of such structured teaching. It could be described as a manipulative, pictured timetable where cards with iconic images depict sequence of activities to be carried out as part of the particular learning-task or the entire school-day. They can be put-on-view or removed according to forthcoming or completed activities. Many children with NDDs are known for their inadequacies in time consciousness and the consequent lack of ability for prompt transition between different activities/sessions. This in turn makes them disoriented and disorganized in carrying out learning tasks. Use of visual reminders as described

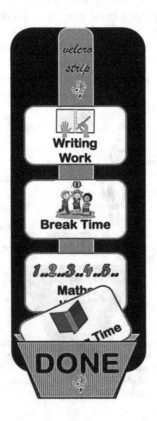

Figure 7.7

above helps them be prepared for commencing or concluding learning actions and activities in time, while becoming conscious of passing time (Hume, 2009; Mesibov et al., 2004).

The instructional sessions need to be custom-scheduled for children with NDDs. Some children with attention deficits, autistic features, and learning disabilities are comfortable working over shorter tasks with meaningfully diverting breaks in-between. In contrast, children with intellectual deficits or motor coordination problems require extended time and practice to master concepts and tasks. Substantial numbers of children with NDDs irrespective of nature of disability are more apt to learn better during specific parts of the day at which time more complex content or demanding tasks can be scheduled (Alberta Learning, 2003; Vaughn and Bos, 2009).

Productive Performance

Subsequent to interactive instruction to acquire meaningful knowledge and useful skills, the next vital consequence in the chain of learning is their productive demonstration. For several reasons, children with NDDs are prevented from attaining this end. First is their inability to focus on the task at hand owing to attention deficit, hyperactivity, or sensory issues. At times this deficiency might be complicated with other deviances like wandering behavior. Another major hurdle in many children with NDDs is insufficient verbal and written communication skills which are predominantly used in conventional assessments. One more difficulty is in cogently organizing ideas for expression, and/or thought process for solving problems. Problems in motor coordination could hinder hand functions for carrying out practical activities demonstrating their knowledge or skills. More elemental problems of access to the different centers of diverse learning activities, and discomfort or incompatibility encountered in adjusting to it might also prevent children with NDDs performing to the best of their ability in spite of good learning. Assistive technology helps with negotiating these problems towards better performance (Reagan, 2012; Sanz-Cervera et al., 2017).

Assistive Aids and Devices

The primary step in the process of children with NDDs demonstrating their learning is to enter the learning environment without struggle and position themselves without strain. Rehabilitation technology offers a wide range of electronically or manually operated mobility aids for moving around barriers that hinder access; from simple canes, crutches and frames, to scooters and wheelchairs for both indoor and outdoor use. Use of these will be further facilitated with lifts/elevators and if feasible automated operatives such as door openers. On reaching their places, the next need is to be positioned comfortably and concentrate in their work to put up advantageous performances. Some children with NDDs with sensory issues are disturbed and distracted by the texture of seating and positioning amid peers. Some others might find the traditional way of seating constraining and might be able to work conveniently when permitted to adopt unconventional positions like standing, sitting at floor level or leaning against the desks/or work tables. A wide range of work surfaces with adjustable height and proximity are available. So are chairs with bulkhead seats providing more space to spread out, comfortable texture, and adaptable height and tilting positions. Other useful accessories are seat inserts for wheel-chairs, side-liers and prone-standers that allow children with NDDs position themselves comfortably for optimal functioning (Ahmad, 2015; Dell et al., 2012; Dikusar, 2019; Pappas, 2012).

After being positioned securely and commencing work on academic tasks, several children with NDDs are deterred owing to deficient or disorganized memory. In such occasions, portable digital work planners like the executive-function reminders in 'Apple watches' come to aid. They remind children of impending work targets, or that it is time to transit from one work or place to another (Arky, 2021). In carrying out the expected work properly, children with NDDs need to understand the nature of performance expected from them and respond appropriately. If the usual verbal or written forms of classroom communication is difficult to follow, speech-to-text interface software enum-erated afore under section on communication, along with talking dictionaries extend significant supports. Subject-specific applications such as 'Math Talk' and talking calculators extend support with illustrated explanations for technical vocabulary and language, and also extended facilities for specialized word-search (Bigby, 2018; Bouck and Flanagan, 2009; Neese, 2021). Employment of afore-described technology for scanning and reading optical characters, recog-nizing voice and/or speech, transcribing speech into text, generating sounds, and synthesizing speech from textual input are facilitative in the productive phase also. They provide for easy convertibility and corroboration between spoken and textual form of information, as well as their visualized representa-tion. This renders class work, assignments and assessments in feasible formats for children with NDDs (Dimian et al., 2018; Izzo et al., 2009; MacArthur et al., 2001; MacArthur and Cavalier, 2004).

Planning and organizing responses might be problematic to some children with NDDs in spite of sound knowledge and sufficient skills in different curricular subjects. In knowledge-based subjects like physical, life and social sciences; dis-crepant executive functioning skills could disrupt orderly organization of infor-mation at hand for effective presentation. In such quandaries, free-form databases and information data managers, along with graphic organizers and/or outlining software help in logically ordering the information into associated clusters under appropriate topics. They eventually enable effective verbal or written presenta-tions/responses enhanced with visual representations. Particularly in struggles to comprehend and correspond with written assignments/assessments, software such as 'Co:Writer, Draft:Builder, VisuWords, etc.' provide prototype blueprints for structuring responses along with procedural prompts for systematic composition. These augmented with specialized word processing software like 'Ginger, Ghotit,

Grammarly', or even mundane applications inbuilt with 'Microsoft Word or Apple Pages' help predict/search words, check spellings and grammar usage in these compositions. Compositely, helping children with verbal deficiencies find exact words to express ideas, organize them in correct order without errors, along with useful auditory feedback to review and further refine their work (Cullen et al., 2008; Englert et al., 2007; Evmenova et al., 2010; Fasting and Halaas, 2005; Handley-More, et al., 2003; MacArthur et al., 2001; Neese, 2021; Rao et al., 2009; Zhang, 2000). 'Clicker 7' and similar applications aid in creating related maps and relevant webs of images that enhance the clarity and comprehensiveness of assignments/presentations. Together these applications help develop better writing skills in children bypassing and/or overcoming hurdles of mechanical writing like legibility, technical skills for spelling and grammar, and complexities of composition/exposition (Batorowicz et al., 2012; MacArthur and Cavalier, 2004; Peterson-Karlan, 2011).

In face of complaints that these supports affect development of independent writing skills in the long run, meta-analyses of research evidences over 25 years allude to the contrary. Systematic use of prompts with programmed weaning was reported to increase motivation and skill for independent expository writing and ingrain methodical steps for compiling/composing information as habitual strategies. Thus, resulting in enhanced vocabulary, its fluent use and improved accuracy in spelling and transcription skills; which in turn contributed to quality performances across all curricular areas (Doughty et al., 2013; Hecker et al., 2002; Lee and Vail, 2005; MacArthur, 2009; Okolo and Diedrich, 2014; Peterson-Karlan, 2011; Tam et al., 2005; Stetter and Hughes, 2010; Wanzek et al., 2006).

Concerning exercises and evaluation in skill-based subjects such as mathematics, software applications like 'Maths Trek 1, 2, 3 and Maths Simulations', and aids like 'graphical multi-function calculators' along with accessories like 'digital maths dictionaries' help children with NDDs to visualize the maths data set before them. This in turn helps better comprehension of the nature of the problems and figure out means to solve them, while digital drills like 'IXL Math' enhance relevant mental maths skills. For many children with NDDs, who frequently err in solving problems owing to disorderly recording of data and/or haphazard execution of solutions; electronic worksheets help align and organize data while reminding the systematic steps to be pursued in solving multistep problems as in 'bodmas' sequence. Still more sophisticated interactive software such as 'Sumdog' helps the teacher in adapting the complexity of problems and questions according to the ability of the children who are taking them. In due course, these various applications alleviate fear of failure and learned helplessness in children with NDDs, while bettering academic self-concept for logical curricular functions as in mathematics (Adcock et al., 2010; Amiripour et al., 2011; Bethell and Miller, 1998; Bouck et al., 2009; Bouck and Flanagan, 2009; Chiang and Jacobs, 2009).

Some children with NDDs might not function optimally or respond satis-factorily owing to constrained motor functions. This inability might arise from varied reasons ranging from deprived sensitivity to tactile-kinaesthetic stimulations, disturbed concentration, deficient physical strength and stamina, and/or disrupted motor coordination. These problems might make difficult and dis-organized, their efforts to manipulate computer input devices which are instrumental in operating many of the advanced assistive technology. Hence, these children might require augmentative or alternate fixtures to the digital devices that can be operated in quick time with minimal effort, while provid-ing most advantageous tactile-kinaesthetic and/or visual feedback to their actions. Useful accessories include 'alternate keyboards' that come with special overlays highlighting character/function of keys with colors/graphics, and also grouping/repositioning keys of similar functions together to overcome diffi-culties in distinguishing the encryptions on keys. For motor difficulties in operating keys and mouse; wands, switches and joysticks manoeuvred with less-complicated movements will be viable. 'Sip-and-Puff Systems like Jouse 3' facilitate these keys, sticks or switches to be manipulated with mouth, cheek, chin or tongue in case of hand/finger movements being severely affected. Even if these minimal movements of other body parts are difficult, alternate applica-tions for operating devices with head movements like 'SmartNav4', and/or eye-ball movements like 'Eye Link, Gaze Point and Smart Eye' that convert these as hands-free mouse movements are available. Voice/speech recognition software described earlier as communication aids also serve as effective opera-tional interface for digital tools. Voice-based operating systems use spoken navigation instructions to operate digital devices, thus enabling children with limited hand functions but intact verbal skills make efficient use of these devices with relative ease. These apart, printers like 'TactPlus' producing embossed and/or textured outputs supply with multisensory instructional materials (Marin et al., 2006; Neese, 2021; Poobrasert, 2017; Rice, 2019; Stanberry and Ras-kind, 2009; Young and MacCormack, 2014).

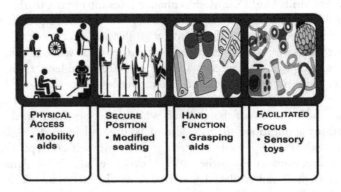

Figure 7.8

Special Supportive Materials

Distracted children with NDDs end with disrupted classroom performances as well as disturbing other children in an inclusive setting. As discussed in the context of supportive surrounding, it is advisable to avoid jarring sights and sounds to facilitate concentration in the academic tasks (Wise, 2017). In instances when these children are distracted by their own self-stimulatory behaviors, a variety of fidgeting toys in the form of spinners and cubes are available to engage their free limbs (Rohrberger, 2011). For children who tend to wander around seeking sensory stimulation, weighted accessories such as jackets, blankets and/or stuffed lap toys filled with heavy beads/stones will provide tactile stimulation reducing their distractive movements (Arky, 2021; Ford-Lanza, 2019). Chairs with strapping or attached lap/work trays also restrict movements away from seating. Some children are incapable of regulating wandering behavior as the un-marked limits for functioning in a large space like classroom with multiple persons around is difficult to perceive. Fixtures like photographs indicating one's seat, floor spaces and boundaries marked with contrast colors provide concrete idea of where to position oneself and work from, and of spaces that are out of bounds (Reagan, 2012; Wise, 2017). Children with NDDs using mobility devices like wheelchairs will require architectural arrangements with wide doorways and passages, ramps, and operatives like switches, latches at reachable level. To help in manual functioning, in the absence of sophisticated digital aids/devices, usual writing tools and other study stationery fitted with grippers and strapping enable sturdy grasp and bolstered sensory feedback when manipulating them (Dikusar, 2019; Rice, 2019; Stanberry and Raskind, 2009).

For children with problems in reading, provision of adequately sized, textured, and appealing textual-cum-visual materials holds their attention as well as conveys information effectively. If too much of diminutively sized textual information, as in textbooks, overwhelms children; the exposure of the amount of reading material at a time can be regulated with help of reading frames. These can be hand-made by cutting out quadrangular openings in the center of hard opaque materials like cardboards; and can be laid over the text to reveal manageable segments of reading information like word/phrase/sentence according to capacity of the child. Sticky notes can be added to summarize verbose information into clear and crisp points. If reading printed material even in regulated amounts is difficult, they can be replaced with alternate reading materials with large-sized, color-coded/highlighted lettering accompanied with relevant images. The surfaces of these images could be variedly textured with diverse materials like cereals, fibre, fabric, grains, etc., as several children with NDDs crave tactile-kinaesthetic feedback from the materials that they handle (Arky, 2021; Rice, 2019; Young and MacCormack, 2014).

Modified Modes of Operation

The key to drawing out appreciable performances from children with NDDs in the mainstream learning environments is flexibility. This applies to both

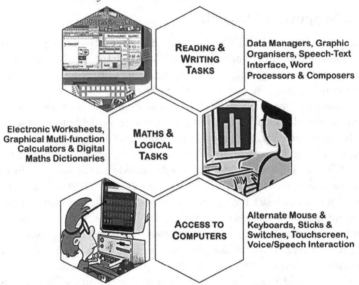

Figure 7.9

teaching input and learning output. The constructive course of drawing and appraising performances has to adopt viable transactional channels, which could be auditory-verbal, visual-print, or tactile-kinaesthetic. In instruction as well as assessment, provisos should be in place to render and/or receive information through any or all three modes optimally utilizing available assistive technology in the process (Kemp et al., 2020; Özdemir et al., 2006).

Depending on attention/concentration span and also processing/performance time which are affected in many children with NDDs, assessment sessions have to be reorganized for shorter/longer durations with refreshing sensory breaks in-between. Following close and careful scrutiny of performances, prompt and constructive feedback will have to be again rendered through multisensory modality. Some widely practised examples for alternate modes of feedback in place of conventional grades/ranks/scores are emoticons, learning ladders, traffic signals, etc. Efforts to draw better performances from children with NDDs at times might involve positively discriminating accommodations in evaluation like preferential seating, additional time, prompter facilities, and avoidance of waiting for turns during which time they might turn distractive. When productive ability is severely limited, more drastic modifications like alternate test formats could be necessary. The major challenge faced in assimilating such flexibilities in an inclusive setting is maintaining parity and providing a level ground for both children with and without disabilities (Arky, 2021; Reagan, 2012; Wise, 2017).

Conclusion

In the lives of children with special needs within and beyond the bounds of school, modern technological advancements have extended immeasurable and indescribable benefits (Cook, 2020; Wallace, 2018). Even while enabling children with NDDs function independently, assistive technology serves to integrate them in the inclusive education process by diminishing differences owing to deficiency or deviancy and increasing their efficiency. Progressively, availability of these technologies is broadening while their applicability is being streamlined even to simple handheld devices. But technology on its own cannot stand up to all challenges arising from disabilities. It is a resourceful tool requiring skilled human resources to put it to best use, that is, confident teachers with pedagogical and technological competence. They should be capable of exploring, experimenting and exploiting assistive technology optimally to derive maximum benefits for children challenged with NDDs and other disabilities. Especially in the instructional front, it has been proved time and again that assistive technology is effective only when combined with efficient instruction. Efficient instruction employing technology is not just teaching in front of the class, but is preceded by thoughtful selection, continued with planned utilization, and sustained with support in the form of necessary monitoring and monetary resources (Lee and Vega, 2005; Nelson, 2006).

In accomplishing this purpose, educators both administrators and teachers need to assume additional responsibilities as technology-coordinators. In educational systems perpetually challenged with limited resources obstructing access to technological advancements, as in India, there is necessity to develop capabilities for need-based choice, cost-effective customization, as well as innovation of indigenous low-technology solutions. Thus, avoiding dependency on externally supported high technology solutions and supports that are usually out of reach to educational functionaries at grassroots (Ault et al., 2013; Marino et al., 2006; Morrison, 2007). Across the world, educators acknowledge the overwhelming possibilities of incorporating technology in instruction, but at once feel overwhelmed by the responsibility to capacitate themselves with skills for exploiting those possibilities. The dread of bearing accountability for creative application and productive execution inhibits optimal utilization of available resources. Many teachers express lack of requisite preparations and provisions within them and without in the educational system and society to undertake the task (Edyburn and Gersten, 2007; Lee and Vega, 2005; Nelson, 2006; Okolo and Diedrich, 2014).

Researches (Ludlow, 2001; Michaels and McDermott, 2003; Nelson, 2006) repeatedly reiterate that teachers' awareness, attitudes, and abilities significantly influence the successful use of assistive technology, and allude to hesitancy among teachers to brace assistive educational technology, owing to lack of preparation. Both pre-service teacher-education programmes and in-service professional enrichment programmes such as workshops are not fully exploited to enhance teacher-capabilities in this front. Even in developed communities as in the USA, it is reported that only one-third of due space is provided for assistive technology in special educational training programmes and still meagre exposure to student-teachers in general education streams (Judge and Simms, 2009; Lee and Vega, 2005). As a remedy planned exposure and experiential training commencing at pre-service stage should continue through in-service enrichment of knowledge and skills. So as to generate empowered teachers capable of coupling technological facilities with context-appropriate instruction for the benefit of all children with or without special needs (Chmiliar and Cheung, 2007; Specht et al., 2007).

In contrast situations of adequacy, supplied with all facets and facilities for sustained use of assistive technology, there is another source of caution. It is that excess and/or tactless use of technology can result in disparaging outcomes turning it into detractor rather than serve as promoter of inclusive learning. Evidences point to possibilities of technology distracting children from learning targets when used as a fancy product rather than as a functional tool (Dell et al., 2012; Donovan et al., 2010). Further even though the primary object of assistive technology is gratifying special educational needs, it could be used as an effective tool to differentiate instruction to meet learning diversities found in mainstream classrooms. And rather than isolated use only for specific students, skills, subjects, or within school, all-encompassing use for every student, across curricula, and permeating beyond school into domestic and social milieu is found to result in far-reaching, favorable consequences (Ahmad, 2015; Nelson, 2006; Okolo and Diedrich, 2014; Specht et al., 2007; Stanberry and Raskind, 2009; Watson et al., 2010).

Technological utilizations should ensure fair play ruling out undue advantage or discrimination of any individual or group of children even for positive purposes. They should be utilized in the best possible way to make growing and learning enjoyable, equitable and effectual for all children in the inclusive learning environment. Sensitive, sensible and seasoned use of assistive technology for educational purposes is reported to help children with NDDs and other disabilities become empowered learners. By minimizing dependency on external human assistance and developing independent study skills, technology builds confidence, boosts learning outcomes and bolsters overall sustenance and success in children with NDDs. These bounties reportedly permeate into children's lives besides and beyond the learning environs, while also benefiting the educational system in realizing maximal outcomes with minimal efforts. To this end, purposeful efforts are imperative to overcome the current gap between potential possibilities and actual utilization owing to lack of conviction and commitment (Burne et al., 2011; Forgrave, 2002; Mull and Sitlington, 2003; Okolo and Diedrich, 2014; Young, 2012).

References

Adcock, W., Luna, E., Parkhurst, J., Poncy, B., Skinner, C., and Yaw, J. (2010). "Effective class-wide remediation: Using technology to identify idiosyncratic math facts for additional automaticity drills." *The International Journal of Behavioural Consultation and Therapy*, 6: 111–123.

Ahmad, F. K. (2015). "Use of assistive technology in inclusive education: Making room for diverse learning needs." *Transcience*, 6(2): 62–77.

Ahn, S. and Hwang, S. (2017). "Cognitive rehabilitation with neurodevelopmental disorder: A systematic review." *NeuroRehabilitation*, 41(4): 707–719, doi:10.3233/NRE-172146.

Alberta Learning. (2003). *Teaching students with autism spectrum disorders.* Edmonton, AL: Alberta Learning.

Allen, A. A., Shane, H. C., and Schlosser, R. W. (2018). "The Echo[TM] as a speaker-independent recognition device to support children with autism: An exploratory study." *Advances in Neurodevelopmental Disorders – Special Issue on Communication Intervention and Assessment*, 2: 69–74, doi:10.1007/s41252-017-0041-5.

American Psychiatric Association. (2014). *Diagnostic and statistical manual of mental disorders* (5th ed.). Arlington, VA: American Psychiatric Publishing.

Amiripour, P., Bijan-zadeh, M. H., Pezeshki, P., and Najafi, M. (2011). "Effects of assistive technology instruction on increasing motivation and capacity of mathematical problem solving in dyscalculia student." *Educational Research*, 2(10): 1611–1618.

Arky, B. (2021). "Parent hacks for special needs kids: Tips for dealing with sensory issues." Retrieved January 25, 2021, from Child Mind Institute: https://childmind.org/article/parenting-hacks-for-special-needs-kids.

Arthur-Kelly, M., Foreman, P., Maes, B., Colyvas, K., and Lyons, G. (2018). "Observational data on socio-communicative phenomena in classrooms supporting students with profound intellectual and multiple disability (PIMD): Advancing theory development on learning and engagement through data analysis." *Advances in Neurodevelopmental Disorders – Special Issue on Communication Intervention and Assessment*, 2: 25–37. doi:10.1007/s41252–41017–0045–0041.

Assistive Technology Act of 2004. (2004) Public Law 108–364 (October 25, 2004).

Ault, M. J., Bausch, M. E., and McLaren, E. M. (2013). "Assistive technology service delivery in rural school districts." *Rural Special Education Quarterly*, 32(2): 15–22.

Bassette, L. A., Bouck, E., Shurr, J., Park, J., and Cremeans, M. (2019). "A Comparison of manipulative use on mathematics efficiency in elementary students with autism spectrum disorder." *Education and Training in Autism and Developmental Disabilities*, 54 (4): 391–405. doi:10.1177/0162643419854504.

Batorowicz, B., Missiuna, C. A., and Pollack, N. A. (2012). "Technology supporting written productivity in children with learning disabilities." *Canadian Journal of Occupational Therapy*, 79(4): 211–224, doi:10.2182/cjot.2012.79.4.3.

Bethell, S. and Miller, N. (1998). "From an E to an A in first year algebra with the help of graphing calculator." *Mathematics Teacher*, 91: 118–119.

Bigby, G. (2018). "Assistive devices for impairment in hearing, voice, speech and language." Retrieved January 25, 2021 from Accessibility Testing: https://dynomapper.com/blog/27-accessibility-testing/463-assistive-devices-for-impairments-in-hearing-voice-speech-and-language.

Blackhurst, A. (2005). "Perspectives on applications of technology in the field of learning disabilities." *Learning Disability Quarterly*, 28(Spring): 175–178. doi:10.2307/1593622.

Bouck E. C., Satsangi, R., Doughty, T. T., and Courtney, W. T. (2014). "Virtual and concrete manipulatives: A comparison of approaches for solving mathematics problems for students with autism spectrum disorders." *Journal of Autism and Developmental Disorders*, 44(1):180–193. doi:10. 1007/s10803–10013–1863–1862.

Bouck, E. C., Bassette, L., Doughty, T. T., Flanagan, S. M., and Szwed, K. (2009). "Pentop computers as tools for teaching multiplication to students with mild intellectual disabilities." *Education and Training in Developmental Disabilities*, 44: 367–380.

Bouck, E. and Flanagan, S. (2009). "Assistive technology and mathematics: What is there and where can we go in special education." *Journal of Special Education Technology*, 24: 24–30.

Bouck, E., Flanagan, S., Miller, B., and Bassette, L. (2012). "Technology in Action." *Journal of Special Education Technology*, 27: 47–57.

Burne, B., Knafelc, V., Melonis, M., & Heyn, P. (2011). *The use and application of assistive technology to promote literacy in early childhood: A systematic review.* Disability and Rehabilitation: Assistive Technology, 6, n.p., doi:10.3109/17483107.2010.522684,207–213.

Chiang, H. and Jacobs, K. (2009). "Effect of computer-based instruction for students self-perception and functional task performance." *Disability and Rehabilitation: Assistive Technology*, 4(2): 106–118. doi:10.1080/17483100802613693.

Chmiliar, L. (2007). "Perspectives on assistive technology: What teachers, health professionals and speech language pathologists have to say?" *Developmental Disabilities Bulletin*, 35(7): 1–17.

Chmiliar, L. and Cheung, B. (2007). "Assistive technology training for teachers: Innovation and accessibility online." *Developmental Disabilities Bulletin*, 35(1): 18–28.

Cook, A. (2020). "Assistive technology in education: Assistive technology for intellectual disabilities." Retrieved December 2, 2020, from Study.com: https://study.com/academy/lesson/assistive-technology-for-intellectual-disabilities.html.

Cullen, J., Richards, S. B., and Frank, C. L. (2008). "Using software to enhance the writing skills of students with special needs." *Journal of Special Education Technology*, 23: 33–44.

Dell, A., Newton, D., and Petroff, J. (2012). *Assistive technology in the classroom: Enhancing the school experiences of students with disabilities* (2nd ed.). Boston, MA: Pearson.

Dikusar, A. (2019). "Educational technology: The use of technology in special education." Retrieved December 2, 2020 from eLearning Industry: https://elearningindustry.com/use-of-technology-in-special-education.

Dimian, A. F., Elmquist, M., Reichle, J., and Simacek, J. (2018). "Teaching communicative responses with a speech generating device." *Advances in Neurodevelopmental Disorders – Special Issue on Communication Intervention and Assessment*, 2: 86–99.

Donovan, L., Green, T., and Hartley, K. (2010). "An examination of one-to-one computing in the middle school: Does increased access bring about increased student engagement?" *Journal of Educational Computing Research*, 42: 423–441, doi:10.2190/EC.42.4.d.

Doughty, T. T., Bouck, E. C., Bassette, L., Szwed, K., and Flanagan, S. (2013). "Spelling on the fly: Investigating a pentop computer to improve spelling skills of three elementary students with disabilities." *Assistive Technology*, 25: 166–175. doi:10.1080/10400435.2012.743491.

Edyburn, D. and Gersten, R. (2007). "Defining quality indicators in special education technology research." *Journal of Special Education Technology*, 22(3): 3–18. doi:10.1177/016264340702200302.

Englert, C. S., Zhao, Y., Dunsmore, K., Collings, N. Y., and Woblers, K. (2007). "Scaffolding the writing of students with disabilities through procedural facilitation: Using an internet-based technology to improve performance." *Learning Disability Quarterly*, 30 (1): 9–29. doi:10.2307/30035513.

Evmenova, A. S., Graff, H. J., Jerome, M. K., and Behrmann, M. M. (2010). "Word prediction programs with phonetic spelling support: Performance comparisons and impact on journal writing for with writing difficulties." *Learning Disabilities Research & Practice*, 25(4): 170–182. doi:10. 1111/j.1540–5826.2010.00315.x.

Fasting, R. B. and Halaas, L. S.-A. (2005). "The effects of computer technology in assisting the development of literacy in young struggling readers and spellers." *European Journal of Special Needs Education*, 20(1): 21–40. doi:10.1080/0885625042000319061.

Ferry, B. (1993).Towards effective teaching strategies with interactive multimedia. Master of Education (Hons.) thesis. Wollongong, New South Wales, Australia: Research Online, University of Wollongong.

Fitzell, S. (2018). "Make your classroom lighting learner friendly." Retrieved August 1, 2017 from susanfitzell.com: http://susanfitzell.com/make-classroom-lighting-learner-friendly.

Ford-Lanza, A. (2019). "Sensory lighting: What helps and what doesn't." Retrieved January 25, 2021 from Harkla: https://harkla.co/blogs/special-needs/sensory-lighting.

Forgrave, K. E. (2002). "Assistive technology: Empowering students with learning disabilities." *The Clearing House: A Journal of Educational Strategies, Issues and Ideas*, 75(3): 122–126. doi:10.1080/00098650209599250.

Gonzalez, J. (2019). "Facial recognition technology allows autistic children to communicate." Retrieved January 25, 2021 from The University Star: www.universitystar.com/news/facial-recognition-technology-allows-autistic-children-to-communicate/article_149d563f-37a9-5d4d-8ea1-297b8d3e3919.html.

Griffin, K. (2018). "Auditory sensitivity: Signs, causes and how to help." Retrieved January 25, 2021 from GriffinOT: www.griffinot.com/auditory-sensitivity-autism-.sensory.

Hamilton, D. R. (2015). "Treatment of neurodevelopmental disorders: Targeting neurobiological mechanisms." *Journal of Developmental & Behavioral Pediatrics*, 36 (6): 425. doi:10.1097/DBP.0000000000000183.

Handley-More, D., Dietz, J., Billingsley, F. F., and Coggins, T. E. (2003). "Facilitating written work using computer word processing and word prediction." *The American Journal of Occupational Therapy*, 57(March–April): 139–151. doi:10.5014/ajot.57.2.139.

Hecker, L., Burns, L., Katz, L., Elkind, J., and Elkind, K. (2002). "Benefits of assistive reading software for students with attention disorders." *Annals of Dyslexia*, 52: 243–272. doi:10.1007/s11881-002-.0015-8.

Hetzroni, O. E. and Shrieber, B. (2004). "Word processing as an assistive technology tool for enhancing academic outcomes of students with writing disabilities in the general classroom." *Journal of Learning Disabilities*, 37(2): 143–154. doi:10.1177/00222194040370020501.

Howard, J. (2016). "How just the right lighting may improve learning in classrooms." Retrieved August 1, 2017 from *The Huffington Post*: www.huffingtonpost.com/entry/lighting-boost-learning-concentration_us_5720cb14e4b0b49df6a9b73e.

Howlin, P., Gordon, R. K., Pasco, G., Wade, A., and Charman, T. (2007). "The effectiveness of Picture Exchange Communication System (PECS) training for teachers of children with autism: A pragmatic, group randomized controlled trial." *Journal of Child Psychology and Psychiatry*, 48(5): 473–481.

Hume, K. (2009). *Steps for implementation: Visual schedules*. Chapel Hill, NC: The National Professional Development Center on Autism Spectrum Disorders, The University of North Carolina.

Illinois University Library. (2020). "Speech disorders: Common assistive technologies." Retrieved January 25, 2021 from Illinois University Library: https://guides.library.illinois.edu/c.php?g=613892&p=4265891.

Institute for the Advancement of Research Education. (2003). "Graphic organizers: A review of scientifically based research." Prepared for the Inspiration Software at AEL.

Izzo, M., Yurick, A., and McArrell, B. (2009). "Supported eText: Effects of text-to-speech on access and achievement for high school students with disabilities." *Journal of Special Education Technology*, 24: 9–20.

Judge, S. and Simms, K. A. (2009). "Assistive technology at the pre-service level." *Teacher Education and Special Education*, 32: 33–44.

Kemp, G., Smith, M., and Segal, J. (2020). "Helping children with learning disabilities." Retrieved January 25, 2021 from Help Guide: www.helpguide.org/articles/autism -learning-disabilities/helping-children-with-learning-disabilities.htm.

Lee, Y. and Vail, C. O. (2005). "Computer-based reading instruction for young children with disabilities." *Journal of Special Education Technology*, 20: 5–18.

Lee, Y. and Vega, L. A. (2005). "Perceived knowledge, attitudes and challenges of AT use in special education." *Journal of Special Education Technology*, 20: 60–63.

Lonkar, H. (2014). "An overview of sensory processing disorder – Honors Theses 2444." Retrieved January 25, 2021 from *Scholar Works at Western Michigan University*: https://scholarworks.wmich.edu/cgi/viewcontent.cgi?article=3437&context=honors_ theses.

Loring, W. and Hamilton, M. (2011). "Visual supports and autism spectrum disorders." Retrieved from Autism Speaks: www.autismspeaks.org/sites/default/files/2018-08/ Visual%20Supports%20Tool%20Kit.pdf.

Ludlow, B. L. (2001). "Technology and teacher education in special education: Disaster or deliverance?" *Teacher Education and Special Education*, 24(2): 143–163. doi:10.1177/ 088840640102400209.

MacArthur, C. A. (2009). "Reflections on research on writing and technology for struggling writers." *Learning Disabilities Research and Practice*, 24(2): 93–103. doi:10.1111/j.1540-5826.2009.00283.x.

MacArthur, C. A., Ferretti, R. P., Okolo, C. M., and Cavalier, A. R. (2001). "Technology applications for students with literacy problems: A critical review." *The Elementary School Journal*, 101(3): 273–301. doi:10.1086/499669.

MacArthur, C. A. and Cavalier, A. R. (2004). "Dictation and speech recognition technology as test accommodations." *Exceptional Children*, 71(1): 43–58, doi:10.1177/ 001440290407100103.

Manitoba Education and Training. (1996). *Success for all learners: A handbook on differentiating instruction – A resource for kindergarten to senior schools*. Winnipeg, MB: Manitoba Education and Training.

Manitoba Education and Training. (2003). *Independent together: Supporting the multilevel learning community*. Winnipeg, MB: Manitoba Education and Training.

Marin, F. A., Dolz, I., Gaya, C., and Martin, M. (2006). "The voice recognition system as a way of accessing the computer for people with physical standards as usual." *Technology and Disability*, 18(3): 161. doi:10.3233/TAD-2006-18301.

Marino, M. T., Marino, E. C., and Shaw, S. F. (2006). "Making informed assistive technology decisions for students with high incidence disabilities." *Teaching Exceptional Children*, 38(6): 18–25.

Mesibov, G. et al. (2004). "Structured teaching." In: *The TEACCH approach to autism spectrum disorders* (pp. 33–49). Boston, MA: Springer. doi:10.1007/978-0-306-48647-0_4.

Michaels, C. A. and McDermott, J. (2003). "Assistive technology integration in special education teacher preparation: Program coordinators' perceptions of current attainment and importance." *Journal of Special Education Technology*, 18(3): 29–44.

Morrison, K. (2007). "Implementation of assistive computer technology: A model for school systems." *International Journal of Special Education*, 22(1): 83–95.

Mull, C. A. and Sitlington, P. L. (2003). "The role of technology in the transition to postsecondary education of students with learning disabilities: A review of the literature." *Journal of Special Education*, 37(1): 26–32. doi:10.1177/00224669030370010301.

Neese, B. (2021). "Assistive technology tools and resources for students with disabilities." Retrieved December 2, 2020 from Teach Thought Staff: www.teachthought.com/tech nology/15-assistive-technology-tools-resources-for-students-with-disabilities.

Nelson, B. (2006). "On your mark, get set, wait! Are your teacher candidates prepared to embed assistive technology in teaching and learning?" *College Student Journal*, 40(3): 485–494.

Okolo, C. M. and Diedrich, J. (2014). "Twenty-five years later: How is technology used in the education of students with disabilities? Results of a state wide study." *Journal of Special Education Technology*, 29(1): 1–20.

Özdemir, P., Güneysu, S. I., and Tekkaya, C. (2006). "Enhancing learning through multiple intelligences." *Journal of Biological Education*, 40(2): 74–78.

Pappas, C. (2012). "Assistive technology for students with disabilities." Retrieved December 2 2020 from eLearning Industry: https://elearningindustry.com/assistive-technology-for-students-with-disabilities.

Peterson-Karlan, G. R. (2011). "Technology to support writing by students with learning and academic disabilities: Recent research trends and findings." *Assistive Technology Outcomes and Benefits*, 7(1): 39–62.

Poobrasert, O. (2017). "Educational assistive technology for students with communication disorders." *Journal of Communication Disorders, Deaf Studies and Hearing Aids*, 5(2): 1–7. doi:10.4172/2375-4427.1000178.

Rao, K. and Meo, G. (2016). "Using Universal Design for Learning to design standards-based lessons." *SAGE Open*, 6(4): 1–12. doi:2158244016680688.

Rao, K., Dowrick, P., Yuen, J., and Boisvert, P. (2009). "Writing in a multimedia environment: Pilot outcomes for high school students in special education." *Journal of Special Education Technology*, 24: 27–38.

Reagan, N. (2012). Effective inclusion of students with autism spectrum disorders. Education Masters Thesis submitted to Ralph C. Wilson, Jr. School of Education. Rochester, NY: Fisher Digital Publications, St. John Fisher College.

Rice, M. (2019). "Assistive technology in the classroom is reimagining the future of education." Retrieved December 2, 2020 from builtinedtech: https://builtin.com/edtech/assistive-technology-in-the-classroom.

Rohrberger, A. (2011). "The efficacy of fidget toys in a school setting for children with attention difficulties and hyperactivity." *Ithaca College Theses*, 330. Retrieved February 11, 2021 from Ithaca College: https://digitalcommons.ithaca.edu/ic_theses/330.

Sanz-Cervera, P., Pastor-Cerezuela, G., González-Sala, F., Tárraga-Mínguez, R., and Fernández-Andrés, M.-I. (2017). "Sensory processing in children with autism spectrum disorder and/or attention deficit hyperactivity disorder in the home and classroom contexts." *Frontiers in Psychology*, 8(1772): 1–12. doi:10.3389/fpsyg.2017.01772.

Schmitt, A. J., McCallum, E., Hennessey, J., Lovelace, T., and Hawkins, R. O. (2012). "Use of reading pen assistive technology to accommodate post-secondary students with reading disabilities." *Assistive Technology*, 24(4): 229–239. doi:10.1080/10400435.2012.659956.

Simacek, J., Pennington, B., Reichle, J.,and Parker-McGowan, Q. (2018). "Aided AAC for people with severe to profound and multiple disabilities: A systematic review of interventions and treatment intensity." *Advances in Neurodevelopmental Disorders – Special Issue on Communication Intervention and Assessment,* 2: 100–115. doi:10.1007/s41252-017-0050-4.

Specht, J., Howell, G., and Young, G. (2007). "Students with special education needs in Canada and their use of assistive technology during the transition to secondary school." *Childhood Education–International Focus Issue,* 83(6): 385–389. doi:10.1080/00094056.2007.10522956.

Stanberry, K. and Raskind, M. H. (2009). "Assistive technology for kids with learning disabilities: An overview." Retrieved December 2, 2020 from *Reading Rockets*: www.readingrockets.org/article/assistive-technology-kids-learning-disabilities-overview.

Stetter, M. E. and Hughes, M. T. (2010). "Computer-assisted instruction to enhance the reading comprehension of struggling readers: A review of literature." *Journal of Special Education Technology,* 25(4): 1–16.

Strangman, N. and Dalton, B. (2005). "Using technology to support struggling readers: A review of the research." In D. Edyburn, K. Higgins, and R. Boone, *Handbook of special education technology research and practice* (pp. 325–334). Whitefish Bay, WI: Knowledge by Design, Inc.

Sturm, J. M. and Rankin-Erickson, J. L. (2002). "Effects of hand-drawn and computer-generated concept mapping on the expository writing of students with learning disabilities." *Learning Disabilities Research and Practice,* 17(2): 124–139. doi:10.1111/1540-5826.00039.

Tam, C., Archer, J., Mays, J., and Skidmore, G. (2005). "Measuring outcomes of word cueing technology." *The Canadian Journal of Occupational Therapy,* 72(5): 301–308. doi:10.1177/000841740507200507.

Taylor, B. (2016). "Augmented reality for special education needs." Retrieved December 2, 2020 from *eLearning Industry*: https://elearningindustry.com/augmented-education-for-special-education-needs.

Thapar, A., Cooper, M., and Rutter, M. (2017). *"Neurodevelopmental disorders."* Lancet Psychiatry, 4(4): 339–346. doi:10.1016/S2215-0366(16)30376-5.

Understood Team. (2017). *Sensory processing issues.* Retrieved January 25, 2021 from Understood for All: https://assets.ctfassets.net/p0qf7j048i0q/77dd9zXK6nXZN1BrWJ2bgb/571188dfe20bf8787af43d15264e44f6/Sensory_Processing_Issues_Fact_Sheet_Understood.pdf.

Vaughn, S. and Bos, C. (2009). *Strategies for teaching students with learning and behavioural problems* (7th ed.). Upper Saddle River, NJ: Pearson.

Wadhera, T. and Kakkar, D. (2018). "Strengthening risk prediction using statistical learning in children with autism spectrum disorder." *Advances in Autism,* 4(3): 141–152. doi:10.1108/AIA-06-2018-0022.

Wadhera, T. and Kakkar, D. (2019). "Eye tracker: An assistive tool in diagnosis of autism spectrum disorders." In S. K. Gupta, S. Venkatesan, S. P. Goswami, and R. Kumar (Eds) *Emerging trends in the diagnosis and intervention of neurodevelopmental disorders* (pp. 125–152). IGI Global. doi:10. 4018/978-971-5225-7004-2.

Wallace, F. (2018). "Assistive technology in education: How e-learning helps students with disabilities." Retrieved December 2, 2020 from *e-Learning Industry*: https://elearningindustry.com/assistive-technology-in-education.

Wanzek, J., Vaughn, S., Wexler, J., Swanson, E. A., Edmonds, M., and Kim, A.-H. (2006). "A synthesis of spelling and reading interventions and their effects on the spelling outcomes of students with LD." *Journal of Learning Disabilities,* 39(6): 528–543. doi:10.1177/00222194060390060501.

Watkins, M. (1989). "Computerized drill-and-practice and academic attitudes of learning disabled students." *Journal of Special Education Technology*, 9: 167–172.

Watson, A. H., Ito, M., Smith, R. O., and Andersen, L. T. (2010). "Effect of assistive technology in a public school setting." *American Journal of Occupational Therapy*, 64 (January–February), 18–29. doi:10.5014/ajot.64.1.18.

Winterbottom, M. and Wilkins, A. (2009). "Lighting and discomfort in the classroom." *Journal of Environmental Psychology*, 29(1): 63–75. doi:10.1016/j.jenvp.2008.11.007.

Wise, R. (2017). "Tips to set up the learning environment for students with ADHD and ASD." Retrieved January 25, 2021 from *Education and Behaviour*: https://educationandbehavior.com/how-to-set-up-the-classroom-for-students-with-autism.

Young, G. (2012). Examining assistive technology use, self-concept and motivation, as students with learning disabilities transit from a demonstration school into inclusive classrooms. Unpublished Doctoral Thesis. London, Ontario, Canada: Western University.

Young, G. and MacCormack, J. (2014). "Assistive technology for students with learning disabilities." Retrieved January 25, 2021 from LD at School: www.ldatschool.ca/assistive-technology.

Zhang, Y. (2000). "Technology and the writing skills of students with learning disabilities." *Journal of Research on Computing in Education*, 32: 467–478.

8 Technology-Driven Interventions for Attention Deficit Hyperactivity Disorder (ADHD)

Tanu Gupta and Pratibha Gehlawat

Introduction

Attention deficit hyperactivity disorder (ADHD) is the most common neurodevelopmental disorder. It is marked with consistent symptoms of inattention, hyperactivity, and impulsivity. These symptoms can be observed in early childhood. Some children might present with hyperactivity during preschool years and become the cause of concern for parents. These symptoms also disrupt the school adjustment and academic achievement of children with ADHD. The presentation of child with ADHD can broadly be divided in to two types, impulsive/hyperactive and poorly self-motivated type (referred to as hyperactive–impulsive type) and inattentive type with learning problems. Majority children might present with a mixture of both types which is known as combined type of ADHD (Guan Lim et al., 2020). The diagnosis of ADHD generally happens in childhood wherein a child presents with symptoms of hyperactivity, inattentiveness and impulsivity. As children grows in age, the symptoms of hyperactivity and impulsivity resolve, however, the symptom of inattentiveness persist and also affect the academic achievement of an individual at later stages of life.

The child with ADHD generally comes to clinical attention owing to learning and academic issues in school. Parents bring the child for consultation owing to the complaints of teachers and their inability to manage the problem behaviors at home. Children with ADHD presents with poor academic performance, learning problems and poor psychosocial adjustment at school (Cortese et al., 2015)

Neuropsychological profiles of children with ADHD have been studied widely, and literature cites evidence for deficits in specific domains. The performance of various subtypes of ADHD were compared in executive function using the Wisconsin Card Sorting Test (WCST) and revealed that ADHD subtypes differ significantly on perseverative responses and perseverative errors on WCST. ADHD-Combined type shows more perseverative responses and perseverative errors than ADHD-Inattentive type (Ahmadi et al., 2014). Pievsky and McGrath (2018) reviewed 34 meta-analyses that compare the neuro-cognitive performance of individuals with ADHD with their peers and

DOI: 10.4324/9781003165569-8

found consistent evidence of poor performance of children with ADHD on different cognitive domains such as reaction time, working memory, vigilance, intelligence, response inhibition, and academic achievement (Pievsky and McGrath, 2018). These deficits can differentiate the performance of children with ADHD from their typically developing peers, as highlighted by a number of studies and systematic reviews.

Importantly, many children can benefit at the same time by using this intervention through technology. Technology-driven interventions can be accessed from home or school that further improve access to care for individuals with ADHD. Individuals with ADHD struggle with inattention, organizational skills deficits, and poor time management and find it difficult to complete tasks. Owing to these difficulties, they find it difficult to remain persistent in their studies and work Upcoming technological advancements (such as apps and computer programs) can be utilized as an asset for children and adults with ADHD as they can help them with their time management and organization skills. Electronic timers can help them to stay organized and finish their tasks on time. In addition, assistive technology used in classroom can improve their focus in class. ADHD-affected children find it difficult to follow instructions, and therefore computer-assisted instructions were found to increase the maths performance of children with ADHD (Mackenzie and Ferrari, 2017).

Technology, when used properly, has the potential to improve focus, productivity, and the academic achievement of children with ADHD.

The Tech Model of ADHD Interventions

Benyakorn et al. (2016) devised a model for technology-based care of individuals with ADHD that broadly categorized care into two categories i.e. direct care and supported care (Benyakorn et al., 2016). Direct care include computerized cognitive training that repeatedly exposes a patient to a task with the purpose to improve the related ability e.g. computerized working memory training program focusses on the improvement of working memory deficits. Supported care provision facilitates a skill with the help of technology like assistive devices used to improve various academic skills or organizational skills. Technology-driven interventions exist on a continuum, wherein they train as well as support the individuals, e.g. the Actigraph commonly used in individuals with ADHD that monitor the motion and sleep parameters and give feedback to the person. By using this motion feedback, individuals with ADHD can achieve better inhibitory control.

Tech models suggest that developers of technology-driven interventions for ADHD should utilize both support and training provisions in their interventions. Effective technology-driven interventions should broadly encompass three components i.e. schedule setting, difficulty matching, and immediate feedback. *Schedule setting* involves goal setting and scheduling to target the issues related to task completion and time management in individuals with ADHD. *Difficulty matching* includes adaptation as per the individual's current level of functioning/skill to maintain the focus and engagement in the given task. It should change, once the individual successfully accomplishes that level with the existing skills. *Immediate feedback*/reinforcement for the performance enhances the motivation and encourages consistent efforts (Benyakorn et al., 2016)

Technology-driven interventions for ADHD

Gamification is a strategy to enhance the motivation and interest for intervention by incorporating the gaming elements into the various given activities. Gamification utilizes different system of rewards, such as badges, points, or level for the participants when they meet their goals (Deterding et al., 2011). It is similar to the star charts that are widely used in behavioral interventions for children with ADHD (Guan Lim et al., 2020)

EpicWin

EpicWin is an app-based on gamified technology; specifically developed for children and adults with ADHD. It helps them in task management by setting a goal and achieves it through role play of an avatar that they choose for themselves. Once they achieve their goal, they get points as rewards which further reinforce their engagement in goal achievement (Epic Win–Level-Up Your Life, n.d.).

MotivAider

Children with ADHD find it difficult to inhibit their response or behavior as per the demand of the situation. Self-monitoring is one such technique that helps them to manage their behavior on a regular basis. MotivAider is a digital devise that utilizes a vibrating element as a tactile prompt as a reminder to return focus on a given task and to inhibit responses to various distractions available in the environment. Such prompts have been found to improve focus, academic performance, and response inhibition in children with ADHD (Legge et al., 2010).

Rescue Time

Individuals with ADHD often struggle with time management. Rescue time is a supported technology-based app that gives a feedback to users about the time that they spend on certain tasks and time spent on procrastinating. By utilizing this feedback, individuals can make appropriate adjustments in their daily routines to effectively manage time. 30/30 is another helpful app for time management that provides reminders every 30 minutes about taking a break and from the given task and assess progress. Users can set timers according to their preferences, and the app will update them about the completion of the time limit (Noreika et al., 2013).

Due

Another commonly used app is Due, which helps individuals with ADHD in scheduling their daily chores and maintaining deadlines. Users can add on the important tasks along with their deadlines in this app, and they receive push notifications as a reminder of the given task and deadline.

Zones of Regulation

Emotional lability has been found to be a major concern for individuals with ADHD. They experience quick transition from one mood state to another. Emotional regulation is one strategy that helps them to deal with their emotional ups and downs. Zones of regulation is a game-based program designed to teach emotional regulation to children with ADHD (Guan Lim et al., 2020). Different colors have been used to define various zones of emotions, such as:

- The Red zone is defined as a zone of intense emotions when we feel out of control, and whenever a child identifies him/herself in the red zone, he has to stop or pause for some time.
- The Yellow zone is defined with less intense emotions which can be controlled so the child has to slow down before reacting.
- The Green zone is defined as a calmer state of mind where a child is focussed and alert, and emotions are under control.
- The Blue zone is defined as a resting area that is activated when people feel tired, bored, or short of energy for work. In this zone, they can just take some time off to themselves to re-energize.

CogMed

Cogmed is a software-based intervention program for working memory training. It entails different visuospatial and verbal tasks targeting specifically the different component of working memory and attention. The intervention can be delivered at home, school or clinical setting through computer or tablet as per the individual's convenience. Computerized working memory training (CWMT) has been shown to improve working memory deficits of individuals with ADHD, but generalizability to other cognitive functions is still questionable (Beck et al., 2010; van der Donk et al., 2015). Literature also quotes mixed findings about CWMT, wherein few studies reported improvement in working memory and ADHD symptoms following CWMT whereas one randomized controlled study found CogMed effective in reducing the distractibility in academic task but no change was observed in parent rated symptoms of ADHD (Klingberg et al., 2005). Similar findings have been reported in a recent meta-analysis by European ADHD guidelines group (Cortese et al., 2015).

Computerized Progressive Attentional Training (CPAT)

CPAT was designed to improve the various components of attention in children with ADHD. It incorporates four types of tasks to enhance sustained, selective, orienting and executive types of attention. This program has various level of difficulty which gets automatically activated as per the performance of the individual user. The efficacy of CPAT has been established in a randomized controlled trial which found significant improvement in attention, hyperactivity and academic performance of children with ADHD post CPAT intervention (Shalev et al., 2007).

Brain Computer Interface-based Attention Training

Brain computer interface (BCI)-based attention training program was developed based on the principles of biofeedback wherein EEG profile of an individual is used to measure the attention of an individual while playing the game and he/she learns to increase attention while playing the game. A BCI-based attention training program is an eight-week program comprised 24 sessions followed by booster sessions every three months. The program was delivered to 20 ADHD children who did not take the medication and found improvement in parent rated symptoms (inattention and hyperactivity/impulsivity) of ADHD (Lim et al., 2012). EEG-based biofeedback systems and neurofeedback therapy have been developed as an alternative treatment modality for ADHD. They are based on the premise that children with ADHD exhibit a specific profile of EEG, and therefore EEG feedback training can target to normalize the specific pattern might result in improvement of certain symptoms (Sterman, 1996). However, these modalities (EEG-based biofeedback, neurofeedback) are being applied in clinical settings regularly, but the evidence of efficacy is still not strong (Gevensleben et al., 2012).

Another BCI and motion sensing technology-based intervention program was developed with the purpose of improving the reading ability of children with ADHD. A fairy tale-based interactive intervention was administered on children with ADHD and assessed brainwaves and motion sensing data during intervention. Findings revealed an improvement in reading and comprehension. The motion sensing data revealed improvements in attention and hyperactivity behavior post-intervention (Park et al., 2019).

Assistive Technology for Children with ADHD

Assistive technology (AT) is defined as any product, equipment, item, software, or system that improves or enhances the functional capabilities of a person with a disability (World Health Organization, n.d.). ATs can improve overall cognitive functioning, including attention, planning, executive functions, and self-regulation among children with ADHD. ATs generally complement the existing interventions and improve the academic achievement of children with ADHD. A number of studies have assessed the efficacy of different ATs for children with ADHD. MOBERO is one such smartphone-based assistive system that encourages independent scheduling of morning and bedtime routines of children with ADHD. MOBERO was found to be effective in improving children's independence for their routines and reducing the parents' frustration level (Sonne et al., 2016). TangiPlan is another AT that targets executive functioning of children with ADHD and facilitates organizational skills, time management, and planning abilities of children with ADHD (Weisberg et al., 2014). Children with ADHD can benefit by using these ATs in their day-to-day life. Various ATs like MotivAider, iSelfcontrol, Time Aids, etc., are available to assist children with disabilities, but research regarding the efficacy of these assistive interventions is more focused on learning disabilities, and little evidence is available for ADHD (Mackenzie and Ferrari, 2017).

Discussion

Today's generation is more attracted to virtual world; therefore, technology-driven interventions can be easily adopted and followed by children with ADHD. Cognitive training with game elements is more engaging for children, and they remain regularly interested in these interventions (Prins et al., 2011). Technology-driven interventions incorporate components of psychoeducation, biofeedback, virtual reality, and neurofeedback to train different cognitive domains, and once children achieve mastery of these tasks, they can then easily apply the virtual learning to real life situations (Lau et al., 2016). Technology-driven interventions provide immediate feedback that leads to early correction of errors, and users remain motivated through continuous rewards, based on their performance. Therefore, the involvement of parents can be effective in delivering digital interventions for children with ADHD. There is a paradigm shift towards delivering interventions through digital modes, owing to their cost effectiveness and convenience for the user. Technology-enabled interventions can be more personalized according to the needs and baseline skill level of the patient.

Conclusion

To conclude, this chapter has highlighted the available evidence of technology-driven intervention for children with ADHD. Literature supports the use of technology-driven interventions in children with ADHD as we have discussed. However, further studies are required to strengthen the existing evidence. In future, work can be done to compare the effectiveness of technology-enabled interventions with other personally delivered behavioral interventions. Researchers can also extend their work towards integrating different components of technology with routine behavioral interventions delivered in clinical settings.

References

Ahmadi, N., Mohammadi, M. R., Araghi, S. M., and Zarafshan, H. (2014). "Neurocognitive Profile of Children with Attention Deficit Hyperactivity Disorders (ADHD): A comparison between subtypes." *Iranian Journal of Psychiatry*, 9(4): 197–202.

Beck, S. J., Hanson, C. A., Puffenberger, S. S., Benninger, K. L., and Benninger, W. B. (2010). "A controlled trial of working memory training for children and adolescents with ADHD." *Journal of Clinical Child and Adolescent Psychology: The Official Journal for the Society of Clinical Child and Adolescent Psychology, American Psychological Association, Division 53*, 39(6): 825–836. doi:10.1080/15374416.2010.517162.

Benyakorn, S., Riley, S. J., Calub, C. A., and Schweitzer, J. B. (2016). "Current State and Model for Development of Technology-Based Care for Attention Deficit Hyperactivity Disorder." *Telemedicine Journal and E-Health*, 22(9): 761–768. doi:10.1089/tmj.2015.0169.

Cortese, S. et al. and European ADHDGuidelines Group (EAGG). (2015). "Cognitive training for attention-deficit/hyperactivity disorder: Meta-analysis of clinical and neuropsychological outcomes from randomized controlled trials." *Journal of the American Academy of Child and Adolescent Psychiatry*, 54(3): 164–174. doi:10.1016/j.jaac.2014.12.010.

Deterding, S., Dixon, D., Khaled, R., and Nacke, L. (2011). "From game design elements to gamefulness: Defining 'gamification'." *Proceedings of the 15th International Academic MindTrek Conference: Envisioning Future Media Environments*, 9–15. https://doi.org/10.1145/2181037.2181040.

Epic Win—Level-Up Your Life. (n.d.). Retrieved 30 January 2021 from www.rexbox.co.uk/epicwin.

Gevensleben, H., Rothenberger, A., Moll, G. H., and Heinrich, H. (2012). "Neurofeedback in children with ADHD: Validation and challenges." *Expert Review of Neurotherapeutics*, 12(4): 447–460. doi:10.1586/ern.12.22.

Guan Lim, C., Lim-Ashworth, N. S. J., and Fung, D. S. S. (2020). "Updates in technology-based interventions for attention deficit hyperactivity disorder." *Current Opinion in Psychiatry*, 33(6): 577–585. doi:10.1097/YCO.0000000000000643.

Klingberg, T. et al. (2005). "Computerized training of working memory in children with ADHD—a randomized, controlled trial." *Journal of the American Academy of Child and Adolescent Psychiatry*, 44(2): 177–186. doi:10.1097/00004583-200502000-00010.

Lau, H. M., Smit, J. H., Fleming, T. M., and Riper, H. (2016). "Serious Games for Mental Health: Are They Accessible, Feasible, and Effective? A Systematic Review and Meta-analysis." *Frontiers in Psychiatry*, 7, 209. doi:10.3389/fpsyt.2016.00209.

Legge, D. B., DeBar, R. M., and Alber-Morgan, S. R. (2010). "The Effects of Self-Monitoring with a MotivAider[R] on the On-Task Behavior of Fifth and Sixth Graders with Autism and Other Disabilities." *Journal of Behavior Assessment and Intervention in Children*, 1(1): 43–52.

Lim, C. G. et al. (2012). "A Brain-Computer Interface-Based Attention Training Program for Treating Attention Deficit Hyperactivity Disorder." *PLoS ONE*, 7(10). doi:10.1371/journal.pone.0046692.

Mackenzie, G. and Ferrari, J. (2017). "The Necessity of Advancing Our Knowledge On Assistive Technologies To Better Support Students With Attention Deficit Hyperactivity Disorder." *Journal of ADHD and Care*, 1(1): 1.

Noreika, V., Falter, C. M., and Rubia, K. (2013). "Timing deficits in attention-deficit/hyperactivity disorder (ADHD): Evidence from neurocognitive and neuroimaging studies." *Neuropsychologia*, 51(2): 235–266. doi:10.1016/j.neuropsychologia.2012.09.036.

Park, K., Kihl, T., Park, S., Kim, M.-J., and Chang, J. (2019). "Fairy tale directed game-based training system for children with ADHD using BCI and motion sensing technologies." *Behaviour & Information Technology*, 38(6): 564–577. https://doi.org/10.1080/0144929X.2018.1544276.

Pievsky, M. A. and McGrath, R. E. (2018). "The Neurocognitive Profile of Attention-Deficit/Hyperactivity Disorder: A Review of Meta-Analyses." *Archives of Clinical Neuropsychology*, 33(2): 143–157. https://doi.org/10.1093/arclin/acx055.

Prins, P. J. M., Dovis, S., Ponsioen, A., ten Brink, E., and van der Oord, S. (2011). "Does computerized working memory training with game elements enhance motivation and training efficacy in children with ADHD?" *Cyberpsychology, Behavior and Social Networking*, 14(3): 115–122. https://doi.org/10.1089/cyber.2009.0206.

Shalev, L., Tsal, Y., and Mevorach, C. (2007). "Computerized progressive attentional training (CPAT) program: Effective direct intervention for children with ADHD." *Child Neuropsychology: A Journal on Normal and Abnormal Development in Childhood and Adolescence*, 13(4): 382–388. doi:10.1080/09297040600770787.

Sonne, T., Müller, J., Marshall, P., Obel, C., and Grønbæk, K. (2016). "Changing Family Practices with Assistive Technology: MOBERO Improves Morning and Bedtime Routines for Children with ADHD." In *Proceedings of the 2016 CHI Conference on Human Factors in Computing Systems* (pp. 152–164). Association for Computing Machinery. doi:10.1145/2858036.2858157.

Sterman, M. B. (1996). "Physiological origins and functional correlates of EEG rhythmic activities: Implications for self-regulation." *Biofeedback and Self-Regulation*, 21(1): 3–33. doi:10.1007/BF02214147.

van der Donk, M. et al. (2015). "Cognitive training for children with ADHD: A randomized controlled trial of cogmed working memory training and 'paying attention in class." *Frontiers in Psychology*, 6. doi:10.3389/fpsyg.2015.01081.

Weisberg, O. et al. (2014). "TangiPlan: Designing an assistive technology to enhance executive functioning among children with ADHD." *Proceedings of the 2014 Conference on Interaction Design and Children*, 293–296. doi:10.1145/2593968.2610475.

World Health Organization. (n.d.). "Assistive devices and technologies." Retrieved 31 January 2021 from www.who.int/disabilities/technology/en.

9 Technology-enabled precision medicine in neurodevelopmental disorders

Pratibha Gehlawat and Tanu Gupta

Introduction

Precision medicine is an approach in healthcare targeted to use different technologies to acquire population-wide data and its application for individually tailored diagnosis and treatment. The main aim is to design and optimize the pathway for diagnosis, intervention, and prognosis by using large biological datasets that capture individual variability in genes, function, and environment. Therefore, precision medicine offers an opportunity to clinicians to personalize preventive as well as treatment-related early interventions to each individual patient. Neurodevelopmental disorders (NDD) are a group of early childhood onset disorders that impair different domains of motor function, higher brain functions, and cognitive development. These usually have a lifelong course and variable prognosis at individual level. Some rare single-gene disorders among NDDs have much severe cognitive and medical consequences. There are higher rates of co-morbidities in NDDs that makes the diagnosis as well as treatment even more challenging. Moreover, there is phenotypic variability between individuals with same diagnosis and also a certain degree of phenotypic overlap between different disorders among NDDs (Coe et al., 2012; Kosmicki et al., 2015; Wall et al., 2012). Thus, the complexities in the diagnosis and treatment of NDDs pave the way for implementation of a precision medicine approach. This group of disorders poses a significant burden on healthcare, and therefore early diagnosis and targeted therapeutic interventions become a healthcare priority to identify those individuals who are likely to benefit most (Mazurek et al., 2019).

Enabling Technology for Precision Medicine

A number of technologies are required in precision medicine to guide personalized diagnosis and treatment for patients. Large biological datasets as well as high-performance computing (HPC) are of utmost important to effectively implement a precision medicine pathway in healthcare. The heart of this strategy is a set of computer algorithms that identify patterns in multidimensional datasets.

Artificial intelligence (AI) applies learning strategies based on classification or pattern recognition to complex input data. This further forms the basis to

DOI: 10.4324/9781003165569-9

predict future datasets that are helpful in early diagnosis as well as treatment outcomes. In simpler form and in the context of clinical scenario, this might be easily understood using examples, i.e. diagnosis can be predicted using the results of pathological specimens, and further staging can be done for the pathological specimen received on a new patient. The available AI algorithms are defined broadly on the basis of whether they are supervised or unsupervised. Some of the methods relevant for clinical practice are evolutionary algorithms, support vectors, neural networks, and random forests:

- Equipment of multiple layers of artificial neuron-based structures with multilayer logistic regression comprises the Neural Network model (Lee, 2001). It consists of an input and output model and a hidden layer of artificial neurons in between the two layers. This is widely used for pattern recognition, classification, etc. that are the common machine learning-related problems.
- EA is an effective optimization model that usually starts from the random assignment of an initial possible solution (known as a population) and progressively applies artificial genetic operators (mutation crossover etc.) to produce a new set of possible solutions in the subsequent generation (Pelikan, 2005). It has the capability to optimize multiple objectives (Gen et al., 2008).

Both neural network-driven machine learning and evolutionary algorithm have shown promising predictive potential (Padovani de Souza et al., 2018). The adaptation of the two models can be done by providing input data in supervised, unsupervised, or semi-supervised models:

- In supervised learning algorithm, the training data helps the algorithm learning a function that maps an input to an output based on known or labelled input-output pairs.
- Unsupervised learning is a type of machine learning that involves unlabelled training data where the input-output relationship is not known and the algorithm infers patterns (or possible solutions) within datasets.
- Semi unsupervised learning is a type of machine learning that involves a mix of known and unknown training data that helps the algorithm to infer input-output relationships.

Another technological advancement termed Neuro-Developmental Engineering (NDE) has been emerging at inter-disciplinary research areas of developmental neuroscience and bioengineering (Campolo et al., 2008). The main aim is to provide novel tools and methods to understand neuro-biology of human brain development, modelling, and quantitative analysis of human behaviour during neurodevelopmental stages and assessment of neuro-developmental milestones. The application of NDE is well acknowledged for early diagnosis, evaluation, and management of NDDs via the development of new clinical protocols and newer generations of educational and interactive toys.

Converging Genomics in Precision Medicine

Precision medicine provides insights into how population-derived biomarkers and proteomic and genetic profiles can be tailor-made for the diagnosis and treatment of an individual. The disorder is thought to be due to a complex interaction of aberrant activities like modifier genes, proteins, cell behaviour, and signalling, etc., and not due to simple linear progression (Li et al., 2015). Thus, new linkages are identified for multi-factorial, complex diseases, and novel treatment approaches are discovered.

A large amount of data related to healthcare has been added, owing to digitization of medical health records in recent decades. "All of Us" and EMERGE network by NIH, USA (Sankar and Parker, 2017); National Health Service, UK (Sheikh et al., 2011); and Electronic Health Record initiatives by Canadian Institutes of Health Research (Gagnon et al. 2014) are some of the world's largest digitization initiatives and electronic health record databases. The application of AI algorithms based on these large digitization efforts have the potential to infer numerous phenotypic correlations and associations and can also be helpful to establish a genotype–phenotype relationship for genetic diseases. However, large-scale digital data should comprise relevant clinical information as well, to model AI algorithms.

Recently, machine learning have been used in DNA sequencing technology to read long stretches of DNA fragments from digital electronic signalling data. The complex structural variants and repetitive regions in the genome can be detected and resolved by long-read technologies. A neural network-based deep learning method to 'call' DNA bases from electronic signal produced by the nanopore flow cells is being specifically used in nanopore sequencing technology. This method can produce mega base long DNA reads and has an accuracy over 98% (Boza et al. 2017). The implication of AI based on large-scale molecular datasets has also been attempted in the clinical classification of genomic variation, based on the splicing code (Xiong et al., 2015), characterization of non-coding variants (Zhou and Troyanskaya, 2015), non-coding RNA (Yi et al., 2018), and DNA/RNA-binding proteins (Alipinahi et al., 2015).

Implementation of Precision Medicine in NDDs

Autism spectrum disorder (ASD) and attention deficit hyperactivity disorder (ADHD) are common, lifelong NDDs. In contrast, there are some individually rare syndromal NDDs that particularly include single-gene disorders. NDD patients present with varying degrees of severity and comorbidity. A relatively smaller number of NDDs such as Fragile X syndrome, Down syndrome, tuberous sclerosis, West syndrome, etc., are diagnosed according to known biological abnormality and diagnostic investigation such as electroencephalography (EEG).

In contrast, most NDDs do not have known biological abnormality and diagnosed as per the presence of threshold symptoms identified by informant history and direct observation. Therefore the diagnostic clarification often becomes indefinitive, because the reliable information as well as expert opinion vary at the individual and clinician level, respectively. Moreover, the clinical picture can also vary over time, owing to the developmental nature of NDDs (Krol and Feng, 2018). Thus, an objective and stable method is necessary to classify individuals with NDDs.

Genomics and Phenotyping in NDDs

All NDDs are considered to be principally genetic in etiology for the implementation of precision medicine (Woodbury-Smith and Scherer, 2018). Major NDDs, along with genetic diagnostic yield, is shown in Table 9.1. A strong, heritable genetic component in ASD is supported by twin and family studies. Also, a lesser phenotype, i.e. Broader Autism Phenotype and ASD tend to run in families. Rare, highly penetrant mutations are found in some individual cases, while some cases are associated with rare genetic syndromes (Uddin et al., 2014; Jiang et al., 2013; Iossifoy et al., 2014; Berry-Krevis, 2014; Curatolo et al., 2015). However, in contrast, most NDDs involves interaction of environmental factors and epigenetic mechanisms with a complex genetic architecture, i.e. multiple genetic variants of variable penetrance (Coe et al., 2012; van Loo and Martens, 2007). Technological developments, both laboratory-based and *in silico*, can be helpful to understand this genetic complexity. The pattern of differentially expressed genes and single nucleotide protein also shows a striking degree of overlap among various NDDs (Grove et al., 2019.) More than 50 genes have been reported that have a strong association with NDDs (Coe et al., 2019). It is important to note that the present clinical genetic diagnostic yield , is about 40% for syndromal NDDs with comorbid Intellectual Disability, and if genome sequencing data are available for the first-generation family members, the genetic diagnostic yield becomes much higher (Wright et al., 2018).

Table 9.1 Prevalence and genetic inheritance of some major NDDs

Prevalence, sex ratio, genetic diagnostic yield (of major NDDs
NDD Prevalence sex ratio (M/F) genetic diagnostic yield
Autism spectrum disorder: 1.69 4:1 >40%
Intellectual disability: 1.7 2:1 >50%
Epilepsy: 1.2 1:1 >45%
Single gene disorders: <1% 1:1 (except X-linked MR) 100%

Source: Centers for Disease Control and Prevention, USA.

Role of Biomarkers

The biomarkers that reflect pharmacodynamic response, treatment response, and target molecular engagement provide efficacy in the early years of children presenting with NDDs.

The clinical examination findings such as dysmorphology, digit ratio, head circumference, face patterns, ear size, cognitive, and behavioural functions, etc., as well as biochemical biomarkers like urine melatonin, blood serotonin, sulphate excretion, etc., can be integrated during routine NDD clinic visits. These biomarkers can be measured during routine clinical care (Wadhera et. al., 2019).

The use of structural and functional neuroimaging has also been found to be widely used in neurological care clinics. Brain function similarities among NDDs are evident from functional magnetic resonance imaging (fMRI) findings. An overlap of the intermediate phenotype between different NDDs (ASD and ADHD, most commonly) have been reported in diffusion tensor imaging studies (Ha et al., 2015). Functional imaging has also been used to elucidate the structures and regions in the brain that are active while performing neuropsychological tasks. However, at a clinical level, the phenotypes differ quite markedly.

Non-invasive techniques such as electro- and magneto- encephalography have recently been considered ideal biomarkers for characterizing NDDs. These have several orders of magnitude with high temporal resolution, the ability to monitor brain activity with high temporal resolution, and provide a direct measure of postsynaptic brain activity. EEG, evoked potentials (auditory, visual, and somatosensory), and eye-tracking indices serve as potential biomarkers for non-syndromic as well as syndromic ASD, Rett syndrome, and intellectual disability (Ewen et al., 2019; Saby et al., 2020).

Transcranial magnetic stimulation of the motor cortex can be used to measure cortical inhibition and excitation when done along with electromyography of the stimulated muscles (Tsubuyama et al., 2019). An emotional facial eye-tracking paradigm is helpful for emotional recognition and social attention through face scanning and pupillometry at a very early stage in ASD (Reisinger et al. 2020). Other biomarker modalities such as autonomic functions and actigraphy are in the process of testing and development. Hence, it is suggested that measurements of biomarkers at multimodal level is more reliable.

Biosensors

Biosensor devices are designed for the multimodal assessment of different perceptual and motor domains for the screening of large number of infants. Instrumented ball, wrist and ankle wearable sensors, audio-video-vestibular cap, etc., include some of the technological approaches for the early diagnosis of NDDs (Campolo et al., 2008). Grasping skills in infants can be assessed through instrumented toy. Spontaneous upper and lower limb movements in premature babies and infants can be measured by wearable sensors. The behaviours in response to audio and visual stimuli are assessed using multimodal caps. Visual eye-trackers are also available that pick eye-gaze deficits and can be considered valid biomarkers for ASD (Wadhera and Kakkar, 2019). The advantage is that these biosensor devices are designed to be operational in ecological scenario and minimally structured environment. These can be used alone or along with other devices.

Precision Therapeutics

The major challenge for NDDs remains application of precision medicine in the treatment part. With the introduction of antisense oligonucleotide therapy and genome editing technologies (i.e. CRISPR/cas9), identification and imitation of cellular phenotype and precise molecular targets has been made possible. (Wang et al., 2015) Eventually, the inhibition of faulty pathways might be done by the target molecules designed by the experimental pathway. Emphasis should be laid on finding the common pathways for the approved drugs in different diseases. An example could be the shared impact of mTOR pathway in epilepsy and tuberous sclerosis (Curatolo et al., 2015; Curatolo et al., 2018)

Challenges and Opportunities for Precision Medicine in NDDs

There exist various challenges in the application of precision medicine in NDDs, owing to hidden large-scale datasets and phenotypic complexities. There are major hurdles that need to be overcome before transforming precision medicine towards healthcare delivery systems, particularly for NDDs. The phenotypic severity and heterogeneity as a result of changing environmental factors in NDDs remains unclear. Post-zygotic mutations owing to the impact of the environment are recently associated with NDDs (Uddin et al., 2017; Lim et al., 2017). Moreover, there are large variations in environmental influences, owing to different geographical locations.

The biggest challenge is the unpredictable nature of progression of NDD over time, as these are not static disorders. Thus, there is considerable amount of within-subject variability in how the disorder evolves over a period of time. This variability of NDD has been neglected in existing research. That the same genetic and neuronal substrate in an individual manifests a wide range of phenotypes during the developmental stages needs to be understood (Uddin, et al. 2017). Thus, to resolve the pattern and variability of disease progression over time, AI algorithms and machine learning can be applied in longitudinal studies.

The challenges are faced from technical aspects too, owing to different methodologies, protocols, and tools. The reproducibility and reliability of the findings varies with experimental settings (Poldrack et al., 2017). Moreover, there are batch effect and technology-specific biases in large omics data (Hoen et al., 2013). The two main issues in AI include a lack of proper training datasets and complexity on interpretability. There is a need for representative

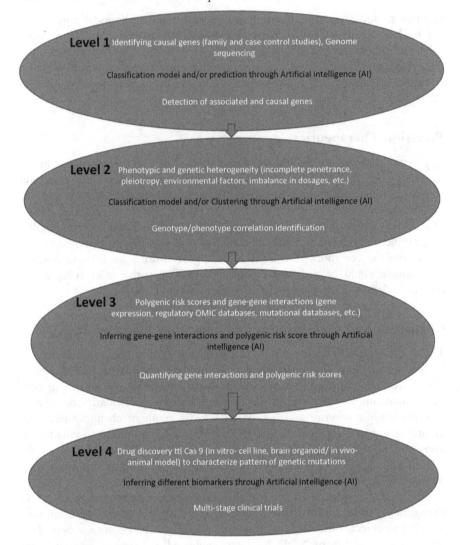

Figure 9.1 Opportunities and challenges for impactful implementation of technology (AI algorithms) in underpinning the complex unresolved mechanisms in NDDs

(both population as well as tissues), more complete biomedical datasets. Therefore, it has been suggested that frontline healthcare staff should play a key role in the paradigm shift promised by precision medicine. Further training should be given to healthcare staff in the strengths and limitations, the interpretation, and translation technology-enabled knowledge, which is clinically relevant and useful for patients with NDDs.

Conclusion

The suite of enabling technologies for precision medicine has provided the ability to identify and monitor various medical disorders. The newer technologies can be helpful in utilizing large databases to search for new therapies, to diagnose disease, and to identify biomarkers and disease progression, etc.

Technological advances like AI and machine learning have already achieved success in the medical field in certain areas like cardiovascular diseases and carcinomas. Likewise, the advances in technology can be helpful to reveal the complexities of NDDs and to give new insight into the diagnosis and management of this group of disorders. The implementation of a precision medicine approach in NDDs will have a great impact on healthcare. The integration of HPC infrastructure managing the multidimensional large emerging datasets with existing and new supervised and unsupervised learning approaches is required to achieve benefits in improving healthcare delivery for individuals with NDDs. There is a need for researchers to take up a more intermediate biologically driven level of phenotype to improvise treatment response and clinical outcomes. The investment needs to be increased in the healthcare sector, in the context of new treatments for NDDs and translational researches. Hence, the development of adequate infrastructure in healthcare becomes a necessity to make professionals experts in knowledge translation. Thus, it is concluded that technology has enabled a precision medicine approach in the medical field, including NDDs. The healthcare sector will achieve long-term benefits from precision medicine by cutting the overall cost of management and improving the health of the population.

References

Berry-Kravis, E. (2014). "Mechanism-based treatments in neurodevelopmental disorders: fragile X syndrome." *Pediatric Neurology*, 50: 297–302.

Boza, V., Brejova, B., and Vinar, T. (2017). "DeepNano: deep recurrent neural networks for base calling in MinION nanopore reads." *PLoS ONE*, 12: e0178751.

Campolo, D. et al. (2008). A Novel Technological Approach Towards the Early Diagnosis of Neurodevelopmental Disorders. 30th Annual International IEEE EMBS Conference Vancouver, British Columbia, Canada, August 20–24, 4875–4878.

Coe, B. P. et al. (2019). "Neurodevelopmental disease genes implicated by de novo mutation and copy number variation morbidity." *Nature Genetics*, 51: 106–116.

Coe, B. P., Girirajan, S., and Eichler, E. E. (2012). "The genetic variability and commonality of neurodevelopmental disease ." *American Journal of Medical and Genetics C Seminars in Medical Genetics*, 160C: 118–129.

Curatolo, P., Moavero, R., and de Vries, P. J. (2015). "Neurological and neuropsychiatric aspects of tuberous sclerosis complex." *The Lancet Neurology*, 14: 733–745.

Curatolo, P., Moavero, R., van Scheppingen, J., and Aronica, E. (2018). "mTOR dysregulation and tuberous sclerosis-related epilepsy." *Expert Review in Neurotherapeutics*, 18: 185–201.

Ewen, J. B. et al. (2019). "Conceptual, Regulatory and Strategic Imperatives in the Early Days of EEG-Based Biomarker Validation for Neurodevelopmental Disabilities." *Frontiers in Integrative Neuroscience*, 21(13): 45.

Gagnon, M. P. et al. (2014). "Electronic health record acceptance by physicians: testing an integrated theoretical model." *Journal of Biomedical Informatics*, 48: 17–27.

Gen, M., Cheng, R., and Lin, L. (2008). *Network Models and Optimization: Multiobjective Genetic Algorithm Approach.* Springer.

Grove, J. et al. (2019). "Identification of common genetic risk variants for autism spectrum disorder." *Nature Genetics*, 51: 431–444.

Ha, S., Sohn, I. J., Kim, N., Sim, H. J., and Cheon, K. A. (2015). "Characteristics of brains in autism spectrum disorder: structure, function and connectivity across the life-span." *Experimental Neurobiology*, 24(4): 273–284.

Hoen, P. A. et al. (2013). "Reproducibility of high-throughput mRNA and small RNA sequencing across laboratories." *Nature Biotechnology*, 31: 1015–1022.

Iossifov, I. et al. (2014). "The contribution of de novo coding mutations to autism spectrum disorder." *Nature*, 515: 216–221.

Jiang, Y. H. et al. (2013). "Detection of clinically relevant genetic variants in autism spectrum disorder by whole-genome sequencing." *American Journal of Human Genetics*, 93(2): 249–263.

Kosmicki, J. A., Sochat, V., Duda, M., and Wall, D. P. (2015). "Searching for a minimal set of behaviors for autism detection through feature selection-based machine learning." *Translational Psychiatry*, 5: e514.

Krol, A. and Feng, G. (2018). "Windows of opportunity: timing in neurodevelopmental disorders." *Current Opinion in Neurobiology*, 48: 59–63.

Lee, H. K. H. (2001). "Model selection for neural network classification." *Journal of Classification*, 18(2): 227–243.

Lim, E. T. et al. (2017). "Rates, distribution and implications of postzygotic mosaic mutations in autism spectrum disorder." *Nature Neuroscience*. 20: 1217–1224.

Mazurek, M. O., Curran, A., Burnette, C., and Sohl, K. (2019). "ECHO Autism STAT: accelerating early access to autism diagnosis." *Journal of Autism and Developmental Disorders*, 49: 127–137.

Padovani de Souza et al. (2019). "Machine learning meets genome assembly." *Briefings in Bioinformatics*, 20(6): 2116–2129.

Pelikan, M. (2005). *Hierarchical Bayesian Optimization Algorithm: Toward A New Generation of Evolutionary Algorithms.* Berlin/Heidelberg: Springer-Verlag.

Poldrack, R. A. et al. (2017). "Scanning the horizon: towards transparent and reproducible neuroimaging research." *Nature Reviews Neuroscience*, 18: 115–126.

Reisinger, D. L. et al. (2020). "Atypical Social Attention and Emotional Face Processing in Autism Spectrum Disorder: Insights From Face Scanning and Pupillometry." *Frontiers in Integrative Neuroscience*, 12(13): 76.

Saby, J. N. et al. (2020). "Evoked Potentials and EEG Analysis in Rett Syndrome and Related Developmental Encephalopathies: Towards a Biomarker for Translational Research. *Frontiers in Integrative Neuroscience*, 28(14): 30.

Sankar, P. L. and Parker, L. S. (2017). "The precision medicine initiative's all of us research program: an agenda for research on its ethical, legal, and social issues." *Genetics in Medicine*, 19: 743–750.

Sheikh, A. et al. (2011). "Implementation and adoption of nationwide electronic health records in secondary care in England: final qualitative results from prospective national evaluation in "early adopter" hospitals." *BMJ*, 343: d6054.

Tsuboyama, M. et al. (2019). "Biomarkers Obtained by Transcranial Magnetic Stimulation of the Motor Cortex in Epilepsy." *Frontiers in Integrative Neuroscience*, 30(13): 57.

Uddin, M. et al. (2014). "Brain-expressed exons under purifying selection are enriched for de novo mutations in autism spectrum disorder." *Nature Genetics*, 46: 742–747.

Uddin, M. et al. (2017). "Germline and somatic mutations in STXBP1 with diverse neurodevelopmental phenotypes." *Neurology Genetics*, 3(6): e199.

van Loo, K. M. and Martens, G. J. (2007). "Genetic and environmental factors in complex neurodevelopmental disorders." *Current Genomics*, 8: 429–444.

Wadhera, T. and Kakkar, D. (2019). "Eye Tracker: An Assistive tool in diagnosis of Autism Spectrum disorders." In: *Emerging trends in diagnosis and intervention in neuro-developmental disorders*. IGI Global.

Wadhera, T., Kakkar, D., Kaur, G., and Menia, V. (2019). "Preclinical ASD screening using Multi-Biometric-Based systems." In: *Design and implementation of health-care Biometric systems*. IGI Global, pp. 185–211.

Wall, D. P., Dally, R., Luyster, R., Jung, J. Y., and Deluca, T. F. (2012). "Use of artificial intelligence to shorten the behavioral diagnosis of autism." *PLoS ONE*, 7(8): e43855.

Wang, P. et al. (2015). "CRISPR/Cas9-mediated heterozygous knockout of the autism gene CHD8 and characterization of its transcriptional networks in neurodevelopment." *Molecular Autism*, 6: 55.

Woodbury-Smith, M. and Scherer, S. W. (2018). "Progress in the genetics of autism spectrum disorder." *Developmental Medicine and Child Neurology*, 60(5): 445–451.

Wright, C. F. et al. (2018). "Making new genetic diagnoses with old data: iterative reanalysis and reporting from genome-wide data in 1,133 families with developmental disorders." *Genetics in Medicine*, 20: 1216–1223.

Xiong, H. Y. et al. (2015). "RNA splicing. The human splicing code reveals new insights into the genetic determinants of disease." *Science*, 347: 1254806.

10 Computational Psychiatry to Bridge the Gap between Data-driven and Theory-Driven Approaches

A Review

Sapumal Ahangama and Indika Perera

1 Introduction

Recent developments in neurological disorder diagnosis and treatment process have notably benefitted from the use of computational methods and software support. Wide acceptance and consideration of computational psychiatry as a mainstream research frontier in the field of neurodevelopmental disorder diagnosis, treatment procedure, and rehabilitation sufficiently warrant the need for reviewing the current state-of-the-art and the key challenges prevailing. This chapter provides insights into the current computational psychiatry practices and suggests enhancements through data analysis to improve the efficacy of current clinical practices.

1.1 Overview of Neurodevelopmental Disorders

Neurodevelopmental disorders (NDDs) are a set of illnesses that are associated with the nervous system leading to the disruption of brain development. This definition covers a wide variety of neurological problems such as Rare Genetic Syndromes, Congenital Neural Anomalies, Schizophrenia, Attention Deficit Hyperactivity Disorder (ADHD), Autism Spectrum Disorder (ASD), Intellectual Disability, Communication Disorders, and Specific Learning Disorders, among many others (Thapar et al., 2017; Brihadiswaran et al., 2019; de Silva et al., 2019a; Meedeniya and Rubasinghe, 2020; Rubasinghe and Meedeniya, 2020). These disorders have been studied extensively by medical practitioners and scientists in the field of neuroscience with substantial progress made towards understanding the link between mechanisms of the brain and nervous system with human behavior (Ferrante et al., 2019).

1.2 Motivation Towards the Study

However, it is noted that incorporating this advanced body of knowledge in actual clinical practices have been extremely challenging and the advances have

DOI: 10.4324/9781003165569-10

not been translated to the same level of success in clinical practice (Ferrante et al., 2019; Huys et al., 2016). A range of reasons has been identified as the root cause of this observation. Firstly, as noted earlier, neuro-developmental diseases have a wide variety and it is inherently complex to correctly classify the diseases and measure treatment outcomes (Thapar et al., 2017). Secondly, mental health depends not only on the functions of the brain and the nervous system alone but is also influenced by the individual's environmental, social and experiential challenges (Huys et al., 2016). These two factors have introduced a multitude of complex variables that are difficult for a clinical practitioner to keep track of.

In this context, computational psychiatry has recently gained much traction in the neuroscience field as a solution to the inherent problems of NDDs in clinical practice (Ferrante et al., 2019; Huys et al., 2016). Compared to traditional approaches of psychiatry medication, computational psychiatry applies an array of computational modelling techniques with interdisciplinary contributions from computer science, mathematics and physics in addition to the knowledge of psychiatry, psychology and neuroscience medical practice (Series, 2020). The recent advances in machine learning algorithms and artificial intelligence, the availability of large training data sets and the advances of computational power, have brought many successes in the field of computational psychiatry (Huys et al., 2016; de Silva et al., 2019b; Ariyarathne et al., 2020; de Silva et al., 2021a; de Silva et al., 2021b; Rubasinghe and Meedeniya, 2020; Haputhanthri et al., 2019; Haputhanthri et al., 2020).

1.3 Background for the Proposed Approach

The computational psychiatry research can be considered in two approaches, namely, data-driven and theory-driven (Bennett et al., 2019). In the data-driven approach, machine learning models are applied in a theoretically agnostic manner to generate predictions based on the given input. In contrast, theory-driven computational psychiatry approaches aim to mathematically explain the under-lying model mechanisms of psychiatric illnesses to ensure the models are rigorous, consistent, and quantitatively explainable (Bennett et al., 2019; Maia et al., 2017).

Owing to the contrasting benefits and limitations of data-driven and theory-driven approaches, recent preliminary studies have suggested the combined use of these two approaches for improved computational psychiatry (Huys et al., 2016). As a simple example, theory-driven approaches can be used in the initial stage to identify the features specifically relevant to a disorder. This avoids the high-dimensionality issues when applying data-driven approaches in the second stage leading to increased efficiency and reliability of the overall model (Frank et al., 2015; Huys et al., 2016; Wiecki et al., 2015). The models used a theory-driven pre-fitted parameter model rather than directly feeding with raw data. It was shown that by following a combined approach, the models had a higher accuracy. As a result, the need for increased engagement between data-driven and theory-driven computational psychiatry research has been highlighted with initial attempts of such integration showing many promising results.

This review article explores the current directions and the achievements of applying machine learning in the field of computational psychiatry. The review would enable better integration of data-driven and theory-driven research approaches which lead to a better understanding of the research and lead to increased applicability of future Computational Psychiatric research in the clinical practice.

2 Research Method

The field of healthcare and medicine is one of the domains that could have the highest return through the application of machine learning models (Rajkomar et al., 2019). This review article will explore the current directions and the achievements of applying machine learning in the field of computational psychiatry. To fulfil these research objectives, we formulated the following systematic research questions (RQ):

RQ1. What are the current directions in data-driven computational psychiatric research?

RQ2. What are the current directions in theory-driven computational psychiatric research?

RQ3. What approaches have research taken to combine data-driven and theory-driven computational psychiatric research to propose hybrid methods?

RQ4. What research direction should be followed to further bridge the gap between computational psychiatric research and clinical application?

Figure 10.1 provides a high-level classification of literature reviewed in the study. With the research question defined, we initiated a formal strategy to search and analyze available empirical research work that is in line with the

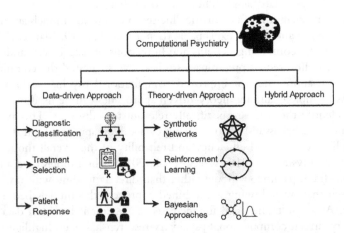

Figure 10.1 High-level classification of computational psychiatric research

research objectives. Prior research (Bennett et al., 2019; Huys et al., 2016) was used as a base to define the search space. Electronic research databases from both Computer Science and Health Care/Medicine such as ACM Digital library, IEEE Xplore, Springer, ScienceDirect, PubMed, etc. were used. The search criteria used for this review were made up of keywords related to computational psychiatric research in conjunction with keywords from the computer science field.

3 Data-driven Approaches

3.1 Data-driven Process

With the availability of clinical data sets, advancement in computation resources and analysis methods, many researchers have opted for data-driven approaches without relying on theoretical-driven hypothesis-based research (Hey et al., 2009; Shih and Chai 2016). A majority of the clinically useful computational psychiatry research has followed the data-driven approach with applications in diagnostic classification, treatment selection and prediction of treatment response as well as understanding relations between symptoms (Huys et al., 2016).

Figure X.2 shows an overall process view of the data-driven approaches. In data-driven approaches, the core intention is to feed the model with available datasets in a theoretically agnostic manner to achieve the highest predictive accuracy as the outcome. However, the output model is a non-interpretable black-box model.

3.2 Diagnostic Classification of Neurological Disorders

The computation psychiatry methods guide the clinical practitioner to make a judgment on the diagnosis. However, the psychiatric disorders show a high level of comorbidity, the case where a patient at times might possess more than a single mental disorder (Meedeniya and Rubasinghe, 2020; Borsboom et al., 2011). As a result, the diagnostic classification of psychiatric diseases uses the machine learning model to handle disorders as a multi-label learning problem, a problem where each example is associated with multiple class labels simultaneously (Zhou and Zhang 2017). Common NDDs such as Alzheimer's disease,

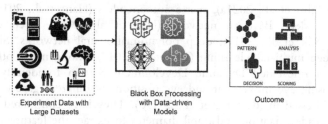

Figure 10.2 Overall process view of the data-driven approaches.

ASD, ADHD, Parkinson's disease, schizophrenia, Obsessive Compulsive Disorder (OCD) are benefited by the recent studies in computational psychiatry, in particular with data analysis and machine learning methods to improve accuracy and reliability of diagnosis, treatment and rehabilitation procedures (Brihadiswaran et al., 2019; de Silva et al., 2019a; Meedeniya and Rubasinghe, 2020).

Many machine learning models have been implemented for psychiatric diagnostic classifications. Examples of classical models are the Support Vector Machines (SVM) in the diagnosis process of psychiatric diseases such as Alzheimer's disease, schizophrenia, major depression, bipolar disorder, presymptomatic Huntington's disease, Parkinson's disease and autistic spectrum disorder (Orru et al., 2012). SVM by far is the most popular method with different varieties of SVM such as linear, non-linear with different kernel and SVM with recursive feature elimination being applied to classify various disorders. In another point of view, Kakkar (2019), has presented an approach to estimate the risk-perception of ASD subjects. This study has used both statistical and SVM techniques to compute neurological performance metrics such as latency and amplitude in the ASD risk-perception estimation process. Moreover, different classification models such as k-nearest neighbor (k-NN), Naive Bayes (NB) (Ebadi et al., 2017; Shao et al., 2012), ensemble methods (Ebadi et al., 2017), random forest (Maggipinto et al., 2017), Binary Gaussian process classifiers (Reinders et al., 2019) and extreme gradient boosting (Dou et al., 2020) are available in the literature.

Neural networks and advanced deep learning models are popular in the diagnostic classification process. The models such as deep belief networks might outperform more standard classification approaches and basic machine learning methods mentioned earlier (Huys et al., 2016). Deep neural networks are effective in capturing higher-order statistical relationships in the context of neuroimaging data that was not possible in shallower neural models (Durstewitz et al., 2019). It has enabled the integration of complementary datasets obtained from multiple brain imaging methods such as functional magnetic resonance imaging (fMRI), structural MRI (sMRI), and positron emission tomography to obtain valuable insights that were otherwise not immediately possible for the clinical practitioners (Durstewitz et al., 2019). Some example scenarios of successful application of deep learning models are the use of fully connected cascaded artificial neural networks (Deshpande et al., 2015), convolutional neural networks (Ariyarathne et al., 2020; de Silva et al., 2021a), sparse autoencoders (Han et al., 2015; Liu et al., 2018), deep Bayesian network (Hao et al., 2015), deep ensemble learning (Suk et al., 2017), deep polynomial neural networks (Shi et al., 2017), deep multi-task learning (Liu et al., 2017) among many others. For instance, a rule-based Dynamic Development System to identify ADHD subjects using eye movement and eye positions of different gaze event type data is addressed in (de Silva et al., 2019b). They have considered the gaze points, saccades, fixation and pupil diameter to extract the features and used decision tree classification.

Another approach to classify fMRI data for ADHD diagnosis support is presented in (Ariyarathne et al., 2020). They have used a seed correlation-based approach to compute the functional connectivity among seeds and brain voxels. The extracted seed correlations from Default Mode Networks (DMN) have been used for the classification process based on Convolution Neural Networks (CNN). This study has identified the most correlated brain areas of ADHD subjects. As an extension, de Silva et al. (2021a) have considered unprocessed fMRI data for ADHD classification using CNN. This study has shown that seed-based correlation gives high classification accuracy values compared to other feature extraction methods such as fALFF and ReHo. They have shown that the neurological disorder classification can be improved by considering different voxels in the brain.

A combination of fMRI and eye movement data has used to support ADHD diagnosis in the tool named ADHD-care (de Silva et al., 2021b). This integrated model has used seed-based correlation in DMN for the feature extraction and CNN for the classification of fMRI data. The aggregated features of fixations and saccades have been used for the feature extraction of eye movement data and ensemble model for the classification. This study is presented in an application named ADHD-Care, which is featured with a rating scale to indicate the severity of ADHD, and can be used as a support tool in clinical practice (ADHD-Care, 2019).

In addition, a generic DSS for neuroimaging data is proposed in (Rubasinghe et al., 2020), to facilitate a single platform for the computational solutions on psychophysiological chronic disorders. Their methodology is based on different pre-processing and learning models applicable to diverse datasets, for better decision making as many neurological disorders share commonalities. The proposed methodology is tested for ADHD with fMRI data using selected classifiers over three types of functional connectivity, as proof of work.

Another DSS named ASDGenus is presented in (Haputhanthri et al., 2019), which has used an EEG based channel optimization classification approach for ASD identification. This study has shown a low-cost approach to diagnosis ASD using a minimum number of EEG channels so that the approach can be easily tested with children. They have applied eye-blink noise filtering and Discrete Wavelet Transform to extract statistical features and a correlation-based approach has been used for feature selection and Random Forest for the classification. As an extension to the previous study, Haputhanthri et al. (2020) have integrated EEG data and thermal imaging data to improve the prediction accuracy of ASD subjects. They have extracted different feature sets and used several learning models such as logistic regression, and multi-layer perceptron algorithms.

3.3 Treatment Selection and Patient Response

Upon classification of the disease, the clinical practitioner is put forward with the issue of treatment selection and the patient's response to the treatment. The clinical practitioner can be assisted to select the appropriate treatment that suits the patient with the problem modelled as a multiclass classification problem (Huys et al., 2016). Also, the ability to predict an individual patient's response to treatment would permit clinicians to have a better understanding of the patient and further plan and modify treatment approach to improve patient outcomes (Huang et al., 2019). However, individual-level personalization of treatment approach and predicting the medication outcome or disease trajectories requires a much deeper understanding of the neurobiological mechanisms of the cognitive and emotional functions of humans across various psychiatric disorders which is much more complicated than disease classification (Koppe et al., 2021).

Although the problem is complex, researchers have made multiple efforts to assist patient treatment selection and treatment response using machine learning with the data-driven approach. For instance, van Loo et al., (2014) used ensemble recursive partitioning and Lasso generalized linear models (GLMs) followed by k-means cluster analysis to predict the variation of the course of depressive disorders. A related study was followed up on patients after 10–12 years of initially reporting to medical assistance on depression to test whether models can accurately predict the reoccurrence of the depression disorder (Kessler et al., 2016). The area under the receiver operating characteristic curve based machine learning models were used, and the results were promising. Further studies have been conducted on predicting the treatment outcome of depression as it has been known that antidepressant treatment efficacy is generally low (Chekroud et al., 2016). The model has identified the top 25 predictors for prediction after the model was fed with all clinical information available.

The use of more advanced machine learning methods has been proposed with the use of neuroimaging data such as Electroencephalography (EEG) data. For example, support vector machines as a classifier have been used to predict the Escitalopram treatment outcome of individuals using EEG data (Zhdanov et al., 2020). EEG data, along with other clinical data, were used with a random forest-based machine learning approach to predict the antidepressant treatment response (Jaworska et al., 2019). Deep learning models using fully connected dense neural networks have also been used for the same problem treatment benefit prediction for treatment selection in depression in recent research which has shown higher accuracies (Mehltretter et al., 2020). However, although the results are promising further continuous research efforts required to strengthen the results. For example, Browning et al. (2020) stress the need for computational assays with improved measurement properties which need to be iteratively optimized and validated continuously in clinically informative studies that would lead to better prediction of treatment outcomes.

3.4 Comparison of Related Studies

A summary of the data types used for data-driven approaches is given in Table 10.1. Data-driven research has predominantly relied on medical imaging datasets, brain signals and clinically collected survey datasets.

Table 10.1 Summary of the data types used in the related studies

Related work	fMRI	MRI	EEG	Radiography	Clinical questionnaires
Ariyarathne et al. (2020)	X				
Han et al. (2015)	X				
Hao et al. (2015)	X				
Rubasinghe et al. (2020)	X				
de Silva et al., (2021b)	X				
Liu et al. (2017)		X			
Reinders et al. (2019)		X			
Dou et al. (2020)		X			
Suk et al. (2017)		X			
Ebadi et al. (2017)		X			
Maggipinto et al. (2017)		X			
Shao et al. (2012)		X			
Zhdanov et al. (2020)			X		
Jaworska et al. (2019)			X		
Haputhanthri et al. (2020)			X		
Zech et al. (2018)				X	
Chekroud et al. (2016)					X
Mehltretter et al. (2020)					X
Kessler et al. (2016)					X
van Loo et al. (2014)					X

Table 10.2 presents the core features, core techniques, and the respective accuracies achieved by data-driven computational psychiatric methods. As observed from the table, the predictive accuracy of a majority of the methods is significantly high. Several techniques have been used in the related literature including SVM, Deep Bayesian Network (DBN), GLM, k-NN, Neural Networks (NN), and CNN.

3.5 Issues with Data-driven Approaches

A major concern with data-driven approaches is the risk taken by healthcare practitioners for relying on theoretically agnostic methods for high-stake healthcare decisions that are traditionally and legally required to drive sound and open judgement (Rudin, 2019). Although data-driven approaches are trained with large datasets, the datasets might not provide comprehensive coverage of the complete

Table 10.2 Summary of the data-driven related work

Related work	Data features	Technique	Accuracy
Ariyarathne et al. (2020)	fMRI features	CNN	85.21%
Han et al. (2015)	fMRI features	Stacked Autoencoders	82.0%
Hao et al. (2015)	fMRI features	DBN	72.7%
Rubasinghe et al. (2020)	fMRI features	SVM, NB, KNN	86.00%
de Silva et al. (2021b)	fMRI features	CNN based ensemble	82.12%
de Silva et al. (2021a)	fMRI features	CNN	85.36%
de Silva et al. (2019b)	Eye movement data	Decision Tree	84.48%
Liu et al. (2017)	Morphological features	CNN	51.8%
Reinders et al. (2019)	Scaler Momentum features	Gaussian Classifier	72.8%
Dou et al. (2020)	Diffusion tensor imaging measures along white matter tracts	SVM	83.7%
Suk et al. (2017)	MRI features	CNN and k-NN based ensemble model	90.3%
Ebadi et al. (2017)	MRI Graph features	CNN and k-NN based ensemble model	83.3%
Maggipinto et al. (2017)	White matter fibre tracts	Random forest	87.0%
Shao et al. (2012)	Brain structural connection network	SVM, k-NN, Naïve Bayes	97.7%
Zhdanov et al. (2020)	EEG signals	SVM	82.4%
Jaworska et al. (2019)	EEG and other clinical data	Random forest	88.0%
Haputhanthri et al., 2020	EEG and thermal images	Logistic Regression	94.00%
Haputhanthri et al. 2019	EEG signals	Random Forest	93.3%
Zech et al. (2018)	Radiographic reports	CNN	99.95%
Chekroud et al. (2016)	Clinical data	Gradient Boost	64.6%
Mehltretter et al. (2020)	Clinical data	NN based	69.0%
Kessler et al. (2016)	Clinical data	NN based	76.0%
van Loo et al. (2014)	Clinical data	GLM	89.0%

set of diseases. This might be the case for rare conditions and diseases in the psychiatry domain which are underrepresented in the datasets. If the datasets do not represent the full set of possible conditions, the models that are trained might be biased leading to incorrect predictions that could misguide the healthcare practitioners (Zech et al., 2018). Another key challenge is the unavailability of representative and large datasets when it comes to training deep learning models, especially in the case of treatment selection and modelling the patient's response (Koppe et al., 2021). A further limitation that needs to be addressed is the need for high computing power with the availability of larger, complex and high dimensional datasets and the increased use of state-of-the-art modelling and simulation techniques on a large scale (Paulus et al., 2016). Also, it has been noted that although no psychiatric application of machine learning currently constitutes standard clinical practice, it is still required to derive proper ethical standards before the applications go mainstream with clinical practice (Starke et al., 2020).

4 Theory-Driven Approaches

4.1 Theory-driven Process

Theory-driven computational psychiatry approaches aim to theoretically explain the underlying model mechanisms of psychiatric illnesses to ensure the models are rigorous, consistent, and quantitatively explainable (Bennett et al., 2019; Maia et al., 2017). The models enable a deeper understanding of the existing psychiatric phenomena and powerful tools for integration with clinical practice (Huys et al., 2016).

Figure 10.3 shows an overall process view of the theory-driven approaches. In these models, the main intuition is to select the independent variables based on an in-depth theoretical analysis of psychiatric literature such that the model can exploit the causal and correlational relationships of independent variables with the outcome variable. As a result, the output models of theory-driven approaches are explainable. These models lead to wider acceptance for clinical application as the models are well-grounded with theory.

Huys et al. (2016) have identified classified theory-driven models as synthetic, algorithmic, and optimal models which are defined as follows. Synthetic models collect data from multiple sources relevant to the disease condition and explore possible interaction effects between these factors through simulations and mathematical analysis with parameters constrained based on scientific literature.

4.2 Synthetic Network Models

As examples of synthetic models, many researchers have explored the relationship between biological abnormalities in the body to behavioral consequences of psychiatric disorders (Mujica-Parodi and Strey, 2020). Each of the research has utilized a parsimonious circuit-based network computational model to identify the interactions between the subsystems of the human body. This networked circuit, for example, integrates neural and psychological frameworks with the systems schematically described with arrows connecting boxes representing the regions associated with different psychological functionality (Mujica-Parodi and Strey, 2020).

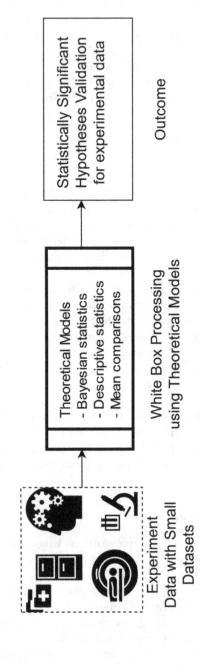

Figure 10.3 Overall process view of the theory-driven approaches

4.3 Reinforcement Learning

It is claimed that reinforcement learning-based mechanisms, architectures, and algorithms developed in recent times have a direct relationship to neural processes in animals (Maia, 2009). Reinforcement learning has been successfully applied to models' multiple psychiatric diseases such as depression (Hamid and Braun 2017; Queirazza et al., 2019; Rothkirch et al., 2017). It also has been noted that the main challenge of the current method of using a theoretical approach to define the states. States defined under laboratory conditions are tractable, but in the real world, the states are continuous and partially observable causing concerns on effective learning and generalization (Hamid and Braun, 2017).

5 Hybrid Approaches

5.1 Hybrid Process

The majority of the studies that have produced clinically useful applications have been theoretically agnostic ML approaches (Huys et al., 2016). However, as noted earlier theoretically driven models will have higher acceptance in the clinical practice as the models are more interpretable. Owing to the limitations of both theory-driven and data-driven approaches, hybrid approaches that combine both theory-driven and data-driven approaches can be advantageous in clinical applications (Huys et al., 2016).

Figure 10.4 shows an overall process view of the hybrid approaches. The first step in hybrid models is to identify theoretically backed independent variables that are directly related to the outcome variable. In the second step, filtered independent variables are applied with data-driven models. As a result, issues that arise owing to the curse of dimensionality can be avoided in hybrid models (Huys et al., 2016). Also, powerful deep learning models enable the extraction of complex non-linear relationships of the data for higher predictive accuracy.

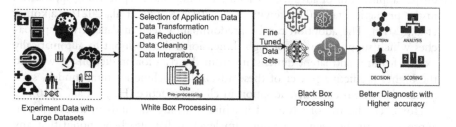

Figure 10.4 Overall process view of hybrid approaches

5.1 Related Studies with Hybrid Approach

Multiple research studies have progressed in this direction in recent times (Brodersen et al., 2014; Frank et al., 2015; Wiecki et al., 2016; Wiecki et al., 2015). Although the studies are at a preliminary stage or a proof of concept stage, the results show a promising direction where overall prediction and classification accuracies have significantly improved.

In a similar direction, a quantitative model was proposed by Puviani and Rama (2016) that lead to the theoretical understanding and derivation of the laws that govern the origin and the dynamics of the placebo response. In addition, Cornblath et al. (2019) show that incorporating theory-driven network modelling in the field of neuroscience with machine learning has led to interpretable results with wider clinical applications. The authors also propose a framework to maximize the transferability of future neuroimaging studies to clinical applications. In a similar direction, Lydon-Staley et al. (2021) demonstrated the advanced capabilities of modelling the brain by aligning theory and assumptions implicit in the analytical clinical approaches with recent advances in machine learning-based model building. Further recent research has also been conducted where theory and hypothesis-driven statistical analysis methods have been first applied to the data before classifying using SVMs resulting in high prediction accuracies (Kakkar, 2019). Introducing another possible direction to hybrid approaches, Krystal et al. (2017) propose discovery-oriented computational psychiatry approaches where machine learning methods are first applied to complex datasets and formalize theories based on the obtained results upon thorough analysis.

6 Discussion

6.1 Current State of Computational Psychiatric Research

In this study, we briefly reviewed the computational psychiatric research segmented as data-driven, theory-driven and hybrid approaches which were the classification followed by Huys et al. (2016). It could be observed that the computational psychiatry research domain has seen multiple innovations with deeper applications of advanced machine learning and deep learning approaches in the prediction tasks (Durstewitz et al., 2019; Koppe et al., 2021; Rajkomar et al., 2019). The adoption can be predominantly seen in data-driven approaches which support the use of high dimensional data as input to automatically extract features and latent dimensions from the data for predictions. Owing to the higher predictive power of these advanced machine learning models, such models have seen extended adoption in clinical practice (Huys et al., 2016).

However, the use of advanced machine learning methods in theory-driven approaches can be seen at a minimum level. It has also been noted that any attempt to interpret black-box type models could perpetuate bad practices and can potentially cause catastrophic outcomes in the healthcare domain (Rudin,

2019). This comes at a cost where theory-driven models have to rely on traditional machine learning approaches such as Bayesian models or regression that have significantly low non-linear modelling capabilities when compared to deeper neural network-based models (Wetzel, 2017). Also, theory-driven approaches inherently require deeper knowledge on the domain expertise in the fields of neuroscience, psychology, and psychiatry. The theory-driven models are predominantly proposed by professionals in these fields. Such professionals might lack the exposure and knowledge on state-of-the-art machine learning research and rely on less advanced and classical machine learning approaches that have less predictive power. As a result, it has been noted that theory-driven approaches have far less clinical application when compared with data-driven approaches (Huys et al., 2016).

Further, the processing of medical data undergoes several challenges when enhanced with technological developments. For example, it is difficult to collect a large set of medial and health care data, owing to the associated ethical consents (Brihadiswaran et al., 2019) (Meedeniya and Rubasinghe, 2020).

6.2 Future Directions

One of the possible research directions is to incorporate several data types for the diagnosis process of computational psychiatry. Other than the questioner based clinical data and medical image scans, it is possible to use gene sequence analysis based on genomics and radiomics sequences to analyze the brain condition (Wijethilake et al., 2020a, Wijethilake et al., 2020b). Moreover, the review presented by Bracher-Smith et al. (2020), have explored the use of genetics to predict psychiatric disorders using learning approaches. Therefore, there are possible directions to analyze gene sequences as well for computational psychiatry research in data-driven approaches.

Moreover, generally, medical image analysis requires high computational power and consumes more time to train deep learning models. It is important to allocate powerful computer resources and assess the possibility of implementing the classification algorithms in parallel (Rajapaksa et al., 2019). Hence, Graphics Processing Unit-based acceleration can be used to speed up the biological computations (Welivita et al., 2017; Welivita et al., 2018). Moreover, the storage and management issues related to big data analytics can be resolved by carefully designed software architectures and engines (Wadhera et al., 2020). Thus, the research of design architectures for the medical image classifications and predictions would increase the processing speed.

Developing a generic framework to classify and predict NDDs is a promising future research area (Rubasinghe and Meedeniya, 2020). The accuracy and performance of such computational DSSs can be improved by applying different deep learning models with parameter tuning and optimizers (Brihadiswaran et al., 2019) (Meedeniya and Rubasinghe, 2020). Also, these medical image data can be classified by integrating both deep learning and probabilistic programming to generate better results (Rubasinghe and Meedeniya, 2019).

Although data-driven approaches have higher prediction accuracy and wider clinical acceptance, extensive application of the models are limited owing to the lack of explanation which is a prime requirement in the medical field since medical diagnosis should be comprehensively justified (Itani et al., 2019). Also, the interpretability of the model leads to a better understanding of the disorder (Maia et al., 2017). A constructive approach that can bridge the gap between data-driven and theoretical approaches as well as to value both the methods is adopting the hybrid approach, where data-driven and theory-driven approaches are used in conjunction (Bennett et al., 2019; Huys et al., 2016).

As evident from our review as well as prior reviews (Huys et al., 2016), the amount of hybrid computational psychiatry research is at the initial stages with minimal attempt. Most of the studies are at the proof-of-concept stage but have shown powerful and promising predictive results (Bennett et al., 2019; Gillan and Whelan 2017; Huys et al., 2016; (de Silva et al., 2021b; Haputhanthri et al., 2020). Their combination of the approaches has been identified to have the potential of improving prognostic accuracy, treatment response prediction, treatment selection, repurposing and monitoring to a greater extent in the field of computational psychiatry (Huys, 2018).

As a result, it is required to further explore computational psychiatry research following a hybrid approach. As noted earlier, computational psychiatry is an interdisciplinary field with contributions from computer science, neuroscience, psychology, and psychiatry (Huys, 2018). Hybrid computational psychiatry will require increased collaborations among these disciplinaries (Gillan and Whelan, 2017). Research collaborations with researchers from neuroscience, psychology and psychiatry will enable the researchers from the computer science domain to better understand the problem as well eliminate the curse of dimensionality issues through the guided selection of independent variables and input data sources (Huys et al., 2016). Also, researchers could explore the use of interpretable deep learning models such that the model output is interpretable (Zhang et al., 2020). Besides, frameworks and tools that support big data management will support the deployment of computational psychiatry research in clinical practice (Wadhera and Kakkar, 2020).

Conclusion

Computational psychiatry has marked its significance in the field of NDD diagnosis and treatment in the recent past. However, as noted above and reported by many, the application of the advancements in the body of knowledge of NDDs in clinical practices have been challenging and have not been translated to the same level of efficacy in clinical use. To explore this disparity in the applied domain and to propose viable enhancements to the current practices this research has formulated a set of research questions as the foundation for the systematic review presented as the outcome. In essence, it is noted that the current directions in computational psychiatry can be further refined into three categories: data-driven approaches, theory-driven approaches, and hybrid approaches.

To answer the query on the current directions in data-driven computational psychiatric research (RQ1) it was revealed that the mainstream orientation has been to incorporate deep learning techniques with larger datasets to build predictive models with higher accuracies and reliability. In contrast, it is apparent that the theory-driven approaches, which initially dominated the computational psychiatric analysis has come to saturation and does not indicate any viable direction or method incorporation for enhancing the current practices (RQ2). This is observed as the used theoretical approaches are fundamental in nature and any possibility to improve the analysis results is limited to obtaining better clinical data in larger quantities. However, it is also noted that such an attempt will not be able to outperform the results of data-driven methods since those are implicitly specialized to work with datasets.

Finally, to recommend approaches to combine data-driven and theory-driven computational psychiatric research to propose hybrid methods (RQ3), it is obvious that the preprocessing of larger datasets to fit with clinical parameters and neurodevelopment domain constraints from theoretical approaches so that quality enhanced and fine-tuned dataset can be used for deep learning models will yield in promising results with higher accuracies and better predictive models. Finally (RQ4), to bridge the gap between computational psychiatric research and clinical application can be identified, in line with the recent research trends into the machine intelligence research frontier. The use of unsupervised learning methods in computational psychiatry can help to improve the analysis results and be closer to the clinical practices threshold levels.

One of the main challenges with current data-driven practices is the isolated datasets limiting the model generalizability. At the same time, clinical datasets require a higher degree of data privacy preservation and access control; therefore the recently introduced federated learning frameworks can help to share the right amount of clinical data without exposing the sensitive information and enable data-driven computational psychiatry analysis in clinical practices with higher generalizability.

References

Ariyarathne, G., De Silva, S., Dayarathna, S., Meedeniya, D., and Jayarathne, S. 2020. "ADHD Identification Using Convolutional Neural Network with Seed-Based Approach for fMRI Data." Proceedings of the 9th International Conference on Software and Computer Applications, pp. 31–35.

Bennett, D., Silverstein, S. M., and Niv, Y. (2019). "*The Two Cultures of Computational Psychiatry.*" *JAMA Psychiatry*, 76(6): 563–564.

Borsboom, D., Cramer, A. O., Schmittmann, V. D., Epskamp, S., and Waldorp, L. J. (2011). "*The Small World of Psychopathology.*" *PloS one* 6(11): e27407.

Bracher-Smith, M., Crawford, K., and Escott-Price, V. (2020). "Machine learning for genetic prediction of psychiatric disorders: a systematic review." *Molecular Psychiatry*.

Brihadiswaran, G., Haputhanthri, D., Gunathilaka, S., Meedeniya, D., and Jayarathna, S. 2019. "*EEG-based processing and classification methodologies for Autism Spectrum Disorder: A Review.*" *Journal of Computer Science*, 15(8): 1161–1183.

Brodersen, K. H.et al. (2014). "Dissecting Psychiatric Spectrum Disorders by Generative Embedding." *NeuroImage: Clinical*, 4: 98–111.

Browning, M. et al. (2020). "Realizing the Clinical Potential of Computational Psychiatry: Report from the Banbury Center Meeting, February 2019." *Biological Psychiatry*, 88:(2): e5–e10.

Chekroud, A. M.et al. (2016). "Cross-Trial Prediction of Treatment Outcome in Depression: A Machine Learning Approach." *The Lancet Psychiatry* 3:(3): 243–250.

Cornblath, E. J., Lydon-Staley, D. M., and Bassett, D. S. 2019. "Harnessing Networks and Machine Learning in Neuropsychiatric Care." *Current Opinion in Neurobiology*, (55): 32–39.

Deshpande, G., Wang, P., Rangaprakash, D., and Wilamowski, B. (2015). "Fully Connected Cascade Artificial Neural Network Architecture for Attention Deficit Hyperactivity Disorder Classification from Functional Magnetic Resonance Imaging Data." *IEEE Transactions on Cybernetics*, 45(12): 2668–2679.

de Silva, S., Dayarathna, S., Ariyarathne, G., Meedeniya, D., and Jayarathna, S. (2019a). "A Survey of Attention Deficit Hyperactivity Disorder Identification Using Psychophysiological Data." *International Journal of Online and Biomedical Engineering*, 15:(13): 61–76.

de Silva, S. et al. (2019b). "A Rule-Based System for ADHD Identification using Eye Movement Data." In: Proceedings of the International Multidisciplinary Engineering Research Conference (MerCon), pp. 538–543, IEEE.

de Silva, S., Dayarathna, S., Ariyarathne, G., Meedeniya, D., and Jayarathna, S. (2021). "fMRI Feature Extraction Model for ADHD Classification Using Convolutional Neural Network." *International Journal of E-Health and Medical Communications*, 12(1): 81–105.

de Silva, S., Dayarathna, S., Ariyarathne, G., Meedeniya, D., Jayarathna, S. and Michalek, A. M. P., 2021. "Computational Decision Support System for ADHD Identification." *International Journal of Automation and Computing*, 18(2): 233–255.

Dou, X.et al. (2020). *Characterizing White Matter Connectivity in Alzheimer's Disease and Mild Cognitive Impairment: An Automated Fiber Quantification Analysis with Two Independent Datasets.* Cortex.

Durstewitz, D., Koppe, G., and Meyer-Lindenberg, A. (2019). "Deep Neural Networks in Psychiatry." *Molecular Psychiatry*, 24(11): 1583–1598.

Ebadi, A. et al. (2017). "Ensemble Classification of Alzheimer's Disease and Mild Cognitive Impairment Based on Complex Graph Measures from Diffusion Tensor Images." *Frontiers in Neuroscience* (11): 56.

Ferrante, M., Redish, A. D., Oquendo, M. A., Averbeck, B. B., Kinnane, M. E., and Gordon, J. A. (2019). "Computational Psychiatry: A Report from the 2017 Nimh Workshop on Opportunities and Challenges." *Molecular Psychiatry*, 24(4): 479.

Frank, M. J., Gagne, C., Nyhus, E., Masters, S., Wiecki, T. V., Cavanagh, J. F., and Badre, D. (2015). "fMRI and EEG Predictors of Dynamic Decision Parameters During Human Reinforcement Learning." *Journal of Neuroscience*, 35(2): 485–494.

Gillan, C. M. and Whelan, R. (2017). "What Big Data Can Do for Treatment in Psychiatry." *Current Opinion in Behavioral Sciences*, (18): 34–42.

Hamid, O. H. and Braun, J. (2017). "Reinforcement Learning and Attractor Neural Network Models of Associative Learning." International Joint Conference on Computational Intelligence. Springer, pp. 327–349.

Han, X., Zhong, Y., He, L., Philip, S. Y., and Zhang, L. (2015). "The Unsupervised Hierarchical Convolutional Sparse Auto-Encoder for Neuroimaging Data Classification." International Conference on Brain Informatics and Health. Springer, pp. 156–166.

Hao, A. J., He, B. L., and Yin, C. H. (2015). "Discrimination of ADHD Children Based on Deep Bayesian Network." In: Proceedings of the IET International Conference on Biomedical Image and Signal Processing, Beijing, pp. 1–6.

Haputhanthri, D., Brihadiswaran, G., Gunathilaka, S., Meedeniya, D., Jayarathna, S., Jaime, M., and Jayawardena, Y. (2019). "An EEG based Channel Optimized Classification Approach for Autism Spectrum Disorder." In Proceedings of the International Multidisciplinary Engineering Research Conference (Mercon), pp. 123–128, IEEE.

Haputhanthri, D. et al. (2020). "Integration of Facial Thermography in EEG-based Classification of ASD." *International Journal of Automation and Computing*, 17(6): 837–854.

Hey, T., Tansley, S., and Tolle, K. (2009). *The Fourth Paradigm: Data-Intensive Scientific Discovery*. Redmond, WA: Microsoft Research.

Huang, X., Gong, Q., Sweeney, J. A., and Biswal, B. B. (2019). "Progress in Psychoradiology, the Clinical Application of Psychiatric Neuroimaging." *The British Journal of Radiology*, 92(1101): 20181000.

Huys, Q. J., Maia, T. V., and Frank, M. J. (2016). "Computational Psychiatry as a Bridge from Neuroscience to Clinical Applications." *Nature Neuroscience*, 19(3): 404.

Itani, S., Rossignol, M., Lecron, F., and Fortemps, P. (2019). "Towards Interpretable Machine Learning Models for Diagnosis Aid: A Case Study on Attention-Deficit/Hyperactivity Disorder." *PloS one*, 14(4): e0215720.

Jaworska, N., de la Salle, S., Ibrahim, M.-H., Blier, P., and Knott, V. (2019). "Leveraging Machine Learning Approaches for Predicting Antidepressant Treatment Response Using Electroencephalography (Eeg) and Clinical Data." *Frontiers in Psychiatry* (9); 768.

Kakkar, D. (2019). "Automatic Detection of Autism Spectrum Disorder by Tracing the Disorder Co-Morbidities." 9th Annual Information Technology, Electromechanical Engineering and Microelectronics Conference: IEEE, pp. 132–136.

Kessler, R. C. et al. (2016). "Testing a Machine-Learning Algorithm to Predict the Persistence and Severity of Major Depressive Disorder from Baseline Self-Reports." *Molecular Psychiatry*, 21(10): 1366–1371.

Koppe, G., Meyer-Lindenberg, A., and Durstewitz, D. (2021). "*Deep Learning for Small and Big Data in Psychiatry.*" *Neuropsychopharmacology*, 46(1): 176–190.

Krystal, J. H. et al. (2017). *Computational Psychiatry and the Challenge of Schizophrenia*. New York, NY: Oxford University Press.

Liu, J., Pan, Y., Li, M., Chen, Z., Tang, L., Lu, C., and Wang, J. (2018). "Applications of Deep Learning to Mri Images: A Survey." *Big Data Mining and Analytics*, 1(1): 1–18.

Liu, M., Zhang, J., Adeli, E., and Shen, D. (2017). "Deep Multi-Task Multi-Channel Learning for Joint Classification and Regression of Brain Status." International conference on medical image computing and computer-assisted intervention. Springer, pp. 3–11.

Lydon-Staley, D. M., Cornblath, E. J., Blevins, A. S., and Bassett, D. S. (2021). "Modeling Brain, Symptom, and Behavior in the Winds of Change." *Neuropsychopharmacology*, 46(1): 20–32.

Maggipinto, T. et al. and Alzheimer's Disease Neuroimaging Initiative (2017). "Dti Measurements for Alzheimer's Classification." *Physics in Medicine & Biology*, 62(6): 2361.

Maia, T. V. (2009). "Reinforcement Learning, Conditioning, and the Brain: Successes and Challenges." *Cognitive, Affective, & Behavioral Neuroscience*, 9(4): 343–364.

Maia, T. V., Huys, Q. J., and Frank, M. J. (2017). "Theory-Based Computational Psychiatry." *Biological Psychiatry*, 82(6): 382–384.

Meedeniya, D. A. and Rubasinghe, I. D. (2020). "A Review of Supportive Computational Approaches for Neurological Disorder Identification." In: T. Wadhera and D.

Kakkar (Eds), *Interdisciplinary Approaches to Altering Neurodevelopmental Disorders*, pp. 271–302. IGI Global.

Mehltretter, J.et al. (2020). "Differential Treatment Benefit Prediction for Treatment Selection in Depression: A Deep Learning Analysis of Star★ D and Co-Med Data." *Computational Psychiatry*, (4): 61–75.

Mujica-Parodi, L. R. and Strey, H. H. (2020). "Making Sense of Computational Psychiatry." *International Journal of Neuropsychopharmacology*, 23(5): 339–347.

Orru, G., Pettersson-Yeo, W., Marquand, A. F., Sartori, G., and Mechelli, A. (2012). "Using Support Vector Machine to Identify Imaging Biomarkers of Neurological and Psychiatric Disease: A Critical Review." *Neuroscience & Biobehavioral Reviews*, 36(4): 1140–1152.

Paulus, M. P., Huys, Q. J., and Maia, T. V. (2016). "A Roadmap for the Development of Applied Computational Psychiatry." *Biological Psychiatry: Cognitive Neuroscience and Neuroimaging*, 1(5): 386–392.

Puviani, L. and Rama, S. (2016). "Placebo Response Is Driven by Ucs Revaluation: Evidence, Neurophysiological Consequences and a Quantitative Model." Scientific reports, 6(1): 1–16.

Queirazza, F., Fouragnan, E., Steele, J. D., Cavanagh, J., and Philiastides, M. G. (2019). "Neural Correlates of Weighted Reward Prediction Error During Reinforcement Learning Classify Response to Cognitive Behavioral Therapy in Depression." *Science Advances*, 5(7): eaav4962.

Rajapaksa, S., Rasanjana, W., Perera, I., and Meedeniya, D. (2019). *GPU Accelerated Maximum Likelihood Analysis for Phylogenetic Inference*, In Proceedings of the 8th International Conference on Software and Computer Applications (ICSCA 2019), ACM, New York, USA, pp. 6–10.

Rajkomar, A., Dean, J., and Kohane, I. (2019). "Machine Learning in Medicine." *New England Journal of Medicine*, 380(14): 1347–1358.

Reinders, A. A. et al. (2019). "Aiding the Diagnosis of Dissociative Identity Disorder: Pattern Recognition Study of Brain Biomarkers." *The British Journal of Psychiatry*, 215 (3): 536–544.

Rothkirch, M., Tonn, J., Köhler, S., and Sterzer, P. (2017). "Neural Mechanisms of Reinforcement Learning in Unmedicated Patients with Major Depressive Disorder." *Brain*, 140(4): 1147–1157.

Rubasinghe, I. D. and Meedeniya, D. A. (2019). "Ultrasound Nerve Segmentation Using Deep Probabilistic Programming." *Journal of ICT Research and Applications*, 13 (3): 241–256.

Rubasinghe, I. D. and Meedeniya, D. A. (2020). "Automated Neuroscience Decision Support Framework." In: B. Agarwal (Ed.), *Deep Learning Techniques for Biomedical and Health Informatics*, pp. 305–326. Elsevier Academic Press.

Rudin, C. (2019). "Stop Explaining Black Box Machine Learning Models for High Stakes Decisions and Use Interpretable Models Instead." *Nature Machine Intelligence*, 1 (5): 206–215.

Series, P. (2020). *Computational Psychiatry: A Primer*. MIT Press.

Shao, J.et al. (2012). "Prediction of Alzheimer's Disease Using Individual Structural Connectivity Networks." *Neurobiology of Ageing*, 33(12): 2756–2765.

Shi, J., Zheng, X., Li, Y., Zhang, Q., and Ying, S. (2017). "Multimodal Neuroimaging Feature Learning with Multimodal Stacked Deep Polynomial Networks for Diagnosis of Alzheimer's Disease." *IEEE Journal of Biomedical and Health Informatics*, 22(1): 173–183.

Shih, W. and Chai, S. (2016). "Data-Driven Vs. Hypothesis-Driven Research: Making Sense of Big Data." *Academy of Management Proceedings*. Briarcliff Manor, NY: Academy of Management, p. 14843.

Starke, G., De Clercq, E., Borgwardt, S., and Elger, B. S. (2020). "Computing Schizophrenia: Ethical Challenges for Machine Learning in Psychiatry." *Psychological Medicine*, 1–7.

Suk, H.-I., Lee, S.-W., Shen, D., and Alzheimer's Disease Neuroimaging Initiative. (2017). "Deep Ensemble Learning of Sparse Regression Models for Brain Disease Diagnosis." *Medical Image Analysis*, (37): 101–113.

Thapar, A., Cooper, M., and Rutter, M. (2017). "Neurodevelopmental Disorders." *The Lancet Psychiatry*, 4(4): 339–346.

van Loo, H. M.et al. (2014). "Major Depressive Disorder Subtypes to Predict Long-Term Course." *Depression and Anxiety*, 31(9): 765–777.

Wadhera, T. and Kakkar, D. (2020). "Big Data-Based System: A Supportive Tool in Autism Spectrum Disorder Analysis." In: *Interdisciplinary Approaches to Altering Neurodevelopmental Disorders*. IGI Global, pp. 303–319.

Welivita, A., Perera, I., and Meedeniya, D. (2017). "An Interactive Workflow Generator to Support Bioinformatics Analysis through GPU Acceleration." In: Proceedings of the IEEE International Conference on Bioinformatics and Biomedicine, IEEE Xplore, Kansas City, MO, USA, pp. 457–462.

Welivita, A., Perera, I., Meedeniya, D., Wickramarachchi, A., and Mallawaarachchi, V. (2018). "Managing Complex Workflows in Bioinformatics - An Interactive Toolkit with GPU Acceleration." *IEEE Transactions on NanoBioscience*, 17(3): 199–208.

Wetzel, S. J. (2017). "Unsupervised Learning of Phase Transitions: From Principal Component Analysis to Variational Autoencoders." *Physical Review E*, 96(2): 022140.

Wiecki, T. V.et al. (2016). "A Computational Cognitive Biomarker for Early-Stage Huntington's Disease." *PLoS One*, 11(2): e0148409.

Wiecki, T. V., Poland, J., and Frank, M. J. (2015). "Model-Based Cognitive Neuroscience Approaches to Computational Psychiatry: Clustering and Classification." *Clinical Psychological Science*, 3(3): 378–399.

Wijethilake, N., Islam, M., Meedeniya, D., Chitraranjan, C., Perera, I., and Ren, H. (2020a). "Radiogenomics of Glioblastoma: Identification of Radiomics associated with Molecular Subtypes." In: Kia, S. M. et al. (Eds), *Machine Learning in Clinical Neuroimaging and Radiogenomics in Neuro-oncology*, vol. 12449. Cham: Springer: Cham, pp. 229–239.

Wijethilake, N., Meedeniya, D., Chitraranjan, C., and Perera, I. (2020b). "Survival prediction and risk estimation of Glioma patients using mRNA expressions." In: Proceedings of the 20th IEEE Conference on Bioinformatics and Bioengineering, USA, pp. 35–42.

Zech, J. R. et al. (2018). "Variable Generalization Performance of a Deep Learning Model to Detect Pneumonia in Chest Radiographs: A Cross-Sectional Study." *PLoS Medicine*, 15(11): e1002683.

Zhang, X., Wang, N., Shen, H., Ji, S., Luo, X., and Wang, T. (2020). "Interpretable Deep Learning under Fire," 29th USENIX Security Symposium (USENIX Security 20).

Zhdanov, A.et al. (2020). "Use of Machine Learning for Predicting Escitalopram Treatment Outcome from Electroencephalography Recordings in Adult Patients with Depression." *JAMA network open*, 3(1): e1918377–e1918377.

Zhou, Z.-H. and Zhang, M.-L. (2017). "Multi-Label Learning." In: Sammut, C. and Webb, G. I. (Eds) *Encyclopedia of Machine Learning and Data Mining*. Boston, MA: Springer.

11 Alzheimer's Disease Diagnosis using Functional and Structural Neuroimaging Modalities

S. De Silva, S. Dayarathna and D. Meedeniya

1 Introduction

1.1 Alzheimer's Disease

Healthcare informatics is an interdisciplinary subject where computer science, information technology, and medical data are amalgamated. There are several branches of this interdisciplinary study which include pathology informatics, imaging informatics, medical informatics, and bioinformatics. Computational algorithms are used intensively in each of these areas to provide reliable, efficient, and effective solutions in medical treatments. Currently, there is a tendency to use Decision Support Systems (DSS) based on deep learning and computer vision techniques as computer-aided diagnosis models to support different neurological disorder diagnosis processes (Basaia et al., 2019; Kruthika et al., 2019; Meedeniya and Rubasinghe, 2020; Wadhera and Kakkar, 2020a).

Alzheimer's disease (AD) is a common neurological disorder among adults around and over 65 years of age. Although the pathology of this disorder is not defined well, more than 60% of dementia conditions are caused by AD. According to the *World Alzheimer's Disease Report* (Prince, 2015), the incidence of AD will grow by 226% by 2050 and will spike especially in South East Asia. Therefore, the study on the AD diagnosis process is an important research direction.

The most notable symptoms of AD include memory loss, gradual decaying of mundane task performance, loss of coordination, and the inability to differentiate between similar objects. This neurodegenerative disease has several progressive stages, where significant changes in the brain occur starting with mild cognitive impairment (MCI), mild, then moderate to severe symptoms of AD (Alberdi et al., 2016). AD's progression as a chronic disease could cause the death of brain cells by the decomposition of plaques created by the Amyloid-beta component. This decomposition causes dysfunction of nerve cells and synapses which results in cell death and ultimately brain shrinkage. Hence early detection and identification of AD are vital to start medical intervention early and reduce the progression of the disease and associated catastrophic conditions.

DOI: 10.4324/9781003165569-11

1.2 Overview of Technology-Enabled Disorder Diagnosis

Neuroimaging data such as Magnetic Resonance Imaging (MRI) and Positron Emission Tomography (PET) scans have been successfully applied to the study of the neurological pathology of fatal diseases like AD (Liu et al. 2018; Basaia et al., 2019). MRI focuses on the study of brain atrophy found in the medial temporal lobe, and PET images focus on the cerebrospinal fluid in the brain. These measures are used to study different aspects of the disease, including the early transitional stage of MCI, disease progression, and classification between AD, MCI, and healthy controls.

Several studies have focussed on the anatomical differences in the brain using the structural MRI (sMRI) data, where the combination of different modalities in neuroimaging would add a new perspective to AD's pathology discovery (Basaia et al., 2019; Liu et al., 2018). Hence, to assist the current usage of sMRI data along with PET images, an amalgamation of different modalities has the potential to develop a novel dimension and build upon it. Therefore, there is a major requirement to generate an objective biological model to classify AD by incorporating structural and functional aspects alike as different modalities in the classification process. Furthermore, the functional connectivity of the brain has studied in other neurological disorders such as autism spectrum disorder (ASD) (Wadhera and Kakkar, 2020b).

1.3 Motivation for the Study

As the pathology of AD is not well defined yet, it is important to research a feasible solution by considering different modalities that cover functional and structural aspects alike. It will be beneficial in the diagnosis process of AD from healthy subjects and to study the patterns in AD progression over time. This will provide precise mechanisms for early detection and prevent severe impacts on adults' lives. As a solution, this chapter explores and proposes a computational model to classify MRI and PET data for the diagnosis of AD. We consider three main deep learning models, namely Capsule neural networks (CapsNets), Dense Net, and Inception V3, and we present the model with the optimal results.

This chapter explores the literature on MRI and PET modalities and associated applications and contributions in AD pathology discovery. The main contribution of this research focuses on neural Inception V3 network architecture, which is described both in theoretical and practical aspects.

2 Technology Enhanced Alzheimer's Disease Diagnosis

2.1 Neuroimaging Data Types for Alzheimer's Disease Diagnosis

2.1.1 Magnetic Resonance Imaging

Magnetic Resonance Imaging (MRI) is a common brain imaging technique that visualizes and examines the anatomy of the brain. Different brain pathological conditions can be identified using MRI images by focusing on abnormalities in brain areas for various neurological aspects (Basaia et al., 2019). MRI represents the interaction between the nuclei of hydrogen atoms in biological tissues. These images can be converted to 3-D brain images in focused areas (Lama et al., 2017, 2018). MRI images are used to detect various brain conditions including structural abnormalities and other neurological chronic diseases (Basaia et al., 2019). Thus, MRI-related experiments are becoming one of the key observations in mental healthcare.

Many studies have focused on using sMRI, where the anatomical differentiation is studied non-invasively for the classification between healthy and AD subjects and to identify the progression of AD (Lin et al., 2018; Lama et al., 2017; Basaia et al., 2019). However, the actual cause of this neurodegenerative disorder can be further studied by the neural activity demonstrated by functional neuroimaging. Hence functional MRI (fMRI) is an ideal way to explore the hidden pathology and patterns in neural activity of these AD subjects. The fMRI images are a presentation of the blood oxygen levels in brain regions referred to as BOLD signals, where it is an underlying representation of the neural activity.

2.1.2 Positron Emission Tomography Scan

Positron Emission Tomography (PET) scan is a test based on imaging data to identify and visualize the functionalities of different human organs and tissues. It uses radioactive tracers to detect the changes in the cellular level. This tracer can either be injected, inhaled, or swallowed, and the special detecting devices are used to identify the higher chemically activated areas corresponding to various diseases using radioactive emissions from the tracer (Gupta et al., 2019). Importantly, PET scans detect cellular level changes in the early stages compared with Computed Tomography (CT) scans and MRI.

As a functional neuroimaging technique, PET scans have been widely used in the field of diagnosis of neurodegenerative diseases. The multidisciplinary combination of machine learning algorithms with the PET scan images is used for early diagnosis and monitoring disease progress (Liu et al., 2018). PET is a nuclear medicine procedure where the metabolic activity of the body cell tissues is measured. This powerful functional imaging technique has been used with different variations of the dosages and has successfully extracted the significant feature maps, following different feature extraction techniques such as return on investment-based and voxel-wise intensity (Liu et al., 2018; Lu et al., 2015).

2.2 Deep Learning Techniques

Deep learning-based algorithms support improving classification accuracy and avoid overfitting compared with machine learning techniques. Convolutional neural networks (CNN) have become a mainstream deep learning technique for object detection and image classification. However, these architectures have mainly focussed on the object existence, hence not considered object localization. Furthermore, the segmentation task becomes complex with the overlapping objects and has low 3-D viewpoint variations. In order to improve performance, CNN architectures introduce more residual layers between the near layers, considering rotational relationships in images. The state-of-the-art neural network architectures such as ImageNet (Deng et al., 2009), DenseNet (Huang et al., 2017), Visual Geometry Group (Simonyan and Zisserman, 2014), and Residual Neural Network (ResNet) have been designed to rely on the convolutional and max-pooling layers, where most of the important information is lost, owing to the dimensionality reduction. In addition, CapsNets were introduced to address the inadequacies of the conventional Artificial Neural Network (ANN) architectures (Sabour et al., 2017).

In this study, the neural network architectures of DenseNet, CapsuleNet, and Inception V3 have been used to compare the model performing results and to identify the most effective model in identifying AD. DenseNet architecture is known for its wide range of applications with neuroimaging (Huang et al. 2017), and Inception V3 is a novel architecture that differs from DenseNet in-terms of the layering (Szegedy et al. 2016) and CapsNets is a novel architecture that has developed the ability to reconstruct the results and produced state-of-the-art results (Sabour et al. 2017) in neuroimaging applications.

2.2.1 Capsule Neural Network

A Capsule neural network (CapsNet) is an ANN with a hierarchical layout, hence in effect representing biological neural relationships (Sabour et al., 2017). The capsules are considered as modules in the brain. CapsNets model relationships among entities and improve learning viewpoint invariants with a reduced set of parameters. Thus, CapsNets have shown state-of-the-art performances in object segmentation in medical images. They use dynamic routing algorithms to identify object features such as orientation, texture, size, and position.

The capsules perform computations on the inputs, representing a nested neural network in each capsule. They convert the results into a vector, which gives a highly informative output, hence does not pass individual neuron activations among layers. Therefore, the vector-based capsules can be replaced by the scalar-based artificial neurons. The length of the output vector of a capsule is used to derive the probability of feature detection, and the direction of the vector length gives the state s_j of the feature such as scale, pose, and location. When a feature moves across an image, the vector length stays stable, and only the direction changes.

The derivation of the prediction vector, $\hat{u}_{j|i}$, is given in Equation 1, where u_i is the pose vector, and W_{ij} is the matrix that translates the rotated vector u_i. Equation 2 gives the calculation of the state s_j in the next higher level as the weighted sum of the matrix multiplication of the output vector, which is the prediction vector from the lower layer. The coupling coefficients define the activation routing between a capsule and all potential parent capsules in the next layer and sum to 1. Here, c_{ij} is the coupling coefficient between the state s_j, and the corresponding lower-level capsule is s_i, hence $\Sigma_i \, c_{ij} \, \hat{u}_{j|i}$ is the sum of the predictions from all capsules in the lower layer. It should be noted that the capsules in the first layer derive from the activation based on the output of the previous convolution layer, hence they do not contain a coupling coefficient.

$$\hat{u}_{j|i} = W_{ij} \, u_i \tag{1}$$

$$s_j = \sum{}_i \, c_{ij} \, \hat{u}_{j|i} \tag{2}$$

Here, the capsule s_j predicts the output of all capsules in the following layer, using its output vector and the coupling coefficient. Hence, it does not directly pass the output vector to all other capsules in the next layer. Instead, the output is forwarded only to the capsule with the largest predicted vector output. Thus, the output prediction of the next layer gets the most fitting capsule for a given high-level feature and updates the coupling coefficient accordingly.

CapsNet addresses the limitations in CNN by considering the routing preferences between capsules and the prediction of next-layer activations. Hence, CapsNet can model strong feature relationships and improve image segmentation.

The CapsNets architecture is designed in such a way that it preserves the proportional and positional information which helps to reconstruct the images from the developed neural network. The newly introduced principal routing by agreement in Capsule architecture helps to execute the prediction in an early stage of the model training, where each capsule layer tries to predict the most appropriate next capsule that should be connected (Sabour, 2017; Kruthika et al., 2019). This architecture enables training with a small number of data points and provides a speedy training experience, as each capsule layer connects to the most appropriate next capsule layer.

2.2.2 Inception V3 Network

Inception V3 architecture is introduced to evacuate the inadequacies of the complex neural architectures in terms of scalability and computational complexity. It has been proposed in such a way that the network can scale up by utilizing its computational resources to the maximum and to provide efficient results from minimal computational power (Szegedy et al., 2016; Vinayak et al., 2020). In order to perform that, the factorized convolutional is enabled instead of linear convolutions and conformed to an aggressive method for regularization. The Inception V3 architecture is known for its generation of high-quality, visual features that are applicable in a plethora of different domains in machine learning (Ding et al., 2019; Vinayak et al., 2020). The high-quality feature set is determined by the application of dimensionality reduction and the parallel design of the Inception modules.

In comparison to other state-of-the-art neural networks, Inception architecture adheres to a unique way of dimensionality reduction method. It gradually reduces the input size without heavily affecting the feature set that it generates in each convolutional layer, by considering more of the correlation structure and dimensionality to support back propagation. This method eliminates the commonly found representational bottlenecks which will result in forfeiting important inherited features in data. Moreover, the balance between the width and depth of the network is handled in this architecture, preventing the model to overfit the training data.

A significant feature in this implementation is that label smoothing regularization appears as an aggressive regularization method. It is determined by defining a margin effect for label dropout during the model training. It further ensures that the maximum unnormalized log probabilities of the class labels have a large gap with the others. It can be represented as a cross entry as in Equation 3 (Szegedy et al., 2016; Géron, 2017).

$$H(\hat{q|},p) = -\sum \_(k=1)\hat{K} \log p(k) \; q\hat{|}(k) = (1-\epsilon)H(q,p) + \epsilon H(u,p) \quad (3)$$

Where p(k) is the probability distribution for the label k (k belongs to {1 .... K}), q(k) refers to ground-truth distribution for the label k, and H is the cross-entropy). This shows that this new regularization method is capable of replacing a single cross-entry loss (H{q,p}) with any other pair of losses.

2.3 Related Studies

Several studies have used machine learning techniques such as Support Vector Machine (SVM) and its derivations, decision tree algorithms including Random Forest, boosting in the AD diagnosis process (Wang et al., 2019). With the available high-dimensional data in massive forms, the most convenient solution directs towards deep learning techniques such as CNNs in 2-D and 3-D formats and deep neural nets.

The combination of multiple modalities including structural and functional MRI along with the PET images provides a novel and powerful union to capture both anatomical and neural activity (Alberdi et al., 2016). This combination of both functional and structural neuroimaging will provide harmonious results, where the AD pathology can be studied in different dimensions using deep learning techniques. Many studies have been focused on using multi-modality in the AD classification process using sMRI and PET. However, the addition of fMRI data into this combination will prove the novelty in our proposed research to explore different perspectives in the pathology of AD.

The advancement of neural network architectures has drawn into efficient training with reduced time and dataset size. Artificial neural networks have been designed to extract features and train the dataset peculiarities as a machine learning model. As fMRI and PET images are highly dimensional, 3-D neural networks have been applied in most of the studies (Lin et al., 2018; Liu et al., 2018; Islam and Zhang, 2019).

The ability of PET to measure the body changes at the cellular level has been efficiently used in the identification of psychiatric disorders by applying various classification algorithms (Nozadi and Kadoury, 2018). An approach of combining modalities of sMRI and PET has been proposed by Gupta et al. (2019) to get the complementary features for the early detection in AD. The obtained results show that the grouping of different modalities performs well compared with using the biomarkers individually for the classification process.

Several recent studies have considered deep neural networks, which enable more information extraction and use two neural networks: one for feature extraction and the other for model training. A content-based image retrieval using the 3-D CapsNets has been implemented by Kruthika et al. (2019) with a model ensemble approach of CNN and CapsNets to improve the overall performance of the early detection of AD. The limitations of CNNs, such as a lack of orientation perspective, have been eliminated by dynamic routing among capsules in CapsNet with a form of vector values compared with the scalar inputs and outputs in CNN. Therefore, an efficient spatial relationship was obtained between image features with proper routing and transformation techniques by covering most of the relevant features compared with CNN.

Table 11.1 states the techniques used for pre-processing, feature extraction, and classification for different dataset types. Some of these techniques include principal component analysis (PCA), CNN), Class Activation Map (CAM), Wasserstein Generative Adversarial Network (WGAN), and Extreme Learning Machine (ELM).

Inception V3-based CNNs have also been widely used in classifying medical images as an effective diagnosis model which is pre-trained on ImageNet dataset. A recent study (Ding et al., 2019) of classifying AD with PET data trained the images on the Inception V3 convolutional model and obtained accuracy of some 90%. Two-dimensional PET images with pre-processing of 16 horizontal brain images placed on a 4 x 4 grid were used to train on Inception V3 with proper regularization techniques. The same learning network has also been used to detect AD with MRI brain images (Vinayak et al., 2020). They showed accuracy of 83% by utilizing the pre-trained Inception V3 model and using its pre-trained weights to get an efficient edge detection compared with other conventionally trained models. (Wang et al., 2019) have proposed an Inception V3 model based on pulmonary image feature extraction by fine-tuning the pre-trained models to extract the features. The classification models were built on Softmax, Logistic, and SVM classifiers and obtained the highest sensitivity and specificity of 95% and 80%, respectively.

However, a limited number of studies have focused on fMRI to support AD classification, owing to the high dimensionality and limited computational

Table 11.1 Summary of the techniques used in related studies

Study	Dataset	Pre-processing techniques							Feature extraction			Classification techniques			
		Normalization	Skull-stripping	Affine registration	Segmentation	Coregistration	Motion Correction	Smoothing	Automatic	PCA	CAM	CNN	Cascading CNN	WGAN	ELM
(Liu et al., 2018)	sMRI, PET	x	x	x					x				x		x
(Basia et al., 2019)	sMRI	x			x	x			x			x			
(Lin et al., 2018)	sMRI	x	x		x	x				x		x			
(Baumgartner et al., 2018)	sMRI	x			x						x			x	
(Duffy et al., 2019)	PET	x							x			x			
(Saraf et al., 2016)	fMRI	x				x	x	x	x			x			
(Lama et al., 2017)	sMRI		x			x				x					

techniques for fMRI modality of brain imaging. Furthermore, the combination of other modalities like PET and fMRI would support a novel method to be used for AD classification along with the sMRI.

3 System Model

3.1 Study Materials

The healthcare data is prone to privacy violations in different aspects where it can lead to patient details, health history where this type of data is considered as a highly sensitive type of data that needs to be handled with much care. The data collection repository Alzheimer's Disease Neuroimaging Initiative (ADNI) is such an initiative where millions of data in different modalities are accessible across the globe. Even though it is a form of open data collection, the entry and maintenance are handled precisely by providing restricted access, notifications on data depreciation, etc.

The datasets considered for this research are from the ADNI database which is available publicly in the web portal (www.loni.ucla.edu/ADNI). It consists of important biomarkers such as genetics, bioinformatics, MRI, neuropathologic, and PET scanning. Hence functional and structural brain activity can be studied using this dataset. ADNI further includes classified datasets on MCI, AD, and control subjects which allows the supervised learning mechanisms on AD subtype identification.

The considered dataset includes 5,121 MRI images and 4,032 PET 2-D images of participants aged between 50 and 89 years. The data include both fMRI and PET scanning data in three different stages of AD. There are 38% AD subjects, 30% MCI subjects, and the remainder are normal subjects in the complete dataset. The remaining percentage of the dataset includes control subjects. A separate unseen test set with one-third of training samples was used for testing purposes. The sample images of the three considered class labels for MRI and PET are shown in Figure 11.1 and Figure 11.2, respectively. In Figure 11.1, the left, middle, and right images show MRI images of a 77-year-old male with AD, a 78-year-old female with MCI, and a 72-year-old female control subject, respectively. In Figure 11.2, the left, middle, and right images

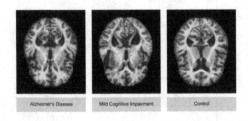

Figure 11.1 Sample MRI data

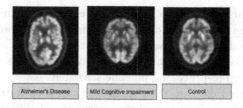

Figure 11.2 Sample PET data

show PET images of three male subjects aged 69 years with AD, MCI, and a control subject, respectively.

The benchmark dataset was obtained from (Salvatore et al., 2015), where 509 patients' data are included. The distribution is marked as per the class label of the trained model as 137 AD subjects, 210 MCI subjects, and 162 control subjects.

3.2 System Process

The proposed solution contains six main steps, including data acquisition, pre-processing, feature extraction, and learning model derivation. As this research supports two modalities of data containing MRI and PET scanning data, pre-processing techniques are applied to each of these modalities. The MRI pre-processing includes skull stripping and normalization, and the PET images are subjected to a pre-processing pipeline consisting of coregistration and segmentation. Then the data is subjected to the application of machine learning and deep learning algorithms such as DenseNet, Inception V3, and CapsuleNet. Each modality of data generates a separate model, and after evaluating and tuning the hyperparameters, the best-performing model is obtained to support the AD classification from healthy subjects.

Figure 11.3 shows the graphical representation of the proposed solution. The neuroimaging data of MRI and PET modalities are first fed into a data pre-

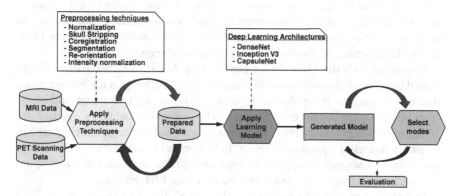

Figure 11.3 High-level process flow of the proposed solution

processing pipeline consisting of data volume normalization, skull stripping, coregistration, segmentation, re-orientation, and intensity normalization. These techniques are predominantly used to reduce the inherent noise in neuroimaging modalities. As these modalities are two different kinds, each modality is passed through the pre-processing pipeline separately.

The pre-processed data are then applied to the deep learning architectures considered. In order to compare the performance of different convolutional architectures, high-performing architectures of DenseNet, Inception V3, and CapsuleNet have been considered in this study. After applying the dataset into the deep learning algorithm, the generated model is used for evaluation using cross-validation, and then the model is selected with the best performance values in terms of accuracy, sensitivity, and specificity.

4 System Methodology

4.1 Data pre-processing

The ADNI MRI dataset consists of a pre-processed subset of data which was reprocessed by FreeSurfer software. The initial pre-processing techniques including bias handling, noise removal, and data standardization have been applied. The raw data is subjected to skull stripping and normalization which ensured that the images are in the same standard scale despite the differences that occurred in the data acquisition. Although the initial dataset supports pre-processing by the vendor, further specialized data pre-processing techniques such as slice time correction, coregistration, and segmentation are used to dissolve the vendor-specific pre-processing and enabled standardization of the dataset.

The MRI data are analyzed using tensor-based morphometry, boundary shift integral method, FreeSurfer processing tool, and tensor-based morphometry-symmetric normalization. Tensor-based morphometry identifies the anatomical differences in regions using the nonlinear distorted regions and their gradients. The boundary shift integral focuses on measuring the cerebral volume changes in the scans. Freesurfer is used to pre-process the data using techniques including intensity normalization, gradient un-wrapping, and non-uniformity elimination and correction. Tensor-based morphometry-symmetric normalization is used to identify the brain structural, cross-sectional, and repeated frames in the scans.

Compared with the MRI dataset provided by ADNI, the PET dataset is supported by a comprehensive pre-processing pipeline. Techniques for denoising and slice time correction are applied as the basic pre-processing techniques, and image coregistration is applied for the PET scans. They are reoriented into a standard size $160 \times 160 \times 96$ voxel image grid, which serves as a standard image to be referred to by all the images of a particular subject. In fact, spatial re-orientation and intensity normalization of scans are applied without any application of non-linear warping or even linear scaling of the brain dimensions in the PET images.

In order to prepare the images for the CNN, the 3-D images were sliced into 2-D images, and to add more variation to the dataset, data augmentation

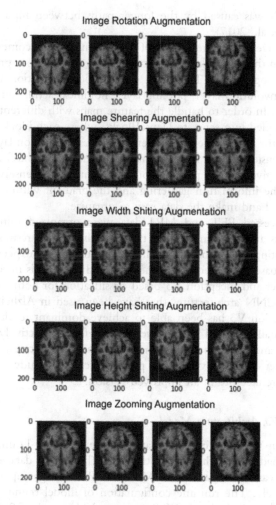

Figure 11.4 Sample image augmentation

was performed. Image rotation, shearing, width and height shifting, and zooming were used as the image augmentation techniques. This processing was carried out by Keras Python library using its image processing tools. A sample series of augmented images of an AD subject, confronted with image rotation, shearing, width, high shifting, and zooming are shown in Figure 11.4.

4.2 Convolutional Neural Network Model

DenseNet architecture is considered as a novel neural network for visual object recognition, with slight differences in the architectural level. The DenseNet was mainly developed to avoid the vanishing gradient problem in neural networks which was caused by the longer paths between input and output layers (Huang et al., 2017).

Generally, in DenseNet the output of the current layer becomes an input to the next layer in the network. It concatenates the outputs from previous layers with composite operations. Therefore, this composite function in DenseNet consists of a convolution layer, pooling layer, nonlinear acting, and batch normalization layer. In order to handle the feature maps with different dimensions, DenseNet is divided into separate DenseBlocks, where each block has different filters but with the same dimensions. DenseNet uses a transition layer to reduce the height dimensions of the images, but the dimensions of the features remain the same. As a given image passes through n number of DenseBlocks with n convolutions, the information gathering and the gradient within the network will be improved and make the data easy to organize.

The pre-processed PET and MRI data were organized using DenseNet neural networks and built models for two modalities. The results in terms of accuracy for testing data in both modalities were not in the expected range for the DenseNet-based classifier. Thus, the proposed research is further extended with CapsuleNet and Inception V3-based classification for both modalities.

Among the CNN architectures that have been used in Alzheimer's disease diagnosis, Inception V3 has been able to achieve dominant results in terms of accuracy. Its parallel-stacked layers have been useful to effectively identify the patterns in data and can then be used in prediction or reconstructing the results. Hence, in order to improve model performance, this study has also used Inception V3 architecture in an improved version.

4.3 Inception V3 Architecture Model

In the Inception V3-based implementation, the extracted 2-D images of shape 160x160 are loaded into the model training. The use of data augmentation techniques increases the number of MRI and PET images up to 5,120 and 6,120, respectively. The runtime configuration of model training includes an n1-high-memory-2 instance, 2vCPU, with a clock speed of 2.2GHz, 13GB RAM and a hard disk size of 64GB. The Anaconda environment is composed of Python 3.0, with CUDA 8.0 as GPU support, and Tensorflow 2.0 is used as an optimization framework for model training.

The Inception V3 network is pre-trained with the ImageNet dataset, which includes general image data of some 14 million images with 1,000 class labels. Then it is modified and fine-tuned with hyperparameter configurations to facilitate training with ADNI datasets. One notable feature of the modified version of the model includes a secondary layer of regularization to support data variations introduced by data augmentation (Goodfellow et al., 2016). Figure 11.5 shows the neural network architecture, which consists of a set of intermediate inception modules and ends with two regularization layers.

The new regularization layer includes an average pooling layer with the pre-trained Inception model supported by a dropout later and a fully connected

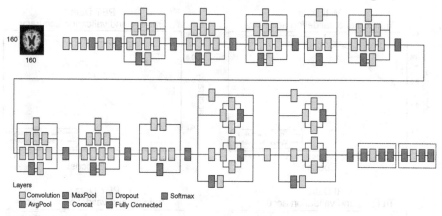

Figure 11.5 Inception V3 architecture (Szegedy et al., 2014)

layer with the ReLu activation function. Furthermore, the second fully connected layer for the class label is applied with a softmax activation function to normalize the output vectors created by the predecessor layers, and it provides the associated probability value for the prediction.

5 Evaluation

The evaluation of the proposed methodology is facilitated by assessing the model evaluation metrics of the individual models generated for each of the data types. The performance of the final system can be further analyzed by measuring the quality metrics in different work settings for model training. Furthermore, the results for each of the neuroimaging modalities considered can be compared with the related work suitable for different modalities. In order to tackle the trade-off with the training and testing data split proportion, cross-validation has been conducted. It has considered k-fold cross-validation in the training and testing where the desired bin size of the cross-validation is considered as 10. The final results are achieved as an average value of each validation iteration of accuracy, sensitivity, and specificity.

The model training graphs are shown in Figure 11.6 for PET and MRI modalities alike. These results show the training accuracy and validation accuracy against the number of epochs, which is the number of passes that the learning algorithm has gone through in the entire training dataset.

Here, the validation accuracy slowly converges to the training accuracy at the same rate where losses are reduced. When the two data modalities are compared in terms of the training cycle statistics, it is evident that the PET dataset is observed with high variations during the training period in comparison with the MRI dataset. A possible cause of this is the high regulation and complexity of the internal hidden neural layers trying to adhere to the dataset properties, where the PET dataset has more feature information compared with

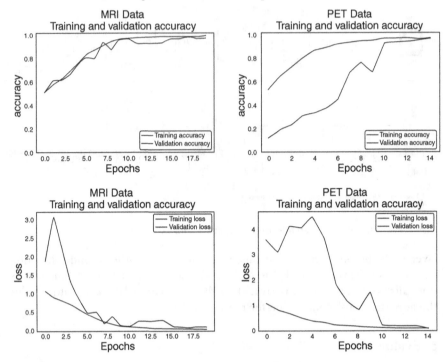

Figure 11.6 Learning curves with the Inception V3 model

the MRI dataset. However, towards the end of the training cycle, it is por-
trayed that the validation PET dataset performance slowly converges with the
training performance in terms of both accuracy and loss.

The accuracy is calculated using the statistics obtained from the model
training as the total correct predictions from the prediction population as a
probability value, which is less than 1.0 as shown in Equation 4.

$$Accuracy = \frac{True\ Positives + True\ Negatives}{True\ Positives + +True\ Negatives + False\ Positives + False\ Negatives} \quad (4)$$

As this is a multiclass classification problem, the categorical cross-entropy is
used as the loss function to calculate the model loss depicted in Equation 5
(Géron, 2017).

$$L(X_i, Y_i) = -\sum_{j=1}^{n} y_{ij} * \log(p_{ij}) \quad (5)$$

Here, Y_i is the one-hot encoded target vector which is the representative
vector $(Y_{i1}, Y_{i2}, ..., Y_{nj})$ of the class label. p_{ij} is the probability of ith element in
the dataset is in the class j.

The evaluation of the learning models is obtained by applying both cross-validations and having the size of one-third of the ADNI dataset as a separate dataset for both MRI and PET modalities. Moreover, important statistical metrics are identified for the evaluation of model performance. Sensitivity and specificity are used as the diagnostic test criteria to evaluate the deep learning model's performance. The derivations of sensitivity and specificity are given in Equation 4 and Equation 5, respectively.

$$Sensitivity = (True\ Positives)/(True\ Positives + False\ Negatives) \quad (4)$$

$$Specificity = (True\ Negatives)/(True\ Negatives + False\ Positives) \quad (5)$$

In this study, the main focus is on MRI and PET datasets in the application of the high-performance learning algorithm Inception V3. In order to highlight the performance with Inception V3 architectures, other state-of-the-art algorithms including DenseNet and CapsuleNet identified that the Inception V3 architecture is capable of delivering reasonably higher results in terms of accuracy, sensitivity, and specificity for MRI and PET modalities alike. The complex and carefully designed layer of the convolution network, and max pooling layers are supported by regularization in comparison to DenseNet and CapsuleNet has been able to identify the associated peculiarities in MRI and PET datasets alike, achieving highly promising results with a 90% confidence level for each of the metrics. The results in Table 11.2 confirm that the Inception V3 deep learning model is capable of distinguishing between the considered AD, MCI, and control groups from the general population.

6 Discussion

6.1 Main contributions

This research mainly contributed to the classification of MCI, AD, and normal controls using different brain imaging modalities. The proposed method has used both MRI and PET modalities to train the classification models on

Table 11.2 Accuracies for MRI and PET modalities

Dataset	Algorithm	Accuracy %	Sensitivity %	Specificity %
MRI	DenseNet	80.88	71.02	62.34
MRI	CapsuleNet	84.88	76.22	70.41
MRI	**InceptionV3**	**96.05**	**87.53**	**80.47**
PET	DenseNet	50.55	44.34	40.84
PET	CapsuleNet	60.12	54.25	49.12
PET	**Inception V3**	**95.49**	**84.12**	**80.18**

different learning algorithms and selected the final model based on the given accuracy levels. For both modalities, the Inception V3 model has given the higher performance values on the testing test. The selected models were enhanced by using different regularization techniques to tune the model and avoid overfitting. The MRI and PET 3-D images were converted to 2-D images before being fed into the neural network model, and data augmentation was performed to add more variation to the dataset. Image rotation, shearing, width and height shifting, and zooming were performed as data augmentation techniques to improve the training dataset.

For MRI modality, inception V3 and CapsNets have given higher performance value in terms of accuracy. One of the key contributions of this study is to obtain higher accuracies using PET and MRI modalities alike, without using hand-crafted features compared to the studies (Ding et al., 2019; Liu et al., 2018) with different crafted features for the model training. Thus, the selected models can be used to learn and extract the relevant features from the images for better performance in classification.

6.2 Comparison with the existing studies

Several studies have been conducted on proposing computational models and techniques for the diagnosis process of different neurological disorders. Different data acquisition, pre-processing, feature extraction techniques, and machine learning-based model have been used in the classification process of the related psychophysiological data such as electroencephalogram signals (Brihadiswaran et al., 2019), fMRI, and eye-movement data (De Silva et al., 2019a; Meedeniya and Rubasinghe, 2020; Haputhanthri et al., 2020). For their part, DSSs facilitate computational support using psychophysiological measurements for the early identification of people with neurological disorders, hence enabling early treatments. Studies have presented technology-based DSS as a variety of neurological disorder conditions such as ASD (Haputhanthri et al. 2019, 2020; Wadhera and Kakkar, 2020a) and Attention Deficit Hyperactivity Disorder (ADHD) (De Silva et al., 2019b; Ariyarathne et al., 2020; De Silva et al., 2021a, 2021b; Rubasinghe et al., 2020), using different machine learning and deep learning-based techniques with different data types.

We have compared the accuracies of the proposed methodology against the existing related studies. As shown in Table 11.3, the proposed methodology obtained accuracy of 96% and 95% for MRI and PET modalities, respectively, with the Inception V3 model. When comparing the obtained accuracies with selected studies for the same modalities with the ADNI dataset, the proposed method has shown significant accuracy for the classification of AD. MRI-related studies have used different sets of features with CNN-based classifiers for the identification process. Among them, CNN-based multimodal correlation and 3D_CapsNet-based classification have shown better accuracy compared with related studies.

However, the proposed architecture, with regularized Inception V3 classifier, has shown a higher accuracy value with the use of a proper data augmentation

Table 11.3 Comparison of existing studies

Related study	PET	MRI	CNN	Accuracy (%)
(Kruthika et al., 2019)	–	x	CapsNet	88.37
(Lin et al., 2018)	–	x	3D CNN	73.04
(Liu et al., 2018)	x	x	3D CNN	82.95
(Islam and Zhang, 2019)	x	–	3D CNN	71.45
(Ding et al., 2019)	x	–	–	92.00
Regularized Inception V3 with MRI data	–	x	**Inception V3**	**96.05**
Regularized Inception V3 with PET data	x	–	**Inception V3**	**95.49**

process to enhance the accuracy level. A similar study (Ding et al., 2019) with the use of Inception V3 architecture trained on the ADNI dataset, obtained accuracy of 92% with higher sensitivity and specificity values. Compared with all the most related studies, the regularized Inception V3-based classifier for PET and MRI modalities performed well in terms of accuracy, sensitivity, and specificity. The reasons for obtaining a comparable higher accuracy level can be categorized into training model selection, model tuning, and feature selection.

6.3 Open Challenges and Future Research Directions

This study focussed on classifying MCI, AD, and control subjects using different modalities and learning algorithms based on machine learning and deep learning. The classification accuracies and processing capabilities can be further improved by applying appropriate different optimizers and fine-tuning the parameters (Brihadiswaran et al., 2019) (Meedeniya and Rubasinghe, 2020).

Furthermore, the proposed deep learning-based classification models can be integrated with probabilistic programming models for a better analysis of the medical image data (Rubasinghe and Meedeniya, 2019). The research can be further extended to support the classification of other stages of mild cognitive disease, including early mild cognitive and late mild cognitive stages. Moreover, different other data types such as genome and radiomics sequence data can be used to enhance the classification process of the data related to brain scans (Wijethilake et al., 2020a; Wijethilake et al., 2020b).

One of another major challenges faced during the model training was the duration to complete the training process. A considerable amount of time was spent on the model training process, but this can be reduced by using proper techniques to utilize hardware utilization. Besides, the parallel implementation of these classification algorithms can be accelerated using a Graphics Processing Unit (Welivita et al., 2017; Welivita et al., 2018; Rajapaksa et al., 2019). Hence, computer-intensive tasks can reduce a considerable amount of processing time.

Most of the medical data analysis studies have limitations such as a lack of benchmark datasets and the ethical issues of processing healthcare data. Moreover, the technology-enabled neurodevelopmental disorder diagnosis process faces challenges such as acquiring large datasets to apply deep learning techniques for building strong relationships, applying in real-world clinical practices, expert knowledge on etiology aspects (Brihadiswaran et al. 2019) (Meedeniya and Rubasinghe 2020). Furthermore, these types of technology-enabled neurodevelopmental disorders diagnosis studies can be extended to a generic model or framework to classify different types of psychophysiological data (Rubasinghe et al., 2020).

7 Conclusion

AD is a common age-related disorder of cognition which is caused mainly by a decline in cognition. A milder degree of AD can be identified as MCI, with a measurable decline in cognition, and has a considerable impact on a person's daily tasks. People with MCI have a higher probability of progressing to the level of AD, and their memory will continue to decline significantly. Thus, MCI can also be identified as an early stage of AD. Therefore, it is important to identify the disease in the early stages to avoid severe impacts in the future.

This study mainly focuses on classifying AD and MCI in control groups with the use of different modalities and classifiers. The pre-processed dataset for the proposed study was obtained from the ADNI data set for PET and MRI modalities. Subjects belong to three main classification groups: AD, MCI, and control groups were selected for training purposes, and the classifiers were tested in unseen testing sets. Different deep learning-related algorithms were used to select the best-performing classifier with proper comparison on accuracy levels obtained for the testing set. The selected algorithms included CapsNet, DenseNet, and Inception V3 architectures. Among them, Inception V3-based architecture produced the highest accuracy for both modalities.

Overall, this study shows that the proposed deep learning-based architecture provides better accuracy in classifying AD, MCI, and control group subjects with MRI and PET images of the brain. Hence, the proposed methodology using well-performing classifiers can be integrated into decision support systems for the identification of AD and further enhanced with the classification of other subcategories with severity score measurements to provide future developments.

References

Alberdi, A., Aztiria, A., and Basarab, A. (2016). "On the early diagnosis of Alzheimer's Disease from multimodal signals: A survey." *Artificial Intelligence in Medicine*, 71: 1–29. doi:10.1016/j.artmed.2016.06.003.

Ariyarathne, G., De Silva, S., Dayarathna, S., Meedeniya, D., and Jayarathna, S., (2020). "ADHD Identification using Convolutional Neural Network with Seed-based

Approach for fMRI Data." *9th International Conference on Software and Computer Applications*, pp. 31–35. doi:10.1145/3384544.3384552.

Basaia, S. and Alzheimer's Disease Neuroimaging Initiative. (2019). "Automated classification of Alzheimer's disease and mild cognitive impairment using a single MRI and deep neural networks." *NeuroImage: Clinical*, 21: 101645. doi:10.1016/j.nicl.2018.101645.

Baumgartner, C. F., Koch, L. M., Can Tezcan, K., Xi Ang, J., and Konukoglu, E. (2018). "Visual Feature Attribution using Wasserstein GANs". *IEEE Conference on Computer Vision and Pattern Recognition*: pp. 8309–8319. doi:10.1109/CVPR.2018.00867.

Brihadiswaran, G., Haputhanthri, D., Gunathilaka, S., Meedeniya, D., and Jayarathna, S. (2019). "EEG-based processing and classification methodologies for Autism Spectrum Disorder: A Review." *Journal of Computer Science*, 15(8): 1161–1183. doi:10.3844/jcssp.2019.1161.1183.

De Silva, S., Dayarathna, S., Ariyarathne, G., Meedeniya, D., and Jayarathna, S. (2019a). "A Survey of Attention Deficit Hyperactivity Disorder Identification Using Psychophysiological Data" *International Journal of Online and Biomedical Engineering*, 15(13): 61–76. doi:10.3991/ijoe.v15i13.10744.

De Silva, S. et al. (2019b). A Rule-Based System for ADHD Identification using Eye Movement Data. In: *International Multidisciplinary Engineering Research Conference (MerCon)*, pp. 538–543, IEEE. doi:10.1109/MERCon.2019.8818865.

De Silva, S.et al. (2021a). "fMRI Feature Extraction Model for ADHD Classification Using Convolutional Neural Network." *International Journal of E-Health and Medical Communications*, 12(1): 81–105. doi:10.4018/IJEHMC.2021010106.

De Silva, S. et al. (2021b). Computational Decision Support System for ADHD Identification, *International Journal of Automation and Computing*, 18(2): 233–255. doi:10.1007/s11633-020-1252-1.

Deng, J., Dong, W., Socher, R., Li, L., Li, K. and Fei-Fei, L. (2009). "*ImageNet: A large-scale hierarchical image database.*" IEEE Conference on Computer Vision and Pattern Recognition, Miami, FL, pp. 248–255. doi:10.1109/CVPR.2009.5206848.

Ding, Y., Sohn, J., Kawczynski, M., Trivedi, H., Harnish, R., and Jenkins, N. (2019). "A Deep Learning Model to Predict a Diagnosis of Alzheimer Disease by Using 18F-FDG PET of the Brain." *Radiology*, 290(2): 456–464. doi:10.1148/radiol.2018180958.

Duffy, I. R., Boyle, A. J., and Vasdev, N. (2019). "Improving PET Imaging Acquisition and Analysis with Machine Learning: A Narrative Review With Focus on Alzheimer's Disease and Oncology." *Molecular Imaging*, 18. doi:10.1177%2F1536012119869070.

Géron, A. (2017). "Hands-On Machine Learning with Scikit-Learn and TensorFlow." In: *Hands-on Machine Learning with Scikit-Learn and TensorFlow*. O'Reilly Media. doi:10.3389/fninf.2014.00014.

Goodfellow, I., Bengio, Y., and Courville, A. (2016). *Deep Learning*. London: The MIT Press.

Gupta, Y., Lama, R., and Kwon, G., (2019). "Prediction and Classification of Alzheimer's Disease Based on Combined Features from Apolipoprotein-E Genotype, Cerebrospinal Fluid, MR, and FDG-PET Imaging Biomarkers." *Frontiers in Computational Neuroscience*, 13(72): 1–18. doi:10.3389/fncom.2019.00072.

Haputhanthri, D. et al. (2019). "*An EEG based Channel Optimized Classification Approach for Autism Spectrum Disorder.*" International Multidisciplinary Engineering Research Conference (Mercon), pp. 123–128. doi:10.1109/MERCon.2019.8818814.

Haputhanthri, D. et al. (2020). "Integration of Facial Thermography in EEG-based Classification of ASD." *International Journal of Automation and Computing*, 17(6): 837–854. doi:10.1007/s11633-020-1231-6.

Huang, G., Liu, Z., Van Der Maaten, L., and Weinberger, K. Q., (2017). *"Densely Connected Convolutional Networks."* IEEE Conference on Computer Vision and Pattern Recognition, Honolulu, HI, 2017, pp. 2261–2269. doi:10.1109/CVPR.2017.243.

Islam, J. and Zhang, Y. (2019). "Understanding 3D CNN Behavior for Alzheimer's Disease Diagnosis from Brain PET Scan."

Kruthika, K. R., Rajeswari, and Maheshappa, H. D. (2019). "CBIR system using Capsule Networks and 3D CNN for Alzheimer's disease diagnosis." *Informatics in Medicine Unlocked*, 14: 59–68. doi:10.1016/j.imu.2018.12.001.

Lama, R. K., Gwak, J., Park, J. S., and Lee, S. W. (2017). "Diagnosis of Alzheimer's disease based on structural MRI images using a regularized extreme learning machine and PCA features." *Journal of Healthcare Engineering*, 2017(5485080): 1–11. doi:10.1155/2017/5485080.

Lin, W. et al. (2018). "Convolutional neural networks-based MRI image analysis for the Alzheimer's disease prediction from mild cognitive impairment." *Frontiers in Neuroscience*, 12: 1–13. doi:10.3389/fnins.2018.00777.

Liu, M., Cheng, D., Wang, K., and Wang, Y. (2018). "Multi-Modality Cascaded Convolutional Neural Networks for Alzheimer's Disease Diagnosis." *Neuroinformatics*, 16(3–4): 295–308. doi:10.1007/s12021-018-9370-4.

Lu, S., Xia, Y., Cai, T., and Feng, D. (2015). *"Semi-supervised manifold learning with affinity regularization for Alzheimer's disease identification using positron emission tomography imaging."* 37th Annual International Conference of The IEEE Engineering in Medicine and Biology Society, Milan, 2015, pp. 2251–2254. doi:10.1109/embc.2015.7318840.

Meedeniya, D. A. and Rubasinghe, I. D., (2020). "A Review of Supportive Computational Approaches for Neurological Disorder Identification." In: T. WadheraandD. Kakkar(Eds), *Interdisciplinary Approaches to Altering Neurodevelopmental Disorders*, pp. 271–302. IGI Global. doi:10.4018/978-1-7998-3069-6.ch016.

Minishima, S., Frey, K. A., Koeppe, R. A., Foster, N. L., and Kuhl, D. E. (1995). "A diagnostic approach in Alzheimer's disease using three-dimensional stereotactic surface projections of fluorine-18-FDG PET." *The Journal of Nuclear Medicine*, 36(7): 1238–1248.

Nozadi, S. and Kadoury, S. (2018). "Classification of Alzheimer's and MCI Patients from Semantically Parcelled PET Images: A Comparison between AV45 and FDG-PET." *International Journal of Biomedical Imaging*, 2018: 1–13. doi:10.1155/2018/1247430.

Prince, M. J. (2015). *World Alzheimer Report 2015: the global impact of dementia: an analysis of prevalence, incidence, cost and trends*, Alzheimer's Disease International. Retrieved from www.alzint.org/u/WorldAlzheimerReport2015.pdf.

Rajapaksa, S., Rasanjana, W., Perera, I., and Meedeniya, D. (2019). *"GPU Accelerated Maximum Likelihood Analysis for Phylogenetic Inference."* 8th International Conference on Software and Computer Applications, New York, USA, pp. 6–10. doi:10.1145/3316615.3316630.

Rubasinghe, I. D. and Meedeniya, D. A. (2019). "Ultrasound Nerve Segmentation Using Deep Probabilistic Programming." *Journal of ICT Research and Applications*, 13 (3): 241–256. doi:10.5614/itbj.ict.res.appl.2019.13.3.5.

Rubasinghe, I. D. and Meedeniya, D. A. (2020). *Automated Neuroscience Decision Support Framework*. In: B. Agarwal (Ed.), *Deep Learning Techniques for Biomedical and Health Informatics*, pp. 305–326. Elsevier Academic Press. doi:10.1016/B978-0-12-819061-6.00013-6.

Sabour, S., Frosst, N., and Hinton, G. E. (2017). "Dynamic routing between capsules." *Advances in neural information processing systems*, 30, 3856–3866. doi:1710.09829.

Salvatore, C. et al. (2018). "MRI Characterizes the Progressive Course of AD and Predicts Conversion to Alzheimer's Dementia 24 Months Before Probable Diagnosis." *Frontiers of Aging Neuroscience*, 24 May 2018. doi:10.3389/fnagi.2018.00135.

Sarraf, S. and Tofighi, G. (2016). *"Deep learning-based pipeline to recognize Alzheimer's disease using fMRI data."* Future Technologies Conference, San Francisco, CA, pp. 816–820. doi:10.1101/066910.

Simonyan, K. and Zisserman, A. (2014). "Very deep convolutional networks for large-scale image recognition."

Szegedy, C., Vanhoucke, V., Ioffe, S., Shlens, J., and Wojna, Z. (2016). *"Rethinking the inception architecture for computer vision."* IEEE conference on computer vision and pattern recognition, Las Vegas, NV, pp. 2818–2826. doi:1512.00567.

Vinayak E. S. S., Shahina, A., and Khan, A. N. (2020). "Detection of Alzheimer's Disease on Brain MRI using Inception V3 Network." *International Journal of Engineering Research & Technology*, 9(10): 17–25.

Wadhera, T. and Kakkar, D. (2020a). "Big Data-Based System: A Supportive Tool in Autism Spectrum Disorder Analysis." *Interdisciplinary Approaches to Altering Neurodevelopmental Disorders*, 303–319. doi:10.4018/978-1-7998-3069-6.ch017.

Wadhera, T. and Kakkar, D. (2020b). "Multiplex temporal measures reflecting neural underpinnings of brain functional connectivity under cognitive load in Autism Spectrum Disorder." *Journal of Neurological Research*, 42(4): 327–337. doi:10.1080/01616412.2020.1726586.

Wang, C.et al. (2019). "Pulmonary Image Classification Based on Inception-v3 Transfer Learning Model." *IEEE Access*, 7, 146533–146541. doi:10.1109/access.2019.2946000.

Welivita, A., Perera, I., and Meedeniya, D. (2017). *"An Interactive Workflow Generator to Support Bioinformatics Analysis through GPU Acceleration."* IEEE International Conference on Bioinformatics and Biomedicine (BIBM), IEEE Xplore, Kansas City, MO, pp. 457–462. doi:10.1109/BIBM.2017.8217691.

Welivita, A., Perera, I., Meedeniya, D., Wickramarachchi, A., and Mallawaarachchi, V., (2018). "Managing Complex Workflows in Bioinformatics - An Interactive Toolkit with GPU Acceleration." *IEEE Transactions on NanoBioscience*, 17(3): 199–208. doi:10.1109/TNB.2018.2837122.

Wijethilake, N., Meedeniya, D., Chitraranjan, C., Perera, I., and Ren, H. (2020a). "Radiogenomics of Glioblastoma: Identification of Radiomics associated with Molecular Subtypes." In: S. M. Kia et al. (Eds), *Machine Learning in Clinical Neuroimaging and Radiogenomics in Neuro-oncology, RNO-AI*, LNCS, vol. 12449. Cham: Springer, pp. 229–239. doi:10.1007/978-3-030-66843-3_22.

Wijethilake, N., Meedeniya, D., Chitraranjan, C., and Perera, I. (2020b). *"Survival prediction and risk estimation of Glioma patients using mRNA expressions."* 20th IEEE Conference on Bioinformatics and Bioengineering (BIBE), USA, pp. 35–42. doi:10.1109/BIBE50027.2020.00014.

12 AviR: Autism Rehabilitation with webVR using Text Classification

Anshu Khurana and Om Prakash Verma

1 Introduction

In 2020 as the coronavirus pandemic spread many nations learnt the importance of focussing on healthcare. Healthcare is now a special concern globally for all countries, especially concerning the future of the countries: that is, our children. The health of an individual might have a connection with a healthy brain. A healthy brain impacts the thinking ability of a person, attitude towards life, happiness, and well-being of a person. Neurodevelopmental disorders (NDD) play an important role in healthcare. The impact of a disorder depends on the stage that it is developed. This abnormality can occur during pregnancy, at birth during childhood, in the perinatal period, and at each stage the impact on a child's behavior is different. One of the most common NDDs is autism spectrum disorder (ASD) (Munson and Pasqual, 2012), which entails problems with social interaction, language, sitting posture and eye contact and can cause a lack of confidence and focus, among other things. ASD is diagnosed when patients confirm at least three of the above symptoms mentioned. Rehabilitation is performed using many conventional clinical therapies and more recently virtual therapies. Consistency therapy can lead to wonderful results in patients (Brady et al., 2013).

The experience of individuals with NDDs can be improved using cognitive behavioral therapy (CBT) as a treatment. CBT is a psychoeducation including a range of techniques consisting of social skill enhancement, learning self-care, and visual aids (Butler et al., 2006). CBT protocols are defined keeping the need of children and adults. Virtual reality cognitive rehabilitation was introduced by (Wang and Reid, 2013) which improves textual recognition and cognitive flexibility in children with autism such as reliable safety tool at a construction site, choosing flowers for a garden and so on. Cognitive and behavioral programs are accessible with the help of virtual reality (VR) to children suffering with autism (Rizzo and Buckwalter, 1997).

One of the emerging technologies, known as VR (Manju et al., 2017), has been proven as an effective tool in the field of healthcare and

DOI: 10.4324/9781003165569-12

rehabilitation (Crocetta et al., 2018). It helps the user by simulating a 3-D environment and communicating with the real surroundings. VR creates sensory experiences such as sight, smells, and sounds. It consists of many technologies, namely: user tracking, stereoscopic delay, and augmented reality, which merges with the real and virtual environment. The other extended tool of VR is webVR (web virtual reality). WebVR is an experimental application programming interface, which enables different applications to interact with VR devices, irrespective of the browser. WebVR is an emerging web virtual technology, as it can run in any browser with all operating systems with or without VR glasses. WebVR applications work using HTML5 with openGL, whereas conventional VR applications work with Unity for specific platforms, which is a complex platform to use. Native VR applications cover only a small distance range, as VR headsets are required. WebVR applications are easily integrated with the Enterprise IT Environment, hence they can be widely and easily incorporated for use in different rehabilitation therapies. WebVR applications are cheaper than native VR application, as these apps can be updated and published in a fraction of a second.

This research presents a new software, AviR, to help in rehabilitation in children to fight a lack of social interaction, language speaking, focus, confidence, and recognition of alphabets. The software includes two games related to text recognition. First, it focuses on the card matching game, CASO, comprising different alphabets in English and Hindi. In the card matching game, children have different cards with sounds and have to recognize the source of the sound. This will help children to recognize the alphabet with sound and to whom it belongs, which increases focus, attention, and cognitive ability. This game is suitable for the age group of four to eight years old children. The second game is the most famous game among children known as 'ATLAS' of countries or places. This game will help children of the age group of four to 18 years old. Many games have already been developed, such as endless reader, which helps in reading skills with the aid of sight words; MITA, which helps to improve cognitive abilities using English, Spanish, German, Arabic, and more. Otismo is a paid-for application which helps children to adapt to speech development, and Commboards lite is another, more expensive, application in which there is a picture assistant with sounds. All the above applications are suitable for children up to the age of five years. The games are designed in such a manner that they will be freely available to the whole world and will attract children suffering from autism as colors attract people suffering from disease. The sounds used in the application will help children to enjoy playing games. These sounds will increase the motivation of patients and enhance happiness in their life. Recognition of sound and letter coordination with sounds will increase focus and hence concentration. The proposed second game where we have used avatars will help patients to communicate confidently in the external world, which will also help in increasing happiness in the life of patients and their families. This particular game, which uses the name of places, helps them to boost their confidence by increasing knowledge and direct communication with avatars. Both the games help to cure patients in a safe and controlled environment. The objectives of the chapter are as follows:

1   The chapter provides a practical application for the rehabilitation for the people suffering from autism spectrum disorder. The tool consists of two fun games and can be played by children up to the age of 18 years.
2   The application will be freely available on Google. (A link is provided below.)
3   The proposed application will help clinical therapists to rehabilitate children sitting in their homes and to check on their progress with rising scores.

2 Related Literature

Autism rehabilitation using VR has been used by therapist for several years now. VR is a 3-D artificial intelligent platform. It gives real-time experiences to the user (Antunes et al., 2017). Many conventional therapies include meditation techniques like mindful meditation (MM) (Crescentini et al., 2016). When VR is implemented for MM, it considers the different states of mind, other physiological factors, and emotional sympathetic activities. The special classroom tool was created by (Nolin et al., 2016) known as clinicalVR. The main aim of this tool is to assess validation by checking the relation existing between the attendant questionnaire sessions and analyzing the effect of age and gender on the performance. Researchers in Cordeil et al. (2016) compared performance using the CAVE automated virtual environment (CAVE) (Pick et al., 2016) and HMD used for immersive collaboration in network connectivity. Participants using HMD performed faster than CAVE. Therefore, HMD was used by a larger number of users. They have used VR for real-time experience, different tasks, and collaborations. CAVE (Pick et al., 2016) is a 3-D environment created using VR. By using CAVE, many operations in the virtual environment were invented, which includes review, creation, and modification. FACE is an interactive application in which a face is constructed using CAD/CAM. It is developed for android platforms, which helps people suffering from autism to identify, learn, and interpret. Therapists help the child with guided therapies to interact with the console. The FACE tool has facial expression tracking protocols, which help to identify deficiencies. Many other analyses have been performed on autistic children. Tanu and Kakkar (2018) and Wadhera and Kakkar (2020b) worked with the help of images and videos to determine the risk of increasing or decreasing autism in children. They analyzed the therapy on a weekly basis for three weeks and concluded that the therapy was impressive. The other tool developed by Wadhera and Kakkar (2019) is an eye tracker for autistic patients. The have developed cognitive tools which focus on eye movement and eye gaze detection using deep learning techniques. Their tool promises to give better results if used by clinicians. The other study of Wadhera and Kakkar (2020b) focussed on risk perception, by analyzing the condition of social interaction and one-to-one interaction. The other main problem of healthcare in Big Data was solved by Wadhera and Kakkar (2020a). They focused on the raw, unstructured, and structured form of data to get stored and how to maintain the data. The authors made the management of all the data easy and specifiable in a way especially for children with ASD. Another study, proposed by Stasolla and Passaro (2020), throws light on the working of autistic children in groups, use of other technologies like touchscreen support, and many more. The authors focussed on the effective training of ASD children.

The use of commercial games for rehabilitation is a new emerging technique, but the re-usability of the game is a major concern (Hocine et al., 2015). Many games developed by t researchers (Malheiros et al., 2016) (de Mello Monteiro et al., 2017) were used for individuals suffering from Down syndrome. The game was related to reaction time consumed while using virtual objects. In other research by (Mousavi Hondori et al., 2016) (Antunes et al., 2017), VR games were provided to autistic children under the supervision of elders, and the researchers studied the impact of games on the improvement of behaviour of autistic children. Another software suite was developed by Mousavi Hondori and Khademi (2014), with some rules to rehabilitate children. The games were developed specially for children with disabilities.

Our games focus mainly on children suffering from ASD. The limitations of the state-of-the-art techniques of following certain rules, expensive VR objects, lack of re-usability, and not being available freely were overcome by our study.

3 Methodology

ASD can be found and diagnosed in children of age group 3−4 years easily via prominent behavioral markers. The games developed prove to be more effective if treated on an child who has been diagnosed early. The disease can easily be diagnosed and rehabilitated, when a child finds it difficult to adapt to a changing environment, feels a lack of confidence, struggles to express their emotional feelings, has a short attention span and lack of focus, among other things (Novak and Morgan, 2019). Our proposed works focusses mainly on the age group from four to 18 years. The use of webVR will enable a virtual environment for students, where they can enjoy real play time in a natural environment. We have used an A-frame framework as the front end for the implementation of our games. The use of html and Java script have made implementation easy. For designing purposes, we have used magicavoxel, which is an integrated platform with an A-frame. All rules were followed while implementing the games, and design components include attractive colors, a friendly environment, and interesting dialogues. Figure 12.2 and Figure 12.3 show screenshots from virtual scenes in both games. We have chosen a green garden environment, as it is soothing for the eyes, and children can feel the freshness of trees. The application user begins with the first game, CASO, and, depending on the scores given by the therapist and Likert scale, the child

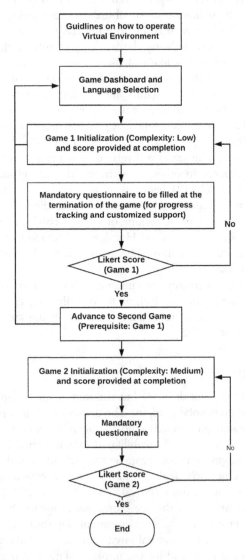

Figure 12.1 Flow process

will play the first game again or jump to the second game. Both a questionnaire and Likert scale are used to analyze the child's performance. The flow of the proposed game is described in Figure 12.1.

3.0.1 CASO

CASO is a card sound game, which displays a card with a sound of an animal. When a card is displayed, a sound can also flash onto the display. When starting the game, the child can select his preferred language from Hindi or English. The child has to select the name matching to the flashing sound on the cards displayed among the four cards. A card on the top displays the initial letter of the flashing sound. A child is prompted to recognize the letter, sound, and name of the origin of sound. The selection of the correct or incorrect card will show a message that the child has marked the correct answer or incorrect answer. The marks or scale of this game will decide whether you will play this game or try the next game. The screenshot of the game is shown in Figure 12.2. Objective: The main purpose of the game is to increase focus, attention span, confidence, and cognitive ability. Improvement in the game scores can be seen after a repetition of four to five times, totally dependent on the severity of the disorder.

3.0.2 ATLAS

Our second game of software, ATLAS, is particularly popular with children. The game features avatars. The first page displays the avatar to be selected. The selection procedure will give the child a choice to play with his/her own choice of friends. Next, when the avatar is displayed, it starts speaking about the place name with a letter chosen by the child from ATLAS. The avatar speaks the place name from the letter and interacts and encourages the child, who is the second player in the game to speak with the other letter. This game increases interaction, focus, and confidence in speaking. When the child gives the correct answer, it encourages the child, and a score is added. The screenshot of the game is shown in Figure 12.3. Objective: The main purpose of the game is to increase confidence to

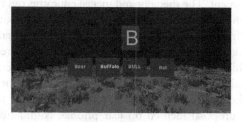

Figure 12.2 Screenshot of CASO game

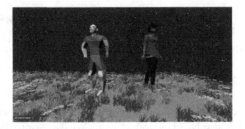

Figure 12.3 Screenshot of ATLAS game

interact socially, make eye contact, increase focus, attention, and verbal ability, while enhancing emotional skills.

The two proposed games are free to use anywhere in the world with the link https://avir.netlify.app. Games are so prepared that it is a collection of sounds, different soothing colors, and a pleasant environment. All these features are added in order to release "happy hormones" in a child, which increases focus and confidence. In the first game, if the child does not reach the appropriate score that is attainable by normal children, then the child repeats the same game. By repeatedly playing the different levels of the games, this leads to improvement in social interaction and other abilities in the physical world.

These games were given to the psychiatry centers, where autistic children were given games to play. Their performance is assessed and marked by the therapist, special educators, and parents.

4 Results and Analysis

Autism rehabilitation when done in clinics follows conventional methods. Conventional therapy believes in the repetition of some physical exercise. These therapies might or might not affect the child in an effective manner. According to Antunes et al. (2017), conventional therapies seem uninteresting to small children.

Thus, games took over the conventional therapies as well. Hence, our proposed model is designed in such a way that child can feel himself to be in different environment, The therapist and special educators can use this software to treat autistic child. The software can be used with or without VR devices. The game can easily be played at home in the supervision of parents. The games can be played again and again until the score of autistic child reaches the score of the normal child. Reaction and responses of therapy is documented by therapist and special educator in a questionnaire form. If the answers are not satisfactory on Likert scale, it is advisable to repeatedly play the first game.

The game proposal focused on fear/phobia, confidence, attention span, focus, social interaction skill and emotions. For the testing phase, games

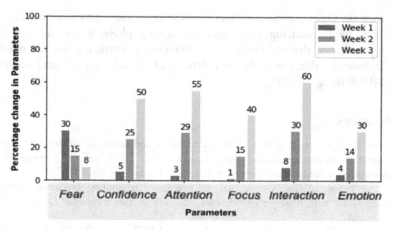

Figure 12.4 Result

were provided at a school and with few families. When the participants were given games to play for the first time, they showed little interest and performance, but after two trials the interest as well as effectiveness increased. The game was played by children for four weeks, twice a week.

The Figure 12.4 analyzes the performance of autistic child after playing games from week 1 to week 4. On x- axis the parameters are taken on which analysis is performed and on y-axis the percentage of improvement is shown. All performance metrics shows the improvement and we have measured the average of all age groups. It can be easily depicted that fear/phobia is decreased to 8% from week 1 to week 4. The interesting part of the game and the major goal of our software is to increase confidence and social interaction. There is an increase from 50% to 60% in both parameters when measured by a therapist based on a questionnaire and survey of the parents. The attention span or sitting time has also shown improvement upto 55%. The effect of software also depends on the age group as well as severity of disorder. It can be stated that in week 1 the results were not improved and not upto the mark. But, after repetition of the games, the progress was analyzed in the improvement of symptoms. Therapist and special educators analyzed and proposed that webVR is beneficial when compared to normal conventional therapy.

4.1 Conclusion

WebVR is an inexpensive method that can be widely used for the treatment of various NDDs. The proposed software provides games for autistic children. Children in general love colors and sounds. Hence, our software can have colorful scenes with different sounds. Our game works well to increase focus, confidence, social communication, and emotional interaction, while reducing fear. After the testing phase, it can be seen that repetition of therapy produces fruitful results. Further scope for research includes working on other deficiencies of an autistic child and on other NDDs using webVR.

References

Antunes, T. P. C. et al. (2017). "Computer classes and games in virtual reality environment to reduce loneliness among students of an elderly reference center: Study protocol for a randomised cross-over design." *Medicine*, 96(10).

Brady, D. I.et al. (2013). "Conceptual and perceptual set-shifting executive abilities in young adults with Asperger's syndrome." *Research in Autism Spectrum Disorders*, 7(12): 1631–1637.

Butler, A. C., Chapman, J. E., Forman, E. M., and Beck, A. T. (2006). "The empirical status of cognitive- behavioral therapy: A review of meta-analyses." *Clinical Psychology Review*, 26(1): 17–31.

Cordeil, M., Dwyer, T., Klein, K., Laha, B., Marriott, K., and Thomas, B. H. (2016). "Immersive collaborative analysis of network connectivity: Cave-style or head-mounted display?" *IEEE Transactions on Visualization and Computer Graphics*, 23(1): 441–450.

Crescentini, C., Chittaro, L., Capurso, V., Sioni, R., and Fabbro, F. (2016). "Psychological and physiological responses to stressful situations in immersive virtual reality: Differences between users who practice mindfulness meditation and controls." *Computers in Human Behavior*, 59: 304–316.

Crocetta, T. B.et al. (2018). "Virtual reality software package for implementing motor learning and rehabilitation experiments." *Virtual Reality*, 22(3): 199–209.

de Mello Monteiro, C. B. et al. (2017). "Short-term motor learning through non-immersive virtual reality task in individuals with Down syndrome." *BMC Neurology*, 17(1): 1–8.

Hocine, N., Gouaïch, A., Cerri, S. A., Mottet, D., Froger, J., and Laffont, I. (2015). "Adaptation in serious games for upper-limb rehabilitation: An approach to improve training outcomes." *User Modeling and User-Adapted Interaction*, 25(1): 65–98.

Malheiros, S. R. P. et al. (2016). "Computer task performance by subjects with Duchenne muscular dystrophy." *Neuropsychiatric Disease and Treatment*, 12: 41.

Manju, T., Padmavathi, S. and Tamilselvi, D. (2017). "*A rehabilitation therapy for autism spectrum disorder using virtual reality*." International conference on intelligent information technologies, 328–336.

Mousavi, H. and Khademi, M. (2014). "A review on technical and clinical impact of microsoft kinect on physical therapy and rehabilitation." *Journal of Medical Engineering*.

Mousavi, H. et al. (2016). Choice of human–computer interaction mode in stroke rehabilitation. *Neurorehabilitation and Neural Repair*, 30(3): 258–265.

Munson, J. and Pasqual, P. (2012). "Using technology in autism research: The promise and the perils." *Computer*, 45(6): 89–91.

Nolin, P. et al. (2016). "Clin- icavr: Classroom-cpt: A virtual reality tool for assessing attention and inhibition in children and adolescents." *Computers in Human Behavior*, 59: 327–333.

Novak, I. and Morgan, C. (2019). "High-risk follow-up: Early intervention and rehabilitation." *Handbook of Clinical Neurology*, 162: 483–510.

Pick, S., Weyers, B., Hentschel, B., and Kuhlen, T. W. (2016). "Design and evaluation of data annotation workflows for cave-like virtual environments." *IEEE Transactions on visualization and Computer Graphics*, 22(4): 1452–1461.

Rizzo, A. A. and Buckwalter, J. G. (1997). "Virtual reality and cognitive assessment." *Virtual Reality in Neuro-Psycho-Physiology: Cognitive, Clinical and Methodological Issues in Assessment and Rehabilitation*, 44: 123.

Stasolla, F. and Passaro, A. (2020). "Enhancing life skills of children and adolescents with autism spectrum disorder and intellectual disabilities through technological supports: A selective overview." In *Interdisciplinary Approaches to Altering Neurodevelopmental Disorders* (pp. 41–62).

Tanu, T. and Kakkar, D. (2018). "Strengthening risk prediction using statistical learning in children with autism spectrum disorder." In: *Advances in Autism*.

Wadhera, T. and Kakkar, D. (2019). "Eye tracker: An assistive tool in diagnosis of autism spectrum disorder." In: *Emerging trends in the diagnosis and intervention of neurodevelopmental disorders* (pp. 125–152). IGI Global.

Wadhera, T. and Kakkar, D. (2020a). "Big data-based system: A supportive tool in autism spectrum disorder analysis." In: *Interdisciplinary approaches to altering neurodevelopmental disorders* (pp. 303–319). IGI Global.

Wadhera, T. and Kakkar, D. (2020b). "Multiplex temporal measures reflecting neural underpinnings of brain functional connectivity under cognitive load in autism spectrum disorder." *Neurological Research*, 42(4): 327–337.

Wadhera, T. and Kakkar, D. (2021). "Modeling risk perception using independent and social learning: application to individuals with autism spectrum disorder." *The Journal of Mathematical Sociology*, 45(4): 223–245.

Wang, M. and Reid, D. (2013). "Using the virtual reality-cognitive rehabilitation approach to improve con- textual processing in children with autism." *The Scientific World Journal*.

13 Future Visions for Deep-Learning-based Approaches for NDDs

Learning from Supervised Brain Tumor Segmentation

Radhika Malhotra, Barjinder Singh Saini and Savita Gupta

Introduction

The interrelationship between brain tumors and neurodevelopmental disorders still remain unclear. The impact of tumors and its treatment on neural development and on behavioral and emotional outcomes have been investigated (Butler and Haser, 2006). Cancer survivors who have been treated primarily with radio-chemotherapy have been shown to exhibit cognitive impairment, including attention deficits and memory deficits (Castellino et al., 2014). The neurobiological changes seen are mostly related to neurotoxic effects of brain tumor which greatly influence the brain structure and function. Moreover, in the case of brain tumors, the tumor's location, in addition to radio-chemotherapy treatment, can influence the neuro-cognitive behavior (Mogavero et al., 2020). As a result, accurate prediction and progression of brain tumors is critical in order to mitigate their detrimental effects on neurodevelopment, which might later lead to neuro developmental disorders at the later stages. Hence for brain image analysis, computer-aided applications have achieved a lot of significance as these techniques assist radiologists with improved treatment-based solutions (Wadhera and Kakkar, 2020b).

The first step towards diagnosing brain tumors is segmentation of the abnormal region from the healthy brain tissues. Segmentation is defined as a simple step in biomedical imaging for selecting the affected area from brain tissues using Magnetic Resonance Imaging (MRI) (Manikandan et al., 2014). Medical Imaging techniques are deployed to provide productive information about morphology of brain tumors. MRI with its multiple sequences like T1, T1 contrast enhanced (T1ce), T2 and T2 Fluid Attenuated Inversion Recovery (T2 FLAIR) are utilized for segmenting tumor and its components. The automatic segmentation of brain tumors is hindered by many challenges such as class imbalance, different sizes of the tumor, scarcity of sufficiently labelled training data (Chaddad et al., 2019), etc. These issues are needed to be addressed effectively. For this, the Medical Image Computing and Computer-Assisted Intervention (MICCAI) society has encouraged work in the area of brain tumors and formulated various brain databases for the community. The aim of this chapter is to give a general review of the recent

DOI: 10.4324/9781003165569-13

trends in the tumor segmentation for the early and accurate prediction of brain tumors in order to overcome its consequences on neurodevelopment. The remaining section of this review is organized as follows. The next part specifies outline of classification of brain tumors, followed by medical image analysis. The following section provides an overview of diagnosing brain tumors using MRI and its sequences with the contribution of deep learning in the area of biomedical imaging. The final part presents the datasets for brain tumor study and an overview of recent deep learning-based tumor segmentation architectures.

Classification of Brain Tumors

The most complicated organ of the human body is the brain, which functions with trillions of cells. In some cases, abnormal cell groups are formed, leading to tumor progression thus affecting the mental and physical well-being of a person concerned. Brain tumors are grouped into two categories: malignant tumors which are cancerous and benign tumors which are non-cancerous. Among these, gliomas are malignant type of tumors and comprise about 80% of total cancerous tumors. The World Health Organization has classified gliomas into four different grades from Grade I to Grade IV, based on the growth rate of abnormal cells as shown in the Figure 13.1. Among these, glioblastoma

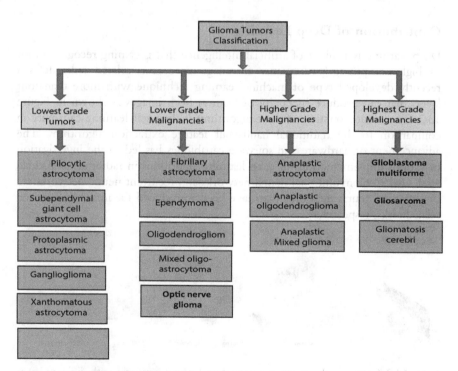

Figure 13.1 Classification of the brain tumors described by American Association of Neurological Surgeons

multiforme is regarded as the most aggressive tumor of the central nervous system (Delgado-López et al., 2016). This tumor falls under the category of grade IV and those affected by it have only a poor median survival rate, of some 12 to 15 months (Xu, 2018).

Medical image analysis

Medical image analysis is the method that is applied for the visualization of the human system. Medical imaging is considered as the most important part in detection and treatment of numerous diseases and helps in representation of different image modalities. It forms a crucial part of the cutting-edge healthcare systems. Computed Tomography, Positron Emission Tomography, Single-Photon Emission Computed Tomography, Magnetic Resonance Spectroscopy and MRI are various available medical imaging techniques which are utilized to impart useful information like morphology, extent and size of the brain tumor (Wadhera and Kakkar, 2020a). Out of these, MRI has proven to be the most widely used imaging modality as it provides detection of soft-tissue contrast and heterogeneity assessment of gliomas. Medical image analysis along with artificial intelligence plays a vital role in tumor detection, segmentation, classification, tumor progression, and many more.

Contribution of Deep Learning

Deep learning is a subset of artificial intelligence that is gaining recognition for its high computing performance in image processing related tasks. It is a recently developed type of machine learning technique with more than four layers that can produce hierarchy of features from images as shown in Figure 13.3. The main attraction of these algorithms is their self-learning capability in comparison to the traditional hand-craft feature extraction algorithms. The advancement of hardware and software capabilities has led to the investigation of various implementations of deep learning algorithms in radiomics (Chaddad et al., 2019). Convolutional neural networks and recurrent neural networks are the types of neural networks that have been introduced for image and speech related tasks, respectively.

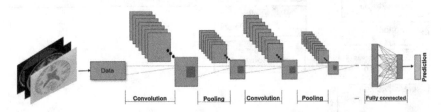

Figure 13.2 General architecture of convolutional neural networks with different layers (Bernal et al., 2019)

Datasets for Brain MRI Analyses

In comparison to various available image or video datasets, datasets for brain tumor analysis are less exhaustive in size. Brain Tumor Segmentation (BraTS) is the most popularly used brain tumor segmentation dataset that is available online. Other available datasets or challenges for brain MRI analyses are discussed below.

BraTS: This brain tumor image segmentation challenge has taken place annually since 2012, along with the MICCAI conference. MRI samples from 19 distinct organizations are included in BraTS datasets for both HGG and LGG patients. Four different MR sequences (T1, T1ce, T2, and T2 FLAIR) with ground truth are incorporated in this dataset. The BraTS 2017 and BraTS 2018 data incorporated the complete survival prediction task along with the segmentation of the tumors. Moreover, BraTS 2019 and the most recent BraTS 2020 incorporated an uncertainty task with survival prediction and automated segmentation of tumor subregions. The summary of various BraTS datasets is provided in Table 13.1.

ISLES: This challenge involves MRI sequences for accessing stroke tumors and their clinical outcome prediction. In this dataset, MR images of patients with acute strokes and their related clinical factors are reported. For ISLES 2016, the available training and testing cases are 35 and 40, respectively.

mTOP: This challenge involves cases of healthy patients as well as patients with traumatic brain injury and emphasize on assessing variations between these two cases. Also, it categorizes the provided data using unsupervised methods into different groups.

MSSEG: The aim of this challenge is to evaluate the participants' recent and progressive segmentation approaches to Multiple Sclerosis data. In total, 38 patients were included in this database which are imaged using 1.5 or 3T MRI scanners.

Deep Learning Approaches in Correlation with Tumor Segmentation

With different levels of abstraction from low-level to high-level, deep learning-based approaches are used to represent information with a hierarchy of multiple processing layers (Nadeem et al., 2020). Qualitative analysis of brain tumors is important for the detection of various neurological diseases and depends greatly on accurate delineation of regions of interest. Segmentation is defined to be labelling of pixels in two-dimensional space or voxels in three-dimensional space. Among all the approaches and techniques for deep learning, Convolutional neural networks (CNN) are one step ahead and are mostly employed for tumor part segmentation (Shboul et al., 2019).

Current CNN architectures based on the processing of data:

Single-path CNN: In a single-path convolutional neural network, a unique path with convolutional and other additional layers like pooling layer, batch

Table 13.1 Summary of BraTS dataset from 2012 to 2020

Datasets	Training samples	Total HGG samples	Total LGG samples	Sequences	Size
BraTS 2012	80	45	35	T1,T1ce,T2,T2 FLAIR	130*170*170
BraTS 2013	30	20	10	T1,T1ce,T2,T2 FLAIR	240*240*155
BraTS 2014	166	130	33	T1,T1ce,T2,T2 FLAIR	240*240*155
BraTS 2015	274	220	54	T1,T1ce,T2,T2 FLAIR	240*240*155
BraTS 2016	274	220	54	T1,T1ce,T2,T2 FLAIR	240*240*155
BraTS 2017	285	210	75	T1,T1ce,T2,T2 FLAIR	240*240*155
BraTS 2018	285	210	75	T1,T1ce,T2,T2 FLAIR	240*240*155
BraTS 2019	285	210	75	T1,T1ce,T2,T2 FLAIR	240*240*155
BraTS 2020	285	210	75	T1,T1ce,T2,T2 FLAIR	240*240*155

normalization, non–linear rectifier units etc. is utilized to process the input data. As the data are processed in one direction, single-path CNNs are computationally efficient and need a smaller number of parameters for training.

Multi-Path CNN: Multi-path CNN can be viewed from two prospects. The first aspect signifies the different scales of the input image that can extract information from various pathways. The input image is scaled at various input dimensions to cope with the different sizes of the tumor (Hao et al., 2020). Multi-scale input at various scales can acquire more features that are beneficial for segmentation and remove redundant information to get the best features. These features are then fused to get the output for processing. Hence multi-scale input adapts more neighborhood information from different angles for improving brain tumor detection. Another aspect of multi-path CNNs might have different pathways or tracks with different parameters like size of convolutional filters, number of convolutional layers, etc. (Aboelenein et al., 2020). These have the capability simultaneously to extract both contextual and global information.

Cascaded CNN: This basically integrates two different CNN networks (Lachinov et al., 2019). To further refine the results, the output of the first network and the initial prediction of class labels are fed to the second CNN. For an instance, (Michal, 2018) utilized two Deep Neural Networks (DNN) in which the first DNN targets the tumorous region and the second network delineates the glioma into its sub-regions. The first DNN used for tumor localization and the second DNN segments tumor into its sub-constituents.

Ensembled CNN: Ensemble methods is a machine learning technique that integrates several base models in order to obtain one optimal predictive model. It is usually comprised of different available architectures that can vary in filter number, model depth, connections, kernel sizes and others (Sun et al., 2019). Ensemble-based techniques use multiple learning algorithms to produce finer predictive performance that can be produced from any of the learning algorithms alone (Cabria and Gondra, 2017). Different model architectures can produce varying performances and behaviour by training different kinds of architectures This can lead to an unbiased generic practice with robust performance.

Challenges to be Addressed: Brain Tumor Segmentation

In the past few years, there has been a major breakthrough in the deep learning models of brain tumor segmentation. Despite this, the state-of-the-art approaches lag satisfactory results, as several challenges related to tumor segmentation need to be addressed effectively. The following challenges are associated with segmentation of brain tumors:

1. *Class Imbalance Issue:* Gliomas are well known for their heterogeneous tumor tissue properties which might challenge the design of automated segmentation techniques. Class imbalance refers to the unequal distribution of the classes in the brain as healthy tissues occupy 98% of brain volume whereas abnormal tissues account for about 1.8% of total brain volume (Zhou et al., 2019). Here are some types of loss functions which are generally utilized in medical image segmentation architectures as shown in Table 13.3 to overcome this problem.

2. *Structural and Location Uncertainty:* The identification and segmentation of brain tumors is challenging, owing to unpredictability in tumor size, shape, and location of tumor cells. The gliomas are characterized by the presence of different cell populations or clones within a tumor (Inda et al., 2014). Therefore, these can develop anywhere inside the brain. Moreover, the HGG sub-regions might also vary in morphology and size. Owing to these structural and location uncertainties, conventional CNN methods cannot attain state-of-the-art results. In order to cope with distinct sizes of the abnormal tissues, multi-path networks are deployed. With multi-model MRIs, multi-path CNNs can extract the contextual information using the symmetric-difference at multi-levels of processing (Nadeem et al., 2020). This type of network processes the input image at different angles or regions in order to overcome the variability in tumor sizes that exist from one patient to another.

3. *Low Contrast and Diffusion:* It is known that multi-channels of MRI are assumed to deliver more image information (Liu et al., 2016). In MRI acquisition, processes like image projection and tomography can lead to poor quality of sliced images (Liu et al., 2020) mostly in low contrast and diffusion. The

Table 13.2 Summary of segmentation methods for brain tumors

Study	Input dimension	Datasets used	Technique	Proposed architecture	Evaluation metric
(Zikic et al., 2014)	2-D	BraTS 2013	Convolutional neural networks (CNN)	Standard CNN structure & Inhomogeneity correction for pre-processing input.	Dice scores Complete 76.3 Core 70.9 Enhancing 67.4
(Hu et al., 2017)	2-D	BraTS 2017	Dilated Convolutional neural networks	Fully convolutional network approach with dilated convolutional kernels for the first time.	Dice scores Complete 0.69 Core 0.617 Enhancing 0.518 Hausdorff Complete 42.79 Core 53.10 Enhancing 87.91
(Brosch et al., 2016)	3-D	MICCAI 2008 and ISBI 2015 challenges	Convolutional neural networks	Deep 3D convolutional networks with encoder, decoder pathways and shortcut connections.	Dice score 68.4 LTPR 74.5
(Pourreza et al., 2018)	3-D	BraTS 2017	Fully Convolutional Network (FCN)	Holistically-Nested Edge Detection (HED) network & intensity normalization using histogram-based method as pre-processing.	Dice scores Complete 0.80 Core 0.55 Enhancing 0.55
(Crimi et al., 2017)	2-D	BraTS 2017	Full resolution residual convolutional neural network (FRRN)	Segmentation using FRRN and exploring dropout using Monte Carlo for uncertainty measurements.	Dice scores Complete 0.874 Core 0.736 Enhancing 0.670 Hausdorff Enhancing 54.791 Complete 8.825 Core 31.332

Study	Input dimension	Datasets used	Technique	Proposed architecture	Evaluation metric
(Hussain et al., 2018)	2-D	BraTS 2015	Convolutional neural network	Utilized four different CNNs for four different modalities and fused to produce a single output map.	Dice for whole tumor 85.46% Accuracy 98.20%
(Zhao and Jia, 2016)	2-D	BraTS 2012 and BraTS 2013	Multi path Convolutional neural networks	Used three different scales of the input image and fuse information from different scales of the inputs.	Accuracy 0.81
(Raza et al., 2017)	3-D	BraTS 2017	Deep convolutional networks (DCN)	3D-UNet and intensity normalization as preprocessing step.	Dice scores Core 0.67 Complete 0.82 Enhancing 0.60 Hausdorff Core 30.66 Complete 11.34 Enhancing 56.4
(Kamnitsas et al., 2017)	3-D	BraTS 2015 and ISLES 2015	Multi-scale Convolutional neural networks	Two convolutional pathways in parallel for multi-scale processing with 3-D fully connected Conditional Random Field.	BraTS 2015: Dice scores Core 0.67 Complete 0.84 Enhancing 0.629 ISLES 2015: Dice score 66 Precision 77 Sensitivity 63
(Li et al., 2017)	2.5-D	BraTS 2017	Multi-path Fully Convolutional Networks	Three multiple branches with fully-convolutional residual network for segmenting brain tumor images	Dice scores Core 0.71 Complete 0.88 Enhancing 0.75
(Zhou et al., 2018)	2-D	BraTS 2017	Convolutional neural networks	Two types of input patches of varying sizes with dual branch convolutional neural network and intensity normalization as preprocessing	Dice scores Core 0.722 Complete 0.88 Enhancing 0.73

Study	Input dimension	Datasets used	Technique	Proposed architecture	Evaluation metric
(Castillo et al., 2018)	3-D	BraTS 2017	Neural Network	Four parallel pathways with residual connections to extract multi-resolution information from input images	Dice scores Core 0.68 Complete 0.88 Enhancing 0.71
(Sedlar, 2018)	2-D	BraTS 2017	Multi-path Convolutional Neural Network	Extracted both local and larger patches for local, symmetry, contextual and spatial information with intensity normalization.	Dice scores Core 0.6938 Complete 0.8436 Enhancing 0.6049
(Chen et al., 2018)	3-D	BraTS 2015	Cascaded Convolutional Neural Networks	Extracted features from deep convolutional layers using cascaded Res-UNet for locating tumor and then tumor sub-regions.	Dice scores Complete 0.85 Active Tumor 0.61 Core 0.72 PPV Complete 0.86 Active Tumor 0.66 Core 0.83
(Casamitjana et al., 2018)	3-D	BraTS 2017	Cascaded Convolutional Neural Networks	Employed a cascaded V-Net architecture in dual step process, firstly localize the tumor area and then delineating different tumor regions.	Dice scores Core 0.637 Complete 0.877 Enhancing 0.71
(Cabezas et al., 2018)	3-D	BraTS 2018	3D U-Net	Deployed an ensemble of 4 architectures namely a U-Net with a dense output (UCNN), U-Net with a fully convolutional output (U-Net) and a dense CNN and Fully Convolutional Networks (FCNNs) with convolutions only.	Dice scores Core 0.717 Complete 0.849 Enhancing 0.667 Hausdorff Core 9.822 Complete 7.765 Enhancing 7.765

Study	Input dimension	Datasets used	Technique	Proposed architecture	Evaluation metric
(Kamnitsas et al., 2018)	3-D	BraTS 2017	Ensemble of different Convolutional Neural Networks	Used ensemble of three different models namely DeepMedic, U-Net and FCN.	Dice scores Core 0.785 Complete 0.886 Enhancing 0.729
(Nuechterlein and Mehta, 2019)	3-D	BraTS 2018	Deep Neural Networks (DNNs)	An ensemble of 26 neural networks with DeepMedic and 3D U-Net as base models. Reported the effect of different initializations, normalizations, batch sizes, etc.	Dice scores Complete 0.894 Core 0.804 Enhancing 0.766 Hausdorff Complete 8.507 Core 8.957 Enhancing 3.992
(Pereira et al., 2016)	2-D	BraTS 2013	Convolutional Neural Networks	Investigated the use of 3*3 kernels for fewer weights in the network and rotating the samples through data augmentation.	Dice scores Complete 0.88 Core 0.83 Enhancing 0.77
(Aboelenein et al., 2020)	2D	BraTS 2018	Hybrid Two-Track U-Net (HTTU-Net)	Utilized two tracks to handle different tumor sizes with first track, focusing on the tumor's form and second track capturing contextual information.	Dice scores Complete 0.865 Core 0.808 Enhancing 0.745
(Hao et al., 2020)	3-D	BraTS 2018	Multi-scale convolutional neural network (MSCNN)	Segmented 2D slices in the coronal, sagittal, and cross-sectional views and fused by averaging method. Used input at different scales to accommodate more neighborhood information.	0.90 for WT using multi-scale integration.

Study	Input dimension	Datasets used	Technique	Proposed architecture	Evaluation metric
(Hussain et al., 2018)	2-D	BraTS 2013 and BraTS 2015	Deep Convolutional Neural Network (DCNN)	Proposed an inception module based on patches to explore the effect of multi-parallel paths.	Dice scores: BraTS 2013 Core 0.89 Complete 0.87 Enhancing 0.92 Dice scores: BraTS 2015 Core 0.87 Complete 0.86 Enhancing 0.9
(Cui et al., 2018)	2-D	BraTS 2015	Cascaded Deep Convolutional Neural Network	Based on tumor localization network to be followed by intratumor classification network with transfer learning technology.	Dice scores Core 0.77 Complete 0.89 Enhancing 0.80
(Isensee et al., 2019)	3-D	BraTS 2018	U-Net	Proposed minor modifications in basic U-Net structure like patch processing, soft dice loss functions, instance normalization etc.	Dice scores Complete 87.81 Core 80.62 Enhancing 77.88 Hausdorff Distances Complete 6.03 Core 5.08 Enhancing 2.90
(Ding et al., 2019)	2-D	BraTS 2015	Residual Networks (Res-Nets)	Proposed Deep Residual Dilate Network with Middle Supervision (RDM-Net) to resolve vanishing gradient issue.	Dice scores Core 0.8347 Complete 0.9037 Enhancing 0.8383
(Zhou et al., 2020)	3-D	BraTS 2015 and BraTS 2017	Deep Convolutional Neural Networks (DNNs)	Proposed One-pass Multi-task Network (OM-Net) to rectify class imbalance problem by integrating different segmentation tasks in single deep model.	Dice scores: BraTS 2015 Complete 87 Core 75 Enhancing 65 Dice scores: BraTS 2017 Complete 0.9071 Core 0.8422 Enhancing 0.7852

Table 13.3 Summary of different loss functions utilized for class imbalance issue

Ref.	Loss function type	Description
(Shelhamer et al., 2017)	Cross-Entropy (CE) loss	Computes the class labels for every pixel separately and then calculate mean for all pixels.
(Milletari, 2016)	Dice Loss (DL)	Estimation of overlap between the predicted mask and actual mask with value ranging from 0–1.
(Sudre et al., 2017)	Generalized Dice Loss (GDL)	Class rebalancing properties and most robust of loss functions.
(Lin et al., 2017)	Focal Loss (FL)	Originally introduced for the detection tasks.

boundary between biological tissues is prone to blur and becomes difficult to detect. These intensity variations limit the automated segmentation algorithms to quantify sufficient information for further processing.

Future Scope of NDDs and Conclusion

Several studies have shown that the initiation and progression of brain tumor have been associated with disintegration of developmental cell signaling pathways. The re-emergence of neurodevelopmental problems in the context of brain tumors underlines many similarities between developmental and therapy mechanisms. So, to make these therapies more feasible, continued investigations and treatment approaches for the different phenotypes of brain tumors should be maintained. But the delineation of tumor sub-compartments or phenotypes is highly reliant on four MRI modalities. Incorporating all of these modalities into a single CNN network is computationally quite complex. As a result, more appropriate methods should be developed that could effectively segment these sub-regions from a set of two or three modalities. Also, the progress of the deep learning approaches is influenced by the choice of pre-processing strategies, hyper-parameters (learning rate, batch size, filter dimensions, initialization, etc.) and post-processing techniques. Therefore, parameter selection plays a vital role in developing model and is quite challenging. Also, the major pitfall of employing these techniques in the medical imaging is small size of the training datasets which might cause generalization errors on unseen datasets. Hence data augmentation strategies which can mimic the divergence in the medical image datasets are much needed. Exploration of other techniques like batch normalization and transfer learning with fine tuning, which could limit the overfitting concerns, are needed. Moreover, deep learning approaches which are derived from unsupervised methods, along with less dependency on the ground truth masks (manual labelling of tumor parts), should be emphasized.

References

Aboelenein, N. M., Songhao, P., Koubaa, A., Noor, A., and Afifi, A. (2020). "HTTU-Net: Hybrid Two Track U-Net for Automatic Brain Tumor Segmentation." *IEEE Access*, 8: 101406–101415. https://doi.org/10.1109/ACCESS.2020.2998601.

Bernal, J., Kushibar, K., Asfaw, D. S., Valverde, S., Oliver, A., Martí, R., and Lladó, X. (2019). "Deep convolutional neural networks for brain image analysis on magnetic resonance imaging: a review." *Artificial Intelligence in Medicine*, 95(November 2016): 64–81. doi:10.1016/j.artmed.2018.08.008.

Brosch, T., Tang, L. Y. W., Yoo, Y., Li, D. K. B., Traboulsee, A., and Tam, R. (2016). "Deep 3D Convolutional Encoder Networks With Shortcuts for Multiscale Feature Integration Applied to Multiple Sclerosis Lesion Segmentation." *IEEE Transactions on Medical Imaging*, 35(5): 1229–1239. doi:10.1109/TMI.2016.2528821.

Butler, R.W. and Haser, J. (2006). "Neurocognitive Effects of Treatment for Childhood Cancer." *Mentally Retardation and Development Disability Research Review*, 12(2): 184–191. doi:10.1002/mrdd.

Cabezas, M. et al. (2018). "Survival prediction using ensemble tumor segmentation and transfer learning." *Radiology*, 13(8): 1–9. http://arxiv.org/abs/1810.04274.

Cabria, I. and Gondra, I. (2017). "MRI segmentation fusion for brain tumor detection." *Information Fusion*, 36(11): 1–9. doi:10.1016/j.inffus.2016.10.003.

Casamitjana, A., Català, M., Sánchez, I., Combalia, M., and Vilaplana, V. (2018). "Cascaded V-Net using ROI masks for brain tumor segmentation." *ArXiv*, 381–391. doi:10.1007/978-3-319-75238-9.

Castellino, S. M., Ullrich, N. J., Whelen, M. J., and Lange, B. J. (2014). "Developing interventions for cancer-related cognitive dysfunction in childhood cancer survivors." *Journal of the National Cancer Institute*, 106(8): 1–16. doi:10.1093/jnci/dju186.

Castillo, L. S., Daza, L. A., Rivera, L. C., and Arbeláez, P. (2018). "Brain Tumor segmentation and parsing on MRIs using multiresolution neural networks." *Lecture Notes in Computer Science (Including Subseries Lecture Notes in Artificial Intelligence and Lecture Notes in Bioinformatics), 10670 LNCS*: 332–343. doi:10.1007/978-3-319-75238-9_29.

Chaddad, A. et al. (2019). "Radiomics in glioblastoma: Current status and challenges facing clinical implementation." *Frontiers in Oncology*, 9(8): 1–9). doi:10.3389/fonc.2019.00374.

Chen, X., Liew, J. H., Xiong, W., Chui, C. K., and Ong, S. H. (2018). "Focus, segment and erase: An efficient network for multi-label brain tumor segmentation." *Lecture Notes in Computer Science (Including Subseries Lecture Notes in Artificial Intelligence and Lecture Notes in Bioinformatics), LNCS*, 11217: 674–689. doi:10.1007/978-3-030-01261-8_40.

Crimi, A.et al. (2017). "Towards Uncertainty-Assisted Brain Tumor Segmentation and Survival Prediction." *Automatic Brain Tumor Segmentation Using Convolutional Neural Networks with Test-Time Augmentation*, 10670(December 2017): 138–149. doi:10.1007/978-3-319-75238-9.

Cui, S., Mao, L., Jiang, J., Liu, C., and Xiong, S. (2018). "Automatic semantic segmentation of brain gliomas from MRI images using a deep cascaded neural network." *Journal of Healthcare Engineering, 2018*(9): 1–14. doi:10.1155/2018/4940593.

Delgado-López, P. D. et al. (2016). "Survival in glioblastoma: a review on the impact of treatment modalities." *Clinical and Translational Oncology*, 18(11): 1062–1071. doi:10.1007/s12094-016-1497-x.

Ding, Y., Li, C., Yang, Q., Qin, Z., and Qin, Z. (2019). "How to Improve the Deep Residual Network to Segment Multi-Modal Brain Tumor Images." *IEEE Access*, 7 (15): 152821–152831. doi:10.1109/ACCESS.2019.2948120.

Hao, J., Li, X., and Hou, Y. (2020). "Magnetic Resonance Image Segmentation Based on Multi-Scale Convolutional Neural Network." *IEEE Access*, 8: 65758–65768. https://doi.org/10.1109/ACCESS.2020.2964111.

Hussain, S., Anwar, S. M., and Majid, M. (2018). "Segmentation of glioma tumors in brain using deep convolutional neural network." *Neurocomputing*, 282: 248–261. doi:10.1016/j.neucom.2017.12.032.

Inda, M., Bonavia, R., and Seoane, J. (2014). "Glioblastoma multiforme: A look inside its heterogeneous nature." *Cancers*, 6(1): 226–239. doi:10.3390/cancers6010226.

Isensee, F., Kickingereder, P., Wick, W., Bendszus, M., and Maier-Hein, K. H. (2019). "No new-net." *Lecture Notes in Computer Science (Including Subseries Lecture Notes in Artificial Intelligence and Lecture Notes in Bioinformatics)*, LNCS, 11384: 234–244. https://doi.org/10.1007/978-3-030-11726-9_21.

Kamnitsas, K.et al. (2017). "Efficient multi-scale 3D CNN with fully connected CRF for accurate brain lesion segmentation." *Medical Image Analysis*, 36: 61–78. doi:10.1016/j.media.2016.10.004.

Kamnitsas, K. et al. (2018). "Ensembles of multiple models and architectures for robust brain tumour segmentation." *Lecture Notes in Computer Science (Including Subseries Lecture Notes in Artificial Intelligence and Lecture Notes in Bioinformatics)*, LNCS, 10670: 450–462. doi:10.1007/978-3-319-75238-9_38.

Lachinov, D., Vasiliev, E., and Turlapov, V. (2019). "Glioma segmentation with cascaded UNet." *Lecture Notes in Computer Science (Including Subseries Lecture Notes in Artificial Intelligence and Lecture Notes in Bioinformatics)*, LNCS, 11384: 189–198. doi:10.1007/978-3-030-11726-9_17.

Lin, T. Y., Goyal, P., Girshick, R., He, K., and Dollar, P. (2017). "Focal Loss for Dense Object Detection." *Proceedings of the IEEE International Conference on Computer Vision*, 2017(October): 2999–3007. doi:10.1109/ICCV.2017.324.

Liu, W., Anguelov, D., Erhan, D., Szegedy, C., Reed, S., Fu, C. Y., and Berg, A. C. (2016). "SSD: Single shot multibox detector." *Lecture Notes in Computer Science (Including Subseries Lecture Notes in Artificial Intelligence and Lecture Notes in Bioinformatics)*, LNCS, 9905: 21–37. doi:10.1007/978-3-319-46448-0_2.

Liu, Z.et al. (2020). *Deep Learning Based Brain Tumor Segmentation: A Survey.* 14(8): 1–21. http://arxiv.org/abs/2007.09479.

Manikandan, S., Ramar, K., Willjuice Iruthayarajan, M., and Srinivasagan, K. G. (2014). "Multilevel thresholding for segmentation of medical brain images using real coded genetic algorithm." *Measurement: Journal of the International Measurement Confederation*, 47(1): 558–568. doi:10.1016/j.measurement.2013.09.031.

Michal, M. (2018). *"Segmenting Brain Tumors from MRI Using Cascaded Multi-modal U-Nets."* BrainLes: International MICCAI Brainlesion Workshop (Vol. 2). Springer International Publishing. doi:10.1007/978-3-030-11726-9.

Milletari, F. (2016). *V-Net: Fully Convolutional Neural Networks for Volumetric Medical Image Segmentation.* 567–573. doi:10.1109/3DV.2016.79.

Mogavero, M. P., Bruni, O., Delrosso, L. M., and Ferri, R. (2020). "Neurodevelopmental consequences of pediatric cancer and its treatment: The role of sleep." *Brain Sciences*, 10(7): 1–15. doi:10.3390/brainsci10070411.

Nadeem, M. W.et al. (2020). "Brain tumor analysis empowered with deep learning: A review, taxonomy, and future challenges." *Brain Sciences*, 10(2): 1–33. doi:10.3390/brainsci10020118.

Nuechterlein, N. and Mehta, S. (2019). "Brain Tumor Segmentation and Tractographic Feature Extraction from Structural MR Images for Overall Survival Prediction."

BrainLes: International MICCAI Brainlesion Workshop (Vol. 2). Springer International Publishing. doi:10.1007/978-3-030-11726-9.

Pereira, S., Pinto, A., Alves, V., and Silva, C. A. (2016). "Brain Tumor Segmentation Using Convolutional Neural Networks in MRI Images." *IEEE Transactions on Medical Imaging*, 35(5): 1240–1251. doi:10.1109/TMI.2016.2538465.

Pourreza, R., Zhuge, Y., Ning, H., and Miller, R. (2018). "Brain tumor segmentation in MRI scans using deeply-supervised neural networks." *Lecture Notes in Computer Science (Including Subseries Lecture Notes in Artificial Intelligence and Lecture Notes in Bioinformatics), LNCS, 10670*: 320–331. doi:10.1007/978-3-319-75238-9_28.

Raza, S. E. A. et al. (2017). "Automatic Brain Tumor Detection and Segmentation Using U-Net Based Fully Convolutional Networks." *Computer Methods and Programs in Biomedicine*, 1(d): 698–706. doi:10.1007/978-3-319-60964-5.

Sedlar, S. (2018). "Brain tumor segmentation using a multi-path CNN based method." *Lecture Notes in Computer Science (Including Subseries Lecture Notes in Artificial Intelligence and Lecture Notes in Bioinformatics), LNCS, 10670*: 403–422. doi:10.1007/978-3-319-75238-9_35.

Shboul, Z. A., Alam, M., Vidyaratne, L., Pei, L., Elbakary, M. I., and Iftekharuddin, K. M. (2019). "Feature-Guided Deep Radiomics for Glioblastoma Patient Survival Prediction." *Frontiers in Neuroscience*, 13(September): 1–17. doi:10.3389/fnins.2019.00966.

Shelhamer, E., Long, J., and Darrell, T. (2017). "Fully Convolutional Networks for Semantic Segmentation." *IEEE Transactions on Pattern Analysis and Machine Intelligence*, 39(4): 640–651.

Sudre, C. H., Li, W., Vercauteren, T., Ourselin, S., and Jorge Cardoso, M. (2017). "Generalised dice overlap as a deep learning loss function for highly unbalanced segmentations." *Lecture Notes in Computer Science (Including Subseries Lecture Notes in Artificial Intelligence and Lecture Notes in Bioinformatics), LNCS, 10553*: 240–248. doi:10.1007/978-3-319-67558-9_28.

Sun, L., Zhang, S., Chen, H., and Luo, L. (2019). "Brain tumor segmentation and survival prediction using multimodal MRI scans with deep learning". *Frontiers in Neuroscience*. doi:10.3389/fnins.2019.00810.

Wadhera, T. and Kakkar, D. (2020a). "Modeling risk perception using independent and social learning: application to individuals with autism spectrum disorder." *Journal of Mathematical Sociology*. doi:10.1080/0022250X.2020.1774877.

Wadhera, T. and Kakkar, D. (2020b). "Multiplex temporal measures reflecting neural underpinnings of brain functional connectivity under cognitive load in Autism Spectrum Disorder." *Neurological Research*, 42(4): 327–337. doi:10.1080/01616412.2020.1726586.

Xu, X. et al. (2018). "The effect of glioblastoma heterogeneity on survival stratification: a multimodal MR imaging texture analysis." *Acta Radiologica*, 59(10): 1239–1246. doi:10.1177/0284185118756951.

Yan, Hu et al. (2017). "Dilated Convolutions for Brain Tumor Segmentation in MRI Scans." *Dilated Convolutions for Brain Tumor Segmentation in MRI Scans, 10670* (December): 138–149. doi:10.1007/978-3-319-75238-9.

Yuexiang, Li et al. (2017). "Deep Learning Based Multimodal Brain Tumor Diagnosis." *Automatic Brain Tumor Segmentation Using Convolutional Neural Networks with Test-Time Augmentation, 10670*(December): 138–149. doi:10.1007/978-3-319-75238-9.

Zhao, L. and Jia, K. (2016). "Multiscale CNNs for Brain Tumor Segmentation and Diagnosis." *Computational and Mathematical Methods in Medicine, 2016*. doi:10.1155/2016/8356294.

Zhou, C., Ding, C., Wang, X., Lu, Z., and Tao, D. (2020). "One-Pass Multi-Task Networks with Cross-Task Guided Attention for Brain Tumor Segmentation." *IEEE Transactions on Image Processing*, 29: 4516–4529. doi:10.1109/TIP.2020.2973510.

Zhou, F., Li, T., Li, H., and Zhu, H. (2018). "TPCNN: Two-phase patch-based convolutional neural network for automatic brain tumor segmentation and survival prediction." *Lecture Notes in Computer Science (Including Subseries Lecture Notes in Artificial Intelligence and Lecture Notes in Bioinformatics), LNCS*, 10670: 274–286. doi:10.1007/978-3-319-75238-9_24.

Zhou, T., Ruan, S., & Canu, S. (2019). A review: Deep learning for medical image segmentation using multi-modality fusion. *Array*, 3–4(May), 1–11. https://doi.org/10.1016/j.array.2019.100004.

Zikic, D., Ioannou, Y., Brown, M., & Criminisi, A. (2014). Segmentation of Brain Tumor Tissues with Convolutional Neural Networks. *Proceedings MICCAI-BRATS, September 2014*, 36–39.

14 Deep Brain Stimulation and Spectral EEG features for Prognosis of Parkinson's Disease and Prevention

Anudruti Singha

1. Introduction

The second most neurodegenerative disorder is Parkinson's disease (PD). Like, Cerebral Palsy (CP), and degenerative tremor (ET), it is a movement disorder that will have clinical features including tremor and gait difficulty. These disorders are often misdiagnosed resulting in a delay in appropriate treatment. Although ET is considered mono-symptomatic, however increasing clinical pieces of evidence explain the complexity of ET involving both motor and non-motor symptoms. Diagnosis of PD could be complex, owing to overlapping symptoms. Among all Parkinson's disease (PD) is the most common degenerative disorder seen in neurological patients. Recently, the researchers are working on the hypothesis that PD is a neurodevelopmental disorder (NDD). In case, it proves in near future, then it would be beneficial to apply the proposed cross-correlation and Independent Component Analysis (ICA) method for electroencephalogram (EEG) channels for early and fast detection of other NDDs lying on the spectrum.

PD is caused as a result of loss of dopamine-generating neurons in the brain. A significant number of these neurons can be found in the substantia region of the brain which is located right above the spinal cord. Loss in these neurons leads to reduced dopamine production. Dopamine is the hormone that is charged with keeping the account of normal body posture and gait. Dopamine loss causes motor symptoms, such as tremor, bradykinesia, rigidity, and hypomimia, together with symptoms of non-motor nature which includes constipation and insomnia. Together all these symptoms are called Parkinsonism symptoms.

Substantia Nigra is the main area where dopamine neuron deficiency occurs prominently in PD. Owing to dopamine deficiency, the nigrostriatal links between Substantia Nigra and Striatum degenerate and produce Lewy bodies. To the extent where Substantia Nigra losses about 80% of its dopamine neuron population the brain losses the motor control of the body. Consequentially, owing to dopamine neuron deficiency, the Thalamus does not get pulses to drive the motion of the body which results in stiffness of muscles.

The root cause of these symptoms and the generation of Lewy bodies is still unknown. Further, research shows that almost 75 percent of people developing

DOI: 10.4324/9781003165569-14

PD have no family history of PD. However, 15 percent are supported with a family history of PD. Different factors can cause the development of PD, i.e. age, some pesticides, gender, heavy metal dust, or gene-mutation. Tremor and rigidity have been characterized as crucial symptoms. The co-occurrence of two of these symptoms is a good indicator of the disease. The PD patients are subject to gait impairment leading to a high risk of falling and related injuries. Individuals suffering from PD are subject to altered gait patterns having an increased cadence, reduced stride length along low walking speed compared to their healthy counterparts. The PD patients suffer from freezing of gait (FOG) and tremor. The FOG can be defined as episodic inability to walk or generate effective movement during one's walk. The FOG can be the result of different clinical conditions such as lock joint, inelasticity, improper nerve conduction, etc.

The chapter highlight the state-of-art in PD treatment procedures in context to Deep Brain Stimulation, and the author's contribution in the development of a novel methodology in support for faster diagnosis of PD with relatable higher accuracy using EEG projections. Further diagnosis and prognosis of PD in support of the EEG signal and its frequency components. A short overview of the future possibilities of the development of intelligent systems to treat or support PD patients have been discussed.

2. Literature Survey

An EEG signal is an electrical signal that is produced by brain nerve potentials. This EEG signal is having a major field of application such as identification of patients with motion imbalance, muscle functioning, and a major part in the contribution of diagnosis of PD (Allen et al., 2010). Simulations using the finite element method are developed and used for the investigation of the electric field (EF) extension of DBS lead designs. However, it is not able to discuss the dipole projections and the origin of Electrical Field Potential around the neurons owing to movement of electric impulses (Brocker and Grill, 2013). The paper helps to describe patient selection, stereotactic implantation, post-operative stimulator programming, and patient care methods. Nevertheless, fails to describe the neurological changes and other tissue damages that might occur owing to DSB (Groiss et al., 2009). New technology such as video, visual perception, auditory stimuli can help in PD treatment. Visual, video and auditory stimuli are subject to the sensational perception of a PD patient. In the worst-case scenario, many patients provide no reaction to external stimuli (Lonini, 2018). The LEAPD algorithm. It uses six-channel EEG leads for data collection. Assuming demographic similarity in EEG signal is quite impractical owing to its high variance in data points (Fahim Anjum et al., 2020). This paper discussed the viability and feasibility to support altered gait patterns using inertial sensors. However, the sensor technology about the article is old dated and can't provide sufficient information and accuracy alone for PD diagnosis (Moon et al., 2020). A Multiple-Instance Learning (MIL) approach. Hereafter implies Deep learning techniques to detect FOG. MIL approach is very useful in the case of data with low variance and low kurtosis. In PD patients the inertial motion sensor data is having a Gaussian nature which can be further reduced (Papadopoulos et al., 2020). The controlled applications of external EF on neuronal cultures are observed in an optimum condition (Stern et al., 2017). The biomarkers are important potential targets for PD diagnosis. However, there are significant failures in investigating the change in EEG power spectrum and its frequency components owing to PD (Tu-Chan et al., 2017). This article helps us to understand field-effect transistor-based biosensors. Guides on the crucial concerns related to devising design and sensor selection methods. The article could have a stronger usage if it would have included Nano-stain gauge sensors, added to the natural and stimulated electron transition methods (Wadhera. et al., 2019). Prior evidence shows that current scientific research in PD diagnosis is still lagging. A major part is still unseen. EEG signal which can provide a high amount of information for Neurological disorders such as PD is not used and not analyzed fruitfully for the mentioned purpose. However, still, a lot of work needs to be done. The present chapter aims to focus on how Deep Brain stimulation, Electrical Field potential, and Dipole formation can help us is PD diagnosis for an earlier stage. A major focus is given on the detection of PD from EEG signals by using different signal processing tools. Moreover, this chapter provides a short and subtle way to develop an assistive device for PD patients.

3. Framework and First Experimental Study

DBS of various basal ganglia nuclei has since developed into a highly effective treatment for several movement disorders. In PD, DBS of the internal Globus pallidus and the subthalamic nucleus (STN) was found to be effective and safe targets.

People suffering from tremors such as PD and CP rely on DBS as a way of treatment. DBS is performed by using an electrical current to target abnormal brain activity. The method triggers blood flow and a series of chemical reactions that lead to the release of neurotransmitters together this function has the potential to make a significant change in PD patients. Neurologists and doctors use the CT scan and MRI of the brain to map out the location for the delivery of the electrical impulses and the region to be targeted. Doctors then implant electrodes using a thin probe lead on the targeted area of the brain. A wire attached to the lead runs through the head, and neck all over to the chest as shown in the X-Ray image of electrode accentuated skull in Figure 14.1. Where the wire attaches to a battery-charged pulse generator, generating electrical impulses, the stimulatory program is activated after a few days of implanting the pulse generator. Each electrode is activated and tested separately. High to low voltage variations are delivered to the STN. After a series of tests that determines the optimal placement, neurosurgeons implant one or more wires, called "leads," inside the brain. The leads are connected with an insulated wire extension to a very small neuro-stimulator (electrical generator) implanted under the person's collarbone, similar to a heart pacemaker.

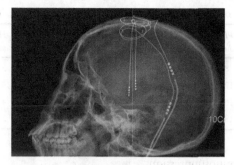

Figure 14.1 X-ray image of electrode positioning in the human skull [12]

Continuous pulses of electric current from the neurostimulator pass through the leads and into the brain. Correspondingly worst and best responses are recorded. However, the method can be flawed under certain circumstances. The patients are kept under certain medications such as levodopa for a period. Effects of the medicated and unmedicated state are measured under Unified Parkinson's Disease Rating Scale (UPDRS). DBS will have no better effect than medicines such as levodopa. Under certain circumstances, the patient might have a risk of developing an infection. High voltage, transmission can damage the brain cells leading to brain stroke or other adverse effects.

An investigation is performed where members were seen under clinical rating scales performed tentatively at gauge (inside one month of a medical procedure), and eight months after STN DBS medical procedure with the trigger on. The seriousness of PD was resolved to utilize the UPDRS, Hoehn and Yahr arranging score, Stand Walk Sit Test (SWST) [13], and the Dyskinesia Rating Scale [14–15] in both the off medicine (PD meds held for 24 h) and taking drugs state where suitable. Table 14.1 given below describes the results for 4 of the patients among all.

A. Patient Selection Criteria in DBS

Inclusion Criteria

- Clinically idiopathic PD
- Significant improvement concerning
- Dopaminergic medication (>30%)
- Refractory motor fluctuations or tremor
- Only minor symptoms during ON-state

Exclusion Criteria

- Biological age over 75 years
- Severe/malignant comorbidity with considerably

Table 14.1 Clinical observations of Patients PD data and rating scales

Patie-nt	Age (yrs)	Sex	PD duration	UPDRS off	UPDRS on	%change (UPDRS)	UPDRS (total)	Hoehn Yahr off (coefficient)	LEDD (mg)
1	64	M	8	32	11	58.2	48	3.0	1470
2	69	F	12	48	12	62.8	66	5.0	1586
3	48	M	10	45	10	67.6	62	4.0	1329
4	77	F	18	46	25	56.9	45	2.0	1633

- Chronic immunosuppression
- Distinct brain atrophy
- Severe psychiatric disorder (Cognitive deficits/dementia, Frontal-dysexecutive syndrome, Manifest Psychosis, Depression, Substance, Abuse, Personality disorder)

B. Side Effects Post DBS Treatment

In the study present below depicts, improvements in cerebral imaging techniques have greatly increased the safety of functional neurosurgery, but surgery-related complications remain a possibility. The most severe complication of DBS surgery is intracerebral haemorrhage (ICH) which is reported to occur in 0.25% (Table 14.2). The degree of haemorrhages varies from asymptomatic ICH to severe ICH resulting in significant and persistent neurological deficits or death. Large variability in the number of postoperative infections ranging from 1.8%−2% of cases is reported. Infections most commonly occur in the area surrounding the pulse generator; The DBS for PD study group, 2001 (Table 14.2). Treatment with systemic antibiotics and local surgical lavation usually suffices, but in severe cases, the implanted device must be removed to

Table 14.2 Complication's statistics after electrode implantation

Year	Number of patients (leads)	Hemorrhage (%)	Infection/erosion (%)	Hardware complications (%)
2003	357	3.1	N/A	N/A
2004	108	N/A	3.8	N/A
2005	119	N/A	3	17.3
2006	78	1.9	3.8	1.3
2006	100	2	4.7	11.5
2007	262	0.2	5.7	13.9
2007	130	6.92	N/A	3.84
2007	319	1.5	4.4	4
2008	103	5.8	6.8	3.9
2009	420	N/A	N/A	4.5
Average		3.06	4.60	7.53

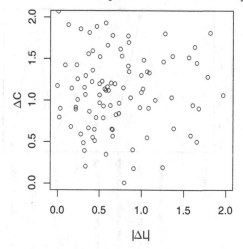

Figure 14.2 Scatter plot of electrode displacement [16]

prevent further spreading of the infection. Other hardware complications include lead breakage or malfunction of the pulse generator. Table 14.2 summarizes the complications related to electrode implantation.

Morishita et. al. (2016), in their article about lead migration inside the skull owing to repetitive head movements as a result of dystonia and Twiddler syndrome, were the risk factors associated with DBS lead migration. Lead migration could, in the majority of cases, be a preventable complication, and careful surgical technique, and possibly an improved lead fixation device, could diminish the incidence of this adverse event. In instances of poor response to DBS therapy, lead localization imaging should be obtained to ensure that the lead is appropriately positioned. Routine lead localization imaging in the early postoperative period, combined with careful evaluation of both clinical effectiveness and thresholds for stimulation-induced adverse effects, might be useful in identifying DBS lead migration cases, and in some cases, could lead to earlier surgical correction. In Figure 14.3, the chart represents the cases in surgery-related as well as hardware-related complications surprisingly mental status decline and deep infections are majorly contributing complications among few others.

4. Framework and Second Experimental Study

EEG signal monitoring is a non-invasive and inexpensive technique to monitor brain health. It is a time-varying, linearly independent signal. The brain generates unique information caring signals from its every region at a given instant of time. EEG signal has a wide range of applications in the diagnosis of Neurophysiological activities. A massive amount of knowledge recorded from even one EEG electrode pair presents an enormous range of information. It is possible to record EEG signals continuously for an extended period of channels;

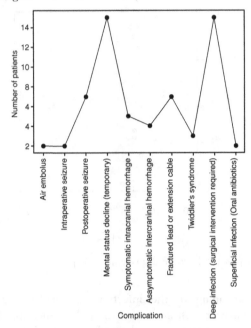

Figure 14.3 Number of cases of post-surgery complications

counting on the appliance, electrode counts can range from single/dual channels. EEG can provide massive temporal resolution, significantly for Parkinson's disease. The EEG can be further classified into five main bands. They are Delta, Theta, Alpha, Beta, and Gamma as shown in Table 14.3.

Symbol	Description
Delta (Δ)	This is a slow, high amplitude band of the EEG wave, comprised of frequencies in between 1 to 3 Hz. These waves are mainly active in children and adults when they are either in stage 3 or stage 4 sleep.
Theta (Ø)	This is classified as a slow activity wave comprising of the frequency range between 3.5 to 7Hz. These band waves represent a day spacey state of mind that is associated with mental inefficiency. It represents the state of mind between sleep and active.
Alpha (α)	This is recognized as a high amplitude band with a frequency of between 7.5 to 13.2 Hz. This waveform is seen in the posterior region of the brain. This is associated with a state of relaxation and represents the brain shifting into an idling gear, waiting to respond when needed. This waveform disappears when the brain shifts back to an alert state of mind.
Beta (β)	This is recognized as the fast-active band of the EEG signal with a frequency range of 14 Hz or greater. It is generally regarded in normal rhythm. According to research beta waveform have a significant role in PD patients. This waveform is attenuated in the region of cortical damage or dis-communication of cortical neurons.

Hypothalamus and Substantia Nigra are the main region of the brain which gets significantly affected owing to Parkinson's disease [18]. Hypothalamus provides a significant contribution to the EEG signal. Studying the EEG signal component of the hypothalamus and Substantia Nigra can provide us with significant insights into Parkinson's disease.

A. Data Acquisition and Processing

The recorder was performed for EEG signal of 23 PD patients and 23 controls, from a study at the Vellore for the training purpose, along with 17 PD patients and 17 controls were performed for testing. Correspondingly, recorded EEG signals from OFF medication conditions for the 23 PD patients from Vellore (India) for, 12 hours after the last dosage of dopaminergic medication. Control participants were demographically matched with PD patients. We gathered EEG data from 63 channels that were common to all datasets as shown in Figure 14.4.

Eye blinks were identified and removed following independent component analysis. Best variance is taken to understand the classification. An EEG of a PD patient comprises of either large-amplitude (450 to 680 microvolt) at 1–3/sec (i.e. synchronized activity) or lower-amplitude (11 to 145 microvolt) at 6–12/ sec (i.e. unsynchronized activity) owing to deficiency in dopamine generation as shown in Figure 14.6.

Similarly, in normal EEG signal, among the normal adult population, the average frequency of the rhythm is 9.7 Hz to 13.2 Hz, and in less than 5%, it is faster than 11.5 Hz or slower than 8.5 Hz Under the stabilized state, the frequency generally varies only about ±0.5 Hz in one recording for a normal EEG signal as shown in Figure 14.6.

B. Data Cleaning

In the figures, the data labelled with blue colour represents the new data after the removal of noise owing to motion artefacts and channel desynchronization, the red colour represents the old data. The EEG data is passed through a linear high pass FIR filter with a transition band between 0.25 Hz to 0.75 Hz. Any channel which is flat for more than 6 seconds is removed. A maximum acceptable high frequency is set to 4 Hz. The minimum acceptable correlation with nearby channels is 0.8. Artefact Subspace Reconstruction bad burst correction is

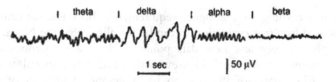

Figure 14.4 Channel location inside the brain [19]

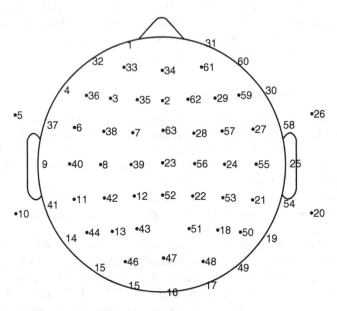

Figure 14.5 Parkinson's EEG after bad data rejection

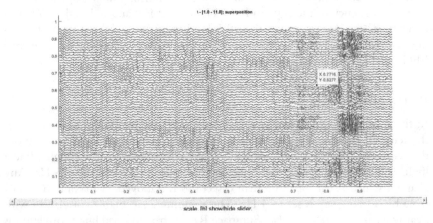

Figure 14.6 Normal healthy EEG after bad data rejection

performed according to the signal requirements. Beta Riemannian distance matrix is used for error estimation. It can be visualized that the Normal healthy EEG graph has very few new data points as there are no motion artefacts owing to normal movements. However, after bad data removal and filtering noise, the EEG graph of PD patients has a significant number of new data points.

C. Biofeedback and Independent Component Analysis

Biofeedback is liable for the development of varying mind states and physical activities, by practically manipulating the brain signal waveforms in desired frequency range by repetitive stimuli. For creating the training simpler, biofeedback methods are often involved. Originally, changes in PD gait patterns are monitored in correlation to the EEG signals. EEG biofeedback or neurofeedback uses EEG signals for feedback input. It is suggested that this learning procedure might help a subject to switch his or her brainwave activity. One of the methods involved in neurofeedback training is that the so-called frequency-following response. The modified signals are further analyzed using ICA. This type of analysis recovers the version of the original signal. ICA makes the output statistically independent by minimizing the mutual information in between the signals, without placing constraints on the orthogonal matrix. ICA decodes the info in a way, on the axis on which the info has maximum independence. According to the central limit theorem, if we take many channel sources independent of each other for EEG recording the distribution will lead to a Gaussian distribution. Having super-Gaussian distribution will result in high Kurtosis, hence achieving the sigma values for every signal component in the EEG will be nearly impossible. The angles are obtained in terms of variance as shown in Equation 1. Where X1(j), X2(j), are the signal acquired from the electrode channel placed over the hypothalamus and substantia nigra respectively. To make it non-Gaussian it starts with the data from the scalp channel and rotates the data in multi-dimensional space is shown within Equation 2. Where U is the ICA source activities, Σ is the Stretching component, $V^\star$ is the Rotational Matrix which can be set according to the degree of freedom of the data, X is the Mixture of obtained EEG, S is the original hypothalamic signal to be acquired. Before rotating the EEG signal the entropy and the joint entropy of the signal is maximized as shown in Equation 3. As higher the entropy, the randomness, and the uniformity increases. Where p(x) is the probability of the signal component at any particular time.

$$Var(\theta) = \sum_{J=1}^{N}[X_1(j) * X_2(j)]\frac{\sin\theta}{\cos\theta} \qquad (1)$$

$$X = (U\Sigma V^*) * S \qquad (2)$$

$$H(X) = -\sum_{x \in X} p(x)log_b p(x) \qquad (3)$$

Every single neuron in the hypothalamus and substantia nigra can be an independent contributor to the EEG signal component for PD patients, but we localized the source which contributes most to the EEG signal component by using an Entropy detection test and the applied a cut-off so that we don't see the components with minimal contributions and high interference. Then with the scalp topography which we obtained from the inverse weight matrix of the ICA, we obtained the source localization using Dipole/Loreto Distributed Source Localization for the signal component from the hypothalamus and substantia nigra respectively. Each neuron has a plus and minus polarity in it, generating an EF. All these neurons in the hypothalamus and substantia nigra generate an EF together which sums up on the scalp. Here ICA creates a spatial filter for each temporally independent source.

Figure 14.7, on the left-hand side, represents the Actual projection and on the right side, it represents the Dipole projection. The residual variance (RV) is computed using the two maps. If the RV is between 0 to 1 the dipole fits it well. A good fit of dipole indicates a healthy EEG. Whereas a high RV indicated a bad fit and provides an optimal indication for PD.

In Figure 14.8 dipole components of a normal person are given. The scalp topography of the person is having one percent and 2 percent RV, respectively, for two subjects. In Figure 14.9 dipole components of a PD patient are given. The RV is very high, ranging to 84 percent. It can be visualized that the components are not localized and are in scattered distribution. The scattered

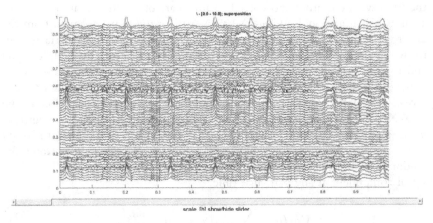

Figure 14.7 Dipole projection

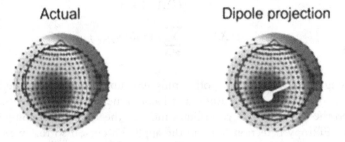

Figure 14.8 Dipole and EF distribution of normal people

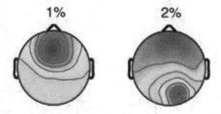

Figure 14.9 Dipole and EF distribution of PD patients

distribution of the dipole components is due to the generation of the disturbed EF. The low dopamine secretion causes reduced electrical propagation and generates propagation delays of electrical impulses because of which scattered dipoles formation takes place. Hence it cannot be modelled using a single dipole.

We aimed to use the whole power spectral density (PSD) of the entire EEG signal rather than the power of individual components. Figure 14.10 and Figure 14.11 show the significant difference in the shape of the mean PSD between normal and PD patients in between a frequency range of 2 Hz to 20 Hz. In Figure 14.10 it can be visualized that there is an upward deflection of the PSD after the mean PDS at 10 Hz, indicating hypothalamic excitation, owing to deep brain stimulation in PD patients. Whereas, in Figure 14.11 the PSD curve keeps a constancy and declines with time, as the person comes to rest. The differences are consistent among the PD and normal subjects and can be verified from the PSD plots.

D. Spectral Analysis

The movement of the electrical charges along the dendrites generates an electrical field potential (EFP). All EFP generated by the multiple neurons gives rise

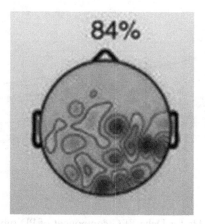

Figure 14.10 PSD of PD patients

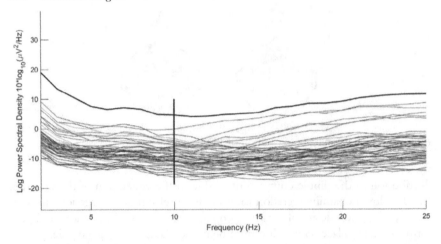

Figure 14.11 PSD of the normal person

to local field potential. Here we assume that the first and second moments of the data distribution are stationary. A significant change in the delta amplitude at about 2 Hz and theta amplitude at around 6 Hz can be observed in PD patients. A prominent spike in the frequency component at 6 Hz can be observed in Figure 14.12. The frequency components in case of PD become slower, incorporated with occipital background slowing. In the statistical observation of absolute theta and alpha amplitude of the EEG spectra the PD subject differed significantly from the controls and can be observed in Table 14.4.

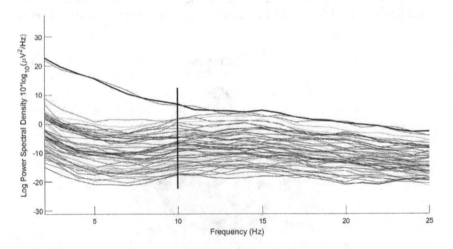

Figure 14.12 PSD at 6Hz for Delta EEG component of PD subject

Table 14.4 Relative amplitude value of the EEG spectral frequency components of PD and control subjects

	PD subject	Control
Delta Amplitude (mV)	15.00 ± 0.72	12.45 ± 0.70
Alpha Amplitude (mV)	44.65 ± 3.20	51.02 ± 1.75
Beta Amplitude (mV)	18.69 ± 1.72	23.09 ± 2.25
Theta Amplitude (mV)	24.75 ± 2.23	17.29 ± 0.26

Then we look at the activity power spectrum components of the hypothalamic and substantia nigra individually for both PD patients and normal persons. We can see that the spectrum is very different in between the two as shown in Figure 14.13, the PD spectrum has a lot of components in high frequency, indicating the instability in movement, and very often these components are transiently active during experiments. A high distortion in the alpha spike is vigilant in the APS of the PD subject. A background slowing in EEG spectral components can also be noticed for PD subjects in comparison to the control group. As it is not possible to visualize multi-dimensional hyperplanes, the validation of it is proofed using quantitative separation of the hyperplanes. The hyperplanes can be identified by principal component analysis (PCA). After identifying the hyperplanes during training, new subjects were classified using vector projections and sub-vector minimization. The projections create a sub-planner projection in a multi-dimensional axis. Deviation in the Magnitude of power in the multi-dimensional axis provides us with a clear differentiation between normal and PD patients.

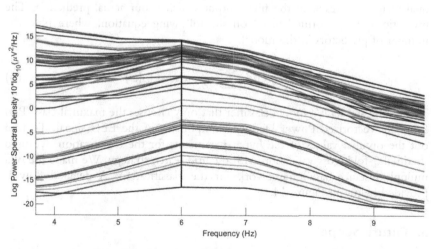

Figure 14.13 APS of PD and normal SUBJECT

E. Classification Model

AdaBoost Classifier with SVM was used to train extracted feature data-frame of EEG data and to make predictions on the training set. The most infamous feature of this algorithm is that it used the relative weight of each element in the dataset, these weights get updated after every step, and so on. The overall inputs become weighted average prediction of all the trees in the Decision Tree Classifier boosted by the Ada-Boost algorithm. This helps us boost the overall accuracy of the model as compared to the highly regularized SVC or Random Forest ensemble method. Let $w^{(i)}$ be the input instance, $\hat{y}_j^{(i)}$ is the prediction of the model over jth training instance of data-frame. The equation below is the weighted error rate of the model.

$$r_j = \frac{\sum\limits_{i=1}^{m} w^{(i)}}{\sum\limits_{i=1}^{m} w^{(i)}} \ \ where \ \hat{y}_j^{(i)} \neq y^{(i)} \tag{4}$$

After computing the weighted error rate of the model, we need to assign predictor weight α_j. The concept works on the fundamental principle of weighted average, as per the learning rate hyperparameter φ the more accurate will be the predictor then more will be its weight to contribute in an overall weighted average of predictions.

$$\alpha_j = \varphi \log \frac{1 - r_j}{r_j} \tag{5}$$

If $\hat{y}_j^{(i)} \neq y^{(i)}$ the instance prediction weight will be updated with $w^{(i)}$ exp $(\alpha_{(j)})$, whereas if the prediction $\hat{y}_j^{(i)} = y^{(i)}$ then the respective weights will be upgraded as per the multiplication factor $w^{(i)}$.

Finally, the AdaBoost algorithm computes the prediction values and individual weights to result in the final output which is our actual prediction. The predictions are performed based on the following equation, where N is the number of predictors in the model.

$$\hat{y}(x) = argmax_k \sum_{j=1}^{N} \alpha_j \ , where \ \hat{y}_j(x) = k \tag{6}$$

The testing model is a model classifier that only chooses the maximal class (PD) from the vectorized Power Density Components of the EEG signal. To find out the optimal values of the hyper-parameters for the classification, we used stratified 5-fold cross-validation with the grid search strategy. We made use of a multiple-instance-based framework for the classification. A detailed flow is provided below in Figure 14.14.

5. Future Scope

Among many gait abnormalities, PD patients significantly suffer from tremors and FOG. The FOG can be defined as the episodic inability to generate

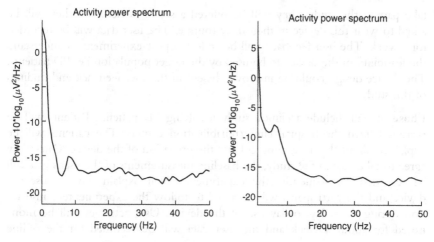

Figure 14.14 Process flow diagram for model

effective stepping during one's walk. Research shows that focused attention and external stimuli or cues can help PD patients to overcome FOG episodes. Auditory, vibratory, visual or other forms of stimuli can help patients to avoid FOG. Application of different sensational stimuli can cause the retention of normal Gait pattern temporarily and can save the person from fall and injuries. However, currently available solutions make use of mainly auditory or visual stimuli. Auditory and visual stimuli are subject to human sensational perceptions and are not that effective. These are certainly ineffective and turmoil in nature for outdoor applications. The approach to our solution is to use Vibratory stimulus or small electrical impulses whenever an abnormal gait pattern is recognized and to restore normal movement pattern for the period. The system can certainly prevent falls and injuries on a large scale. The system can be provided with additional alarm notification and tracking system, to track the patient's location. If the patient undergoes a fall or an injury even after the use of an assistive device, the guardian of the patient will get notification together with the location of the patient.

The entire process is divided into three phases:

Phase 1: will include the design and development of a low-cost and portable device to monitor one's activity. For this, a battery-operated/self-powered, micro-controller-based system will be developed for the target-specific application. Also, this device will be enabled with wireless connectivity such as wifi or Bluetooth connectivity. Further, this device will be enabled to offer vibratory stimuli to the user based on the detection of FOG. The device will be replicated and these devices will be attached to the user's upper limb and or lower limb on each side. Also, the device will be enabled to connect and transfer the recorded data to the cloud for creating a log file of the user activities.

Phase 2: healthy individuals will be recruited for a feasibility study (pilot study) related to the device developed in Phase 1. Once the user provides consent to take part in the study, they will be offered a set of devices and they will be asked to wear this device in their daily routine. The user data will be recorded for a week. The user feedback will be collected post-experiment to understand the feasibility of the device to be used by the target population i.e. PD patients. The device design could be improved based on the user feedback and findings of this study.

Phase 3: will include a clinical study involving PD patients. Patients will be recruited from the hospital/clinic/rehabilitation centers. The patients will be explained about the study protocol and the operation of the device. Once they agree to take part in the study, the baseline measurements of the user's gait will be recorded. Subsequently, the experimenter will explain how to use the device and the participants will be asked to follow the experimenter's instruction during their day-to-day use of the device. User activities will be monitored for about a week and the user data will be recorded for the offline

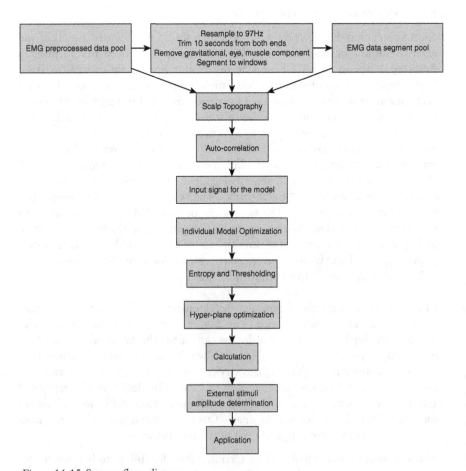

Figure 14.15 System flow diagram

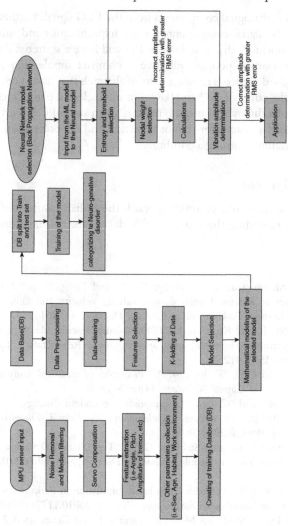

Figure 14.16

analysis. Also, the user's gait-related measures will be recorded post experiments. The user's daily routine details, medication details and feedback related to the device will be collected post-experiment.

6. Conclusion

The work proposed a novel approach to detect PD activity over the EEG channels, which is a minimum possible examination and widely available. The proposed algorithm detects and segregates channels that exhibit some similarity. It removes the left alfa signal components from the EEG signal. Further decomposes it down into the signal components for the hypothalamus and substantia nigra. The chapter concludes that people with PD will have a scattered dipole on their scalp, whereas normal people will have a compact dipole. Experiments have shown that a good choice is to select pairs of channels that have a cross-correlation coefficient in the range of 0.73 and 0.87. For each selected pair of channels, ICA is performed, and a differential measurement is given using PCA. Furthermore, the chapter proposed a system for tremor detection and fall prevention using inertial sensors and machine learning algorithm.

Acknowledgment

I would like to show our gratitude towards the Indian Institute of Technology Bangalore for providing the most valuable dataset for the experimentations.

References

Allen, N. E., Sherrington, C., Canning, C. G., and Fung, V. S. (2010). "Reduced muscle power is associated with slower walking velocity and falls in people with Parkinson's disease." *Parkinsonism and Related Disorders*, 16: 261–264.

Chae, J., Sheffler, L. and Knutson, J. (2008). "Neuromuscular electrical stimulation for motor restoration in hemiplegia." *Topics in Stroke Rehabilitation*, 15(5): 412–426. doi:10.1310/tsr1505-412.

Brocker, D. T. and Grill, W. M. (2013). "Principles of electrical stimulation of neural tissue." *Handbook of Clinical Neurology*, 11(6): 3–18.

Fahim Anjum, M. et al. (2020). "Linear predictive coding distinguishes spectral EEG features of Parkinson's disease." *Parkinsonism & Related Disorders*, 79: 79–85. doi:10.1016/j.parkreldis.2020.08.001.

Goetz, C. G., Nutt, J. G., and Stebbins, G. T. "The Unified Dyskinesia Rating Scale: Presentation and clinimetric profile." *Movement Disorders*, November 2018. doi:10.1002/mds.22341.

Groiss, S. J. et al. (2009). "Review: Deep brain stimulation in Parkinson's disease." *Therapeutic Advances in Neurological Disorders*, pp. 379–391. doi:10.1177/1756285609339382.

Kakkar, D. (2018). A Study on Machine Learning Based Generalized Automated Seizure Detection System. 8th International Conference on Cloud Computing, Data Science & Engineering (Confluence) (pp. 769–774).

Lonini L. et al. (2018). "Wearable sensors for Parkinson's disease: which data are worth collecting for training symptom detection models." *NPJ Digital Medicine*, 1(1): 64.

Moon, S., Song, H. J., Sharma, V. D. et al. (2020). "Classification of Parkinson's disease and essential tremor based on balance and gait characteristics from wearable motion sensors via machine learning techniques: a data-driven approach." *Journal of NeuroEngineering and Rehabilitation*, 17: 125. doi:10.1186/s12984-020-00756-5.

Morishita, M.A., Higuchi, K. S., Yoshio, T., Hiroshi, A. and Tooru, I. (2016). "Changes in Motor-Related Cortical Activity Following Deep Brain Stimulation for Parkinson's Disease Detected by Functional Near Infrared Spectroscopy: A Pilot Study." *Frontiers in Human Neuroscience*. doi:10.3389/fnhum.2016.00629.

Papadopoulos, A.et al. (2020). "Detecting Parkinsonian Tremor From IMU Data Collected in-the-Wild Using Deep Multiple-Instance Learning ." *IEEE Journal of Biomedical Health Informatics*, 24(9): 2559–2569. doi:10.1109/JBHI.2019.2961748.

Skorvanek, M. et al. (2017). "Differences in MDS-UPDRS Scores Based on Hoehn and Yahr Stage and Disease Duration." *Movement Disorders*, 4: 536–544. doi:10.1002/mdc3.12476.

Stern, S., Rotem, A., Burnishev, Y., Weinreb, E., and Moses, E. (2017). "External Excitation of Neurons Using Electric and Magnetic Fields in One- and Two-dimensional Cultures." *Journal of Visualized Experience*, 2017(123): 54357. doi:10.3791/54357.

Tu-Chan, A. P., Natraj, N., Godlove, J., Abrams, G., and Ganguly, K. (2017). "Effects of somatosensory electrical stimulation on motor function and cortical oscillations." Journal of NeuroEngineering Rehabilitation, 14(1): 113. doi:10.1186/s12984-017-0323-1.

Wadhera, T. and Kakkar, D. (2020a). "Conditional entropy approach to analyze cognitive dynamics in autism spectrum disorder." *Neurological Research*, 42(10): 869–878.

Wadhera, T. and Kakkar, D. (2020b). "Big Data-Based System: A Supportive Tool in Autism Spectrum Disorder Analysis." In: *Interdisciplinary Approaches to Altering Neurodevelopmental Disorders* (pp. 303–319). IGI Global.

Wadhera, T., Kakkar, D., Wadhwa, G. et al. (2019). "Recent Advances and Progress in Development of the Field Effect Transistor Biosensor: A Review." *Journal of Electronic Materials*, 48: 7635–7646. doi:10.1007/s11664-019-07705-6.

Xie, Y., Meng, X., Xiao, J., Zhang, J., and Zhang, J. (2016). "Cognitive changes following bilateral deep brain stimulation of subthalamic nucleus in Parkinson's disease: a meta-analysis." *BioMed Research International*, 2016: 3596415.

15 A Hybrid Deep Model with Concatenating Framework of Convolutional Neural Networks for Identification of Autism Spectrum Disorder

Sumit Kumar and Shallu Sharma

1 Introduction

Autism spectrum disorder (ASD) is a neurodevelopmental disorder (NDD) that causes problems with social interaction and communication. Restricted, repetitive, and stereotypical behaviour are the most common clinical manifestations demonstrated by people who suffered from ASD (Faras, Al Ateeqi, and Tidmarsh, 2010; Lauritsen 2013). Lack of concentration, anxiety, depression, motor, and sensory problems are various difficulties that can be experienced by ASD patients, as well as comorbidities with other NDDs like dyslexia (Ogundele, 2018). As a matter of fact, the majority (but not all) of people with ASD require lifetime care and support, as ASD begins in childhood and tends to persist in adolescence and adulthood (Lord, Elsabbagh, Baird, and Veenstra-Vanderweele, 2018; WHO, 2021). Numerous people are the sufferer of ASD all over the world. The incidence rate of ASD is increasing at an extremely high rate. According to WHO, one in every 160 children has ASD (WHO). In this context, earlier diagnosis of ASD can help people in sustaining a better life by assisting clinicians in following the optimal therapeutic strategies for ASD patients. Plenty of efforts have already been taken in the past by researchers and clinicians working in the domain of neuroscience which helped us by developing a better understanding related to the aetiology of the disease in the brain (Jones, Hanley, and Riby, 2020; Rane et al., 2017; Wadhera and Kakkar, 2019; Wadhera and Kakkar, 2020; Werkman et al., 2020). Despite this advancement, the actual cause of ASD is still unknown. A reliable and efficient diagnosis of ASD as early as possible can be made at the age of two by utilizing a combination of the current standardized diagnostic assessment data for infants and toddlers (Control and Prevention, 2020; Zwaigenbaum, Brian, and Ip, 2019). In addition, the early indication for ASD is determined by analyzing the structural changes in the brain using magnetic resonance imaging (MRI), which play a significant role in comprehending the mechanism of ASD (Ismail et al., 2016; Nanglia, Kumar, and Luhach, 2019; Zhang et al., 2018). MRI is a non-invasive technique of neuroimaging and assists in predicting the patient's outcome by offering potential markers or features.

DOI: 10.4324/9781003165569-15

Machine learning and deep learning algorithms-based automated systems are gaining attention for creating new device applications in the field of artificial intelligence. Especially in healthcare systems, the implementation of emerging deep learning paradigms helps in providing a potential to raise productivity, consistency, and quality of treatment. A large community of researchers, engineers and academicians are continuously investigating the new machine learning algorithms to employ them in designing automated systems for applications ranging from object detection to medical diagnosis. Machine learning is a subset of 'Artificial Intelligence' which learns from the data. It analyzes the existing patterns in the data and responds to a situation for which they have not been explicitly programmed (Mehra, 2018; Wadhera and Kakkar, 2020; Wadhera, Kakkar, Kaur, and Menia, 2019). More and more people are interacting with the systems that are based on machine learning, for example, biometric systems, 'Alexa' (the voice recognition system), self-driving cars and 'Google Suggest' or 'Autocomplete'. In addition, machine learning is aiding the development of automated and effective systems in the field of computer vision, which includes object detection, facial expression recognition, human pose estimation, crowded scene analysis, and medical image analysis. In spite of noteworthy advancement in the diagnosis of a variety of diseases, such as cancer (Nanglia, Kumar, Mahajan, Singh, and Rathee, 2020; Nanglia, Mahajan, Rathee, Kumar, and Informatics, 2020; Sharma and Mehra, 2020), neuronal disorders (Ahmed, Mohamed, Zeeshan, and Dong, 2020; Del Rey et al., 2018), NDDs are still a worldwide problem. Therefore, the development of efficient and affordable approaches for early detection, diagnosis, and treatment is urgently needed to treat NDDs.

Contributions

In this chapter, experimental work has been performed systematically and leads to the following contributions:

1   A hybrid approach is applied to extract the features from the brain MRI images using deep learning models and analyzed the classification performance for the developed classification model based on accuracy, precision, sensitivity, f1-score, and receiver operating characteristic (ROC) to identify the potential of proposed classifier in the classification of the ABIDE dataset.
2   In addition, we have employed different techniques of affine transformations for data augmentation to avoid the problem of overfitting as well as to enlarge the dataset for extracting discernible features from the images for better training of the classifier.
3   We have also compared the performance of the proposed classifier with the existing state-of-the-art classifier for ABIDE dataset classification for a coherent comparison.

2. Relevant Studies

ABIDE data have previously been used by many researchers but in different manners. (Nielsen et al., 2013) utilized the functional MRI data of the Autism Brain Imaging Data Exchange (ABIDE) database to classify ASD and healthy control subjects based on brain connectivity measurements. They computed the BOLD signal for the 964 subjects from non-overlapped grey matter which was segmented by utilizing the mask (SPM8 mask grey.nii). A total of 7,266 regions of interest (ROIs) were generated from the considered data, and a connectivity square matrix of size 7,266×7,266 was computed by determining a correlation coefficient for every pair of the ROIs. A general linear model was fit to each group i.e. ASD and healthy control to associate the connectivity matrix with subject-related variables: age, gender, and handedness. However, the differences between the data sites were the major challenge with the ABIDE dataset, owing to variability in scanners, scanning parameters, and utilized protocols. This challenge was then addressed by using the difference between one site's mean value for the connection and another site's mean value for the same connection. For the left-out subject, the actual value for each connection was then subtracted from the estimated values obtained from the ASD model and the healthy control model. The average of this subtraction across all 7,266 ROIs was computed, and the average values of ROIs were added up. Positive values were classified as ASD and negative values, as controls. The authors obtained an accuracy rate of 60% for the classification of ASD versus healthy controls. Abraham et al., 2017 achieved the highest accuracy rate, of 67%, by building participant-specific functional connectivity matrices (connectomes) for the full ABIDE dataset. In the present study, we aimed to improve the accuracy obtained from functional MRI data by implementing the designed classification model from only the structural MRI data of the ABIDE dataset.

3 Material and Methodology

3.1 Autism Brain Imaging Data Exchange (ABIDE) Dataset

The main aim behind the creation of the ABIDE dataset was to overcome the scarcity of large and comprehensive databases related to MRI images of ASD (Heinsfeld, Franco, Craddock, Buchweitz, and Meneguzzi, 2018). The motive behind the sharing of the database on the public front is to encourage researchers and machine learning engineers to develop an automatic classification system for ASD diagnosis. Martino and Mostofsky (Mertz, 2017) laid the foundation for this database by collaborating with 17 international sites. The ABIDE database contains 1,112 digitized MRI images in Nifty format, collected from 539 ASD patients and 573 from typical controls of ages 7–64 years. Hence, the database is broadly classified into two categories: ASD (A) and Control (C). In the present study, we are performing a binary classification of

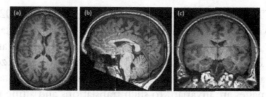

Figure 15.1 Illustration of MRI Images in ABIDE Dataset: (a) Axial, (b) Sagittal, and (c) Coronal

MRI images. The whole dataset is divided 80:20 for training and testing of the classifier. An illustration of available MRI data is depicted in Figure 15.1. Images in the training set for both the classes are equal (which is 432), and the testing set having 100 images per class.

3.2 Pre-processing

In this section, we have elaborated the process that has been performed on all the MRI images to enhance the quality of data. Bias-Correction, image de-noising, ACPC detection and alignment are the methods that we have implemented to convert the input raw data into a more understandable and suitable format for feature extraction. In this context, BRAHMA using free-surfer has been employed to process the ABIDE data (Pai et al., 2020). The input images are corrected to remove low-frequency intensity inhomogeneities using the Non-Parametric Non-Uniform Intensity Normalization (N4ITK) algorithm implemented using the ANTs toolbox, resulting in a bias-corrected image. The bias–corrected images are filtered using ANTs, with Adaptive Non-Local Means filtering, providing a denoised image. The denoised images are processed to identify the AC and the PC landmarks with the AC-PC line being used to align the image. The ACPC locations are detected using the MIPAV and ATRA toolboxes.

3.3 Data-augmentation

Augmentation is a process in which information preserving transformations are applied to the image samples for improving the ability of generalization (Shorten and Khoshgoftaar, 2019). The problem of overfitting can also be avoided by employing the data augmentation techniques which often confronted, owing to an imbalanced dataset (Kellenberger, Marcos, and Tuia, 2018; Sharma and Mehra, 2020). The available techniques of data augmentation can be broadly categorized into two classes: basic image manipulations and deep learning approaches. Basic image manipulations techniques consist of random erasing, mixing images, colour space transformation, elastic transformation, pixel-level transformation, and geometric transformation (Lee, Zaheer, Astrid, and Lee, 2020). The techniques which fall under the deep learning approaches are adversarial training, neural transfer style and GAN data augmentation (Tran, Tran, Nguyen, Nguyen, and Cheung, 2021). The incorporation and evolution of the new approaches of data-augmentation are highly imperative but the safety of application is equally important at that time for preserving the label information. For MRI images, rotation, zooming, cropping, flipping, and translations are the safest techniques for data augmentation because these images are invariant to such translations and affine transformations (Andersson and Berglund, 2018). In this chapter, we have opted for a real-time mode of data augmentation for memory management and performed using the ImageDataGenerator module from the Keras framework. Hence, random affine transformations have been applied to the images.

4 Fundamental Framework

The efficient implementation of the proposed hybrid deep learning approach has been conducted to improve the classification performance with minimum computational cost and training time (see Figure 15.2). The major rationale behind the use of the hybrid deep learning approach is to get the full benefit of both the considered deep neural networks. The network training starts by initializing the weights of the network using the Xavier initializing scheme. As per the Xavier initialization scheme, the variance of the activations is the same across every layer which further helps in preventing the problem of vanishing gradient. The algorithms are designed to receive all the training instances from an unknown function for solving the supervised machine learning problems, defined as:

$$k = f(l) \quad (1)$$

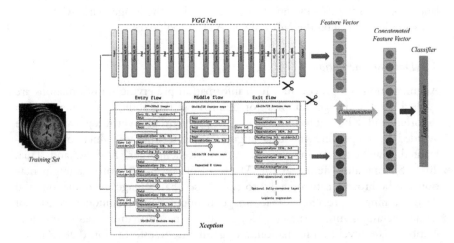

Figure 15.2 Schematic for the training protocol of VGG16 and Xception hybrid model for the classification of ASD from typical control.

where 'k' is the class label and 'l' is the feature vector. The algorithm then searches for the function 'g' through a space of hypotheses function 'H'. In the present work, we have considered two well-known CNN architectures namely, VGG16 and Xception. However, the selection of the VGG16, as well as the Xception model, is based on a previous work done by Shallu et. al in which the network was utilized for binary classification and multiclassification of the histopathological images (Kumar and Sharma, 2021; Mehra, 2018). The experimental analysis has been demonstrated that a pre-trained VGG16 network and the Xception model performed far better than VGG19 and ResNet50 in the classification of the histopathological images when employed as a feature extractor. Owing to this fact, a hybrid architecture of the VGG16 and the Xception model has been reconsidered to obtain optimum performance for the classification of ABIDE data. Further, a conventional classifier i.e. Logistic Regression is appended on the last fully-connected layer for a final decision.

4.1 Training Details

The proposed hybrid model is implemented using the Keras and Tensorflow frameworks. The specification of the system is as follows: ThinkPad E470 (i7) | 8 GB RAM, and NVIDIA GeForce 940MX the Graphic Card. Furthermore, we have considered Adam optimizer for achieving the best performance of the classifier (Sharma, Mehra, and Kumar, 2020). Here, the pre-existing VGG16 and the Xception model consist of 115,185,088 parameters and 20,861,480 parameters, respectively. These parameters are trained on the features extracted from the two classes of ABIDE dataset with a learning rate and scheduling rate of 10^{-6} and 0.912, respectively.

5 Results and Discussion

In this section, the performance of the proposed hybrid deep learning model is compared for the classification of ABIDE dataset. A balanced training set of 432 images (per class) is considered for the training of the model and the testing set of 100 images (per class) is utilized to compute the classification performance of the model.

5.1 Classifier's Performance Evaluation

The results obtained with the designed hybrid deep learning model are evaluated based on various performance evaluation parameters such as accuracy, sensitivity, precision, and f1-score. In this context, the value for the considered evaluation metrics is computed. The proposed hybrid model with logistic regression classifiers achieved an accuracy of 84.53% besides a sensitivity, precision and f1-score of 84.53%, 89%, 90%, and 89%, respectively. Furthermore, the performance of the developed hybrid model is compared with the results of the existing state-of-the-art and shown in Table 15.1.

Table 15.1 Comparison of the proposed and existing state-of-the-art technique with 5-fold-cross-validation of the ABIDE dataset

Classifier	Accuracy	Sensitivity	Precision	F1-score	Specificity	Reference
Random Forest	0.63	0.69	————	————	0.58	(Ho, 1995)
Support Vector Machine	0.65	0.68	————	————	0.62	(Vapnik, 1998)
Deep Neural Network	0.70	0.74	————	————	0.63	(Heinsfeld et al., 2018)
Proposed Model	0.84	0.89	0.90	0.89	————	Present Work

It has been observed from Table 15.1 that the proposed approach has the potential to surpass the existing approach of classification for ABIDE data classification with a significant margin. The evaluation of all models is based on a 5-fold cross-validation schema where the data from all 17 sites are rolled into one. Here, we have also reported the value of precision and f1-scores besides the accuracy and sensitivity of the proposed classifier. The confusion matrices and corresponding ROC curve in conjunction with an area under the curve for the developed models under the optimized hyper-parameters configuration are presented in Figure 15.3.

6 Conclusion

This chapter has represented the feasibility of hybrid deep learning models for the classification of ABIDE dataset. Apart from feasibility, the reliability of the classification performance has also been affirmed by this experimental study. The developed hybrid deep learning model is compared with the existing

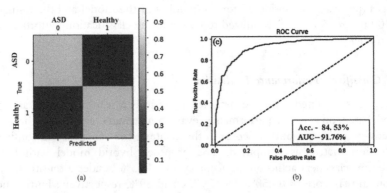

Figure 15.3 An illustration of the performance evaluation metrics (a) Confusion matrix, and (b) ROC with AUC for the testing set

conventional machine learning model and deep neural network. It has been observed through the experimental study that the hybrid deep learning model provides a significant performance in comparison to the conventional machine learning algorithm. However, a comparable performance is achieved with the simple deep neural network.

In the foreseeable future, different combinations of the existing deep learning model can be employed and compared to select the best hybrid model for the classification of the ABIDE dataset to identify between ASD and controls. Moreover, the effect of different weight initialization schemes and transfer learning methods can be analyzed to further improve network performance.

References

Abraham, A. et al. (2017). "Deriving reproducible biomarkers from multi-site resting-state data: An Autism-based example." *Neuroimage, 147*: 736–745.

Ahmed, Z., Mohamed, K., Zeeshan, S., and Dong, X. J. D. (2020). *Artificial intelligence with multi-functional machine learning platform development for better healthcare and precision medicine.*

Andersson, E. and Berglund, R. (2018). Evaluation of data augmentation of MR images for deep learning. Lund University.

Control, C. F. D. and Prevention. (2020). "Screening and diagnosis of autism spectrum disorder for healthcare providers." Centers for Disease Control and Prevention, Atlanta.

In: Del Rey, N. L.-G.et al. (2018), *Advances in Parkinson's disease: 200 years later. Frontiers in Neuroanatomy, 12*, 113.

Faras, H., Al Ateeqi, N., and Tidmarsh, L.. (2010). "Autism spectrum disorders." *Neuron, 30*(4): 295–300.

Heinsfeld, A. S., Franco, A. R., Craddock, R. C., Buchweitz, A., and Meneguzzi, F. J. N. C. (2018). "Identification of autism spectrum disorder using deep learning and the ABIDE dataset." *NeuroImage: Clinical, 17*: 16–23.

Ho, T. K. (1995). Random decision forests. Paper presented at the Paper presented at the Proceedings of 3rd international conference on document analysis and recognition.

Ismail, M. M.et al. (2016). "Studying autism spectrum disorder with structural and diffusion magnetic resonance imaging: a survey." Frontiers in Human Neuroscience, *10*: 211.

Jones, E. K., Hanley, M., and Riby, D. (2020). "Distraction, distress and diversity: Exploring the impact of sensory processing differences on learning and school life for pupils with autism spectrum disorders." Research in Autism Spectrum Disorders, 72: 101515.

Kellenberger, B., Marcos, D., and Tuia, D. (2018). "Detecting mammals in UAV images: Best practices to address a substantially imbalanced dataset with deep learning." Remote Sensing of Environment, 216: 139–153.

Kumar, S. and Sharma, S. (2021). "Sub-classification of invasive and non-invasive cancer from magnification independent histopathological images using hybrid neural networks." *Evolutionary Intelligence*, 1–13.

Lauritsen, M. B. J. E. (2013). "Autism spectrum disorders." *European Child Adolescent Psychiatry*, 22(1): 37–42.

Lee, J.-H., Zaheer, M. Z., Astrid, M., and Lee, S.-I. (2020). Smoothmix: a simple yet effective data augmentation to train robust classifiers. Paper presented at the Paper presented at the Proceedings of the IEEE/CVF Conference on Computer Vision and Pattern Recognition Workshops.

Lord, C., Elsabbagh, M., Baird, G., and Veenstra-Vanderweele, J. (2018). "Autism spectrum disorder." *The Lancet*, *392*(10146), 508–520.

Mehra, R. (2018). Automatic magnification independent classification of breast cancer tissue in histological images using deep convolutional neural network. Paper presented at the Paper presented at the International Conference on Advanced Informatics for Computing Research.

Mehra, R. andSharma, S. (2018). "Breast cancer histology images classification: Training from scratch or transfer learning?" *ICT Express*, 4(4): 247–254.

Mertz, L. J. I. (2017). "Sharing data to solve the autism riddle: An interview with Adriana Di Martino and Michael Milham of ABIDE." *IEEE Pulse*, 8(6): 6–9.

Nanglia, P., Kumar, S., and Luhach, A. K. (2019). "Detection and analysis of lung cancer using radiomic approach." In: *Smart Computational Strategies: Theoretical and Practical Aspects* (pp. 13–24): Springer.

Nanglia, P., Kumar, S., Mahajan, A. N., Singh, P., and Rathee, D. (2020). "A hybrid algorithm for lung cancer classification using SVM and Neural Networks." *ICT Express*.

Nanglia, P., Mahajan, A. N., Rathee, D. S., Kumar, S. and Informatics. (2020). "Lung cancer classification using feed forward back propagation neural network for CT images." *International Journal of Medical Engineering and Informatics*, 12(5): 447–456.

Nielsen, J. A. et al. (2013). "Multisite functional connectivity MRI classification of autism: ABIDE results." *Frontiers in Human Neuroscience*, 7: 599.

Ogundele, M.(2018). "Behavioural and emotional disorders in childhood: A brief overview for paediatricians." World Journal of Clinical Pediatrics, 7(1): 9.

Pai, P. P. et al.(2020). "BRAHMA: Population specific t1, t2, and FLAIR weighted brain templates and their impact in structural and functional imaging studies." *Magnetic Resonance Imaging*, 70: 5–21.

Rane, S., Jolly, E., Park, A., Jang, H., and Craddock, C. J. R. I.. (2017). "Developing predictive imaging biomarkers using whole-brain classifiers: Application to the ABIDE I dataset." *Research Ideas and Outcomes*, 3: e12733.

Sharma, S., Mehra, R., and Kumar, S. (2020). "Optimised CNN in conjunction with efficient pooling strategy for the multi-classification of breast cancer." *IET Image Processing*.

Sharma, S. and Mehra, R. (2020). "Conventional machine learning and deep learning approach for multi-classification of breast cancer histopathology images—a comparative insight." *Journal of Digital Imaging*, 33(3): 632–654.

Sharma, S. and Mehra, R. (2020). "Effect of layer-wise fine-tuning in magnification-dependent classification of breast cancer histopathological image." *The Visual Computer*, 36(9): 1755–1769.

Shorten, C. and Khoshgoftaar, T. (2019). "A survey on image data augmentation for deep learning." *Journal of Big Data*, 6(1): 1–48.

Tran, N.., Tran, V., Nguyen, N., Nguyen, T., and Cheung, N. (2021). "On data augmentation for GAN training." *IEEE Transactions on Image Processing*, 30: 1882–1897.

Vapnik, V. (1998). "The support vector method of function estimation." In: *Nonlinear Modeling* (pp. 55–85). Springer.

Wadhera, T. and Kakkar, D. (2019). "Eye Tracker: An Assistive Tool in Diagnosis of Autism Spectrum Disorder." In: *Emerging Trends in the Diagnosis and Intervention of Neurodevelopmental Disorders* (pp. 125–152). IGI Global.

Wadhera, T. and Kakkar, D. (2020). "Big Data-Based System: A Supportive Tool in Autism Spectrum Disorder Analysis." In: *Interdisciplinary Approaches to Altering Neurodevelopmental Disorders* (pp. 303–319). IGI Global.

Wadhera, T. and Kakkar, D. (2020). "Conditional entropy approach to analyze cognitive dynamics in autism spectrum disorder." *Neurological Research*, 42(10): 869–878.

Wadhera, T., Kakkar, D., Kaur, G., and Menia, V. (2019). "Pre-Clinical ASD Screening Using Multi-Biometrics-Based Systems." In: *Design and Implementation of Healthcare Biometric Systems* (pp. 185–211). IGI Global.

Werkman, M. et al. (2020). "The moderating effect of cognitive abilities on the association between sensory processing and emotional and behavioural problems and social participation in autistic individuals." *Research in Autism Spectrum Disorders*, 78: 101663.

World Health Organization. (2021). "Autism spectrum disorders." Retrieved from www.who.int/news-room/fact-sheets/detail/autism-spectrum-disorders.

Zhang, W. et al. (2018). "Revisiting subcortical brain volume correlates of autism in the ABIDE dataset: effects of age and sex." *Psychological Medicine*, 48(4): 654.

Zwaigenbaum, L., Brian, J. A., and Ip, A. J. P. (2019). "Early detection for autism spectrum disorder in young children." *Paediatric Child Health*, 24(7): 424–432.

Index

Please note that page references to Figures will be in **bold**, while references to Tables are in *italics*. NDDs stand for "neurodevelopmental disorders".

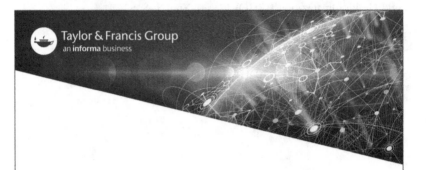

Printed in the United States
by Baker & Taylor Publisher Services